NOV, 7

OCT 1 1 20

Nursing

Oxford Handbook of Cancer Nursing
Edited by Mike Tadman and Dave Roberts

Oxford Handbook of Cardiac Nursing
Edited by Karen Rawlings-Anderson and Kate Johnson

Oxford Handbook of Children's and Young People's Nursing
Edited by Alan Glasper, Gillian McEwing, and Jim Richardson

Oxford Handbook of Gastrointestinal Nursing
Edited by Christine Norton, Julia Williams, Claire Taylor,
Annmarie Nunwa, and Kathy Whayman

Oxford Handbook of Mental Health Nursing
Edited by Patrick Callaghan and Helen Waldock

Oxford Handbook of Midwifery
Janet Medforth, Susan Battersby, Maggie Evans, Beverley Marsh, and
Angela Walker

Oxford Handbook of Nursing Older People
Edited by Beverley Tabernacle, Marie Honey, and Annette Jinks

Oxford Handbook of Nurse Prescribing
Sue Beckwith and Penny Franklin

Oxford Handbook of Primary Care and Community Nursing
Edited by Vari Drennan and Claire Goodman

Oxford Handbook of Respiratory Medicine
Edited by Terry Robinson and Jane Scullion

Oxford Handbook of
Respiratory Nursing

Edited by

Terry Robinson
Specialist Respiratory Nurse, Harrogate and District NHS
Foundation Trust

Jane E. Scullion
Respiratory Nurse Consultant, University Hospitals of
Leicester

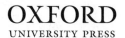

OXFORD
UNIVERSITY PRESS

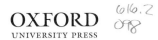

616.2
098

OXFORD
UNIVERSITY PRESS

Great Clarendon Street, Oxford OX2 6DP

Oxford University Press is a department of the University of Oxford.
It furthers the University's objective of excellence in research, scholarship,
and education by publishing worldwide in

Oxford New York

Auckland Cape Town Dar es Salaam Hong Kong Karachi
Kuala Lumpur Madrid Melbourne Mexico City Nairobi
New Delhi Shanghai Taipei Toronto

With offices in

Argentina Austria Brazil Chile Czech Republic France Greece
Guatemala Hungary Italy Japan Poland Portugal Singapore
South Korea Switzerland Thailand Turkey Ukraine Vietnam

Oxford is a registered trade mark of Oxford University Press
in the UK and in certain other countries

Published in the United States
by Oxford University Press Inc., New York

British Library Cataloguing in Publication Data
Data available

Library of Congress Cataloguing in Publication Data
Data available

Typeset by Cepha Imaging Private Ltd., Bangalore, India
Printed in China
on acid-free paper by
Asia Pacific Offset

ISBN 978–0–19–922623–8

10 9 8 7 6 5 4 3 2 1

Foreword

The practice of modern medicine is changing rapidly and nursing roles have developed to meet this challenge. Whilst much of the world is still affected by acute or infectious illnesses, there has been an increasing focus on chronic diseases that are now prevalent even in developing countries. Chronic respiratory disease continues to make a prominent contribution to global ill health and cannot be ignored. Most major respiratory diseases cannot be cured but have to be managed to limit their impact on the patient and their families. This approach requires the collaboration of several healthcare disciplines as well as the active involvement of the patient and their relatives. The emphasis on moving healthcare closer to the patient's home will inevitably mean that nurses in particular will have greater involvement in routine and unscheduled care.

In this book on the nursing of respiratory disorders it is evident that the reader is invited to acquire knowledge and skills specific to acute and chronic respiratory diseases that will help them understand and manage the patient effectively. This book seeks to provide the common knowledge base for the nurse professional who is developing an enthusiasm for the provision of first-class respiratory care. The chapter authors in this welcome book have all demonstrated their commitment and enthusiasm to the care of people with lung disease. They have also all contributed to the practical development of innovative respiratory services and aim to share that experience with the reader. They are justly proud of their achievements but understand that they must spread the word to be even more effective.

Mike Morgan
Consultant Respiratory Physician
Chairman of the British Thoracic Society
July 2008

Acknowledgements

We would like to offer our grateful thanks to the following relatives, friends and colleagues for their support, advice and guidance on various sections of the book.

Mrs Sharon Haggerty, Mr John Robinson, Dr Tony Fennerty, Dr Claire Taylor, Mrs Shona Shires, Ms Sarah Howard.

And to all our contributors for their patience and hard work.

Preface

The multitude of respiratory diseases present a considerable burden on healthcare resources, the economy, and particularly on individual patients and their carers. In the United Kingdom (UK) one in five deaths occur as the result of respiratory disease with more deaths occurring from this group of disease than from coronary heart disease or the non-respiratory cancers. The UK death rate from respiratory disease is also one of the highest in Europe, estimated to be around twice the European (EU) average, and it appears that this burden is increasing, which contrasts sharply to coronary heart disease where the overall relative burden falls year on year. Around one in eight admissions to the acute sector are as a consequence of respiratory disease. It also places a heavy burden on primary care, with many consultations both at the surgery and in the patient's home.

This handbook was put together to give a practical, reliable and useful guide to practitioners interested in some of the more common respiratory conditions affecting adults, recognizing that respiratory patients present in all specialties and in a variety of settings. This is therefore a useful book for anyone from the interested novice to the experienced practitioner. It can give quick facts or can be read in a more in-depth style

Written in the style of previous Oxford Handbooks, the book appears in topics which are also cross-referenced to other relevant sections within the book. It is up-to-date and written by experienced practitioners within the specialty, directly involved in patient care. A glossary at the end provides a useful adjunct to the topics. Given the breadth and range of respiratory conditions it is not an exhaustive guide, but it does look at the more common presenting problems with their care, management and treatment. Each chapter is useful as a stand-alone text and is presented with further reading rather than being referenced throughout.

Terry Robinson and Jane Scullion
July 2008

Contents

Detailed contents

Contributors

Iain Armstrong
Nurse Consultant, Royal
Hallamshire Hospital, Sheffield

Nicola Bell
Lung Cancer Nurse Specialist
Harrogate District Foundation
Trust, North Yorkshire, UK

Dave Burns
National Training Manager,
Respiratory Education UK,
Liverpool

Malcolm Cocksedge
Senior Tuberculosis Nurse
Specialist, Bart's and the London
NHS Trust, UK and Chair of
the Royal College of Nursing
Tuberculosis Forum

Alison Conway
Respiratory Nurse Practitioner,
University Hospitals of Leicester

Liz Darlison
Consultant Nurse, Mesothelioma
UK and University Hospitals of
Leicester

Bernadette Donaghy
Cystic Fibrosis Nurse Specialist,
Glenfield Hospital, Leicester

Jane French
Nurse Consultant in Respiratory
Medicine, Papworth Hospital NHS
Foundation Trust, Cambridge

Sharon Haggerty
Head of Adult Services (North),
Chester Le Street Community
Hospital, Durham

Theresa Harvey
Specialist Respiratory
Physiotherapy Practitioner,
Glenfield Hospital, Leicester

Jane Leyshon
Head of Academic Studies,
Education for Health, Warwick
and Respiratory Specialist Nurse,
Primary Care

Lorna McLaughlan
Community Respiratory Nurse
Specialist, Ashton Leigh and Wigan
PCT

Pauleen Pratt
Consultant Nurse, Critical Care
University Hospitals of Leicester

Robert Pretorius
Consultant in Critical Care and
Anesthesia, University Hospitals
of Leicester NHS Trust, Glenfield
Hospital, Leicester

Samantha Walker
Director of Education and
Research, Education for Health,
Warwick and Hon. Senior Lecturer
(nonclinical), University of
Edinburgh

Abbreviations

6MWT	6-minute walk test
ABG	arterial blood gases
ACBT	active cycle of breathing technique
ACE	angiotensin-converting enzyme
ADR	adverse drug reaction
AFB	acid-fast bacilli
AIDS	acquired immune deficiency syndrome
ALI	acute lung injury
AMS	acute mountain sickness
ANCA	antinuclear cytoplasmic antibody
ANA	antinuclear antibody
ANF	atrial natriuretic factor
ARDS	acute respiratory distress syndrome
ARNS	Association of Respiratory Nurse Specialists
ASM	airway smooth muscle
β_2	β_2 agonist
BAC	bronchial alveolar cell
BCG	Bacillus Calmette-Guérin
BHR	bronchial hyper-reactivity
BLF	British Lung Foundation
BMI	body mass index (kg/metres^2)
BNF	British National Formulary
BOOP	bronchiolitis obliterans-organizing pneumonia
BP	blood pressure
BPM	breaths per minute
BSAC	British Sub-Aqua Club
BTS	British Thoracic Society
cAMP	cyclic adenosine monophosphate
CAP	community-acquired pneumonia
CBT	cognitive behavioural therapy
CF	cystic fibrosis
CFC	chloroflourocarbon
CFRD	cystic fibrosis-related diabetes
CFTR	cystic fibrosis transmembrane conductance regulator
CHF	congestive heart failure
CHART	continuous hyperfractionated accelerated radiotherapy

CHM	Commission on Human Medicines
CHP	chronic hypersensitivity pneumonitis
CO	carbon monoxide
CO_2	carbon dioxide
COPD	chronic obstructive pulmonary disease
COSHH	Control of Substances Hazardous to Health
CPAP	continuous positive airway pressure
CRP	C-reactive protein
CT	computerized tomography
CTPA	computerized tomography pulmonary angiography
CURB	confusion, urea, respiratory rate, blood pressure
CVA	cerebral vascular accident
CVS	cardiovascular system
CVS	chorionic villus sampling
CXR	Chest X-ray
DIOS	distal intestinal obstruction syndrome
DLCO	CO diffusing capacity
DOT	directly observed therapy
DPI	dry powder inhaler
DPLD	diffuse parenchymal lung disease
DVLA	Department of Vehicle Licensing Authority
DVT	deep vein thrombosis
$ECCO_2R$	extra corporeal carbon dioxide removal
ECG	electrocardiograph
ECMO	extra corporeal membrane oxygenation
ECOG	European Cooperative Oncology Group
EDRTB	extreme drug-resistant tuberculosis
EDS	excessive daytime sleepiness
EPAP	expiratory positive air presssure
EPP	Expert Patients' Programme
ERA	endothelin receptor antagonists
ERV	expiratory reserve volume
ESR	erythrocyte sedimentation rate
ETA	endothelin receptor type A
ETB	endothelin receptor type B
EU	European Union
FBC	full blood count
FEV_1	forced expiratory volume in 1 second
FiO_2	fractional inspired oxygen
FRC	functional residual capacity
FVC	forced vital capacity

GCS	Glasgow Coma Scale
GMS	General Medical Services
GP	General Practitioner
GPIAG	General Practice Airways Group
GPwSI	General Practitioner with a Special Interest
H_2A	H_2 receptor antagonists
HACE	high altitude cerebral oedema
HADS	hospital anxiety and depression scale
HaH	hospital at home
HAPE	high altitude pulmonary oedema
Hb	haemoglobin
HCO_3	bicarbonate
HDU	high dependency unit
HEF	high efficiency filters
HFA	hydrofluoroalkane
HIB	*Haemophilus influenza* B
HIV	human immunodeficiency virus
HOCF	home oxygen consent form
HOOF	home oxygen order form
HRCT	high-resolution computerized tomography
IC	inspiratory capacity
ICS	inhaled corticosteroids
ICU	intensive care unit
IgE	immunoglobulin E
IgG	immunoglobulin G
IgA	immunoglobulin A
IgM	immunoglobulin M
IMIG	International Mesothelioma Interest Group
IMPRESS	IMProving and Integrating RESpiratory Services in the NHS
INR	international normalized ratio
IPAP	inspiratory positive air pressure
IPF	idiopathic pulmonary fibrosis
IPPV	intermittent positive pressure ventilation
IRV	inspiratory reserve volume
ITU	intensive therapy unit
IV	intravenous
IVC	inferior vena cava
JVP	jugular venous pressure
LABA	long-acting beta agonist
LAM	lymhangioleiemyomatosis

LDH	lactate dehydrogenase
LMW	low-molecular weight
LRTI	lower respiratory tract infection
LTOT	long-term oxygen therapy
LTRA	leukotrine receptor antagonists
LVF	left ventricular failure
LVRS	lung-volume reduction surgery
LVS	large volume spacer
MAI	*Mycobacterium avium intracellular*
MDRTB	multi-drug-resistant tuberculosis
MDT	multidisciplinary team
MEF	Mid-expiratory flow
MHRA	Medicines and Healthcare Products Regulatory Agency
MPAP	mean pulmonary artery pressure
MRC	Medical Research Council
MRSA	methicillin-resistant *Staphylococcus Aureus*
MTB	*Mycobacterium tuberculosis*
N	nitrogen
NCA	neutrophil chemotactic activity
NHS	National Health Service
NICE	National Institute for Health and Clinical Excellence
NiPPV	non-invasive positive pressure ventilation
NIV	non-invasive ventilation
NMC	Nurses and Midwives Council
NP	Nurse Practitioner
NRT	nicotine replacement therapy
NSAID	non-steroidal anti-inflammatory drugs
NSCLC	non-small cell lung cancer
NSIP	non-specific interstitial pneumonia
O_2	oxygen
OPD	outpatient department
OSA	obstructive sleep apnoea
OT	occupational therapist
OTC	over the counter
$PaCO_2$	partial pressure of arterial carbon dioxide
PACS	Picture Archiving and Communication System
PAF	platelet-activating factor
PAH	pulmonary arterial hypertension
PaO_2	partial pressure of arterial oxygen
PCI	prophylactic cranial irradiation

PCO	primary care organizations
PCT	Primary Care Trust
PCV	packed cell volume
PCWP	pulmonary capillary wedge pressure
PE	pulmonary embolism
PEEP	positive end expiratory pressure
PEF	peak expiratory flow
PEFR	peak expiratory flow rate
PET	positron emission tomography
PGI2	epoprostenol
PH	pulmonary arterial hypertension
PI	pancreatic insufficiency
PICU	paediatric intensive care unit
PMDI	pressurized meter dose inhaler
PO_2	oxygen tension
PPI	proton pump inhibitor
RADS	reactive airway dysfunction syndrome
RAST	radioallergosorbent test
RBC	red blood cell
RCN	Royal College of Nursing
RF	rheumatoid factor
RSV	respiratory synactial virus
RV	residual volume
RVC	relaxed vital capacity
SaO_2	arterial oxygen saturation
SARS	severe acute respiratory syndrome
SCLC	small cell lung cancer
SCUBA	self-contained underwater breathing apparatus
sIgE	specific immunoglobulin E
SIRS	systemic inflammatory response syndrome
SOB	shortness of breath
SPAP	systolic pulmonary artery pressure
SVC	slow vital capacity
SVS	small volume spacer
SWT	shuttle walk test
TB	tuberculosis
TENS	transcutaneous nerve stimulation
TLC	total lung capacity
TNF	tumour necrosis factor
TNM	tumour, nodes, metastasis

TTE	transthoracic echocardiogram
TV	tidal volume
UDV	União do Vegetal
UIP	usual interstitial pneumonia
UK	United Kingdom
VALI	ventilator-associated lung injury
VAP	ventilator-associated pneumonia
VAS	visual analogue scale
VATS	video assisted thorascopic surgery
VC	vital capacity
VQ	ventilation perfusion
Vt	tidal volume
WBC	white blood cell count
WHO	World Health Organisation
XDRTB	extreme drug-resistant tuberculosis

Chapter 1

Introduction

Overview and causes of respiratory diseases

Overview

Respiratory diseases are one of the most common forms of ill-health. They affect about eight million people in the United Kingdom (UK); one person in every family on average.

There are more than thirty conditions that can affect the lungs and/or airways and impact on a person's ability to breathe. These diseases are a leading cause of hospitalization and death.

Major respiratory diseases include infective lung diseases such as tuberculosis and pneumonia; obstructive lung diseases such as asthma and chronic obstructive pulmonary disease (COPD); restrictive lung diseases such as interstitial lung disease; pulmonary vascular diseases such as pulmonary hypertension and pulmonary embolism along with many others.

Respiratory health problems have a major impact on the daily lives of people everywhere, accounting for a significant amount of morbidity, disability and mortality. People with lung disease can experience severe restrictions on their mobility and ability to undertake day-to-day activities, such as getting dressed or cooking a meal.

Causes of respiratory disease

Whilst some respiratory diseases are closely related to smoking; COPD
and lung cancer for example, it is important to stress that there is a wide
variety of other factors which impact on lung health. These include:

- Viral lung infections in childhood
- Inadequate lung development in childhood
- Passive smoking
- Air pollution
- Occupational exposure to materials such as dust, asbestos fibres and
  other irritant particles
- Poor nutrition
- Social deprivation including poor housing and homelessness
- Genetic factors.

The specific causes of the most common respiratory diseases will be
discussed in the individual chapters in this book.

Mortality and morbidity

Mortality

Respiratory disease is the second biggest killer globally after cardiovascular diseases. Out of 68 million deaths worldwide in 2020, 11.9 million will be caused by lung diseases. Respiratory disease kills one person in five in the UK, and accounts for more deaths each year than coronary artery disease or non-respiratory cancer. Unlike other chronic diseases, deaths from respiratory disease do not appear to be falling.

Data from the World Health Organisation (WHO) shows that death rates from diseases of the respiratory system in the UK are higher than both the European average and the European Union (EU) average. This difference is particularly marked for females: death rates from respiratory disease for females in the UK are about three times higher than those for females in France and Italy.

A higher proportion of respiratory disease deaths are caused by social inequality than by any other disease. Almost a half of all deaths (44%) are associated with social class inequalities, compared with 28% of deaths from ischaemic heart disease.

Men aged 20–64 employed in unskilled manual occupations are around 14 times more likely to die from COPD, and 9 times more likely to die from tuberculosis than men employed in professional roles.

Mortality by type of respiratory disease

- Respiratory cancers—30% of respiratory deaths
- Pneumonia—29% of respiratory deaths
- COPD—23% of respiratory deaths.

The remaining approximatley 20% of deaths are caused by a range of respiratory diseases including cystic fibrosis, tuberculosis, and acute respiratory infections.

Morbidity

Respiratory disease is the most commonly reported long-term illness in children and the third most commonly reported in adults. Many of the eight million people with respiratory disease in the UK suffer considerable personal discomfort.

Rates of self-reported respiratory morbidity vary with socio-economic status. In 2004 about 40% more men and women in routine and manual occupations reported long-term respiratory conditions than those in managerial and professional jobs.

Lung disease has a multiple impact on patients and their carers, as well as the NHS. This impact on the NHS includes the following areas:

Inpatient hospital treatment

- There were over 845,000 inpatient admissions for respiratory disease in NHS Hospitals in England during 2004/05. This represents nearly 7% of all admissions
- Of these, more than 550,000 were emergency admissions—13% of all emergency admissions
- Respiratory disease accounts for 5.2 million bed days, nearly 10% of all hospital bed days.

Consultations in general practice

- There are nearly 24 million consultations in general practice due to respiratory disease in the UK per year
- Nearly one in five males and one in four females consulted a GP for a respiratory complaint in the UK in 2004
- The most commonly reported illnesses in babies and children are lung-related—asthma is one of the commonest single causes of admission to hospital among children.

Drug treatment

- About 51 million prescriptions were dispensed in England in 2004, for the prevention and treatment of respiratory disease
- Just about half of these were for bronchodilators used in the treatment of asthma and COPD, corticosteroids now account for over a quarter of respiratory drugs (📖 p.391)
- Respiratory prescriptions account for 7% of all prescribed drugs in the whole of the UK.

Costs of respiratory disease

Lung disease not only causes much individual suffering, but it also has a major economic impact. Respiratory disease costs the NHS and society £6.6 billion, £3 billion in costs to the care system, £1.9 billion in mortality costs and £1.7 billion in illness costs per annum. The British Thoracic Society's (BTS) document, the burden of lung disease[1] published in 2006 gave the following costs of respiratory disease in 2004 in the UK:

• 24 million consultations with GPs—at a cost of £501 million to primary care
• An estimated one million admissions a year for respiratory disease in the UK—at a suggested cost of £1,496.4 million to secondary care
• £975.3 million—spent on prescribed respiratory drugs
• Nearly 25 million certified sickness absence days in 2002/2003 related to respiratory disease—amounting to an estimated £1,728.5 million of lost production due to respiratory disease
• These figures do not include days lost from self-certified sickness, and so they under-estimate the true cost of respiratory disease.

1. British Thoracic Society (2006) The burden of lung disease, 2nd edn.

Why work in respiratory nursing?

A career in respiratory medicine or thoracic surgery?

Working in the specialty of respiratory medicine and thoracic surgery offers an interesting, diverse and wide ranging choice of excellent opportunities for an appealing and fulfilling career. The specialty includes over thirty different medical conditions of which some are common and some relatively rare so there is ample opportunity to subspecialize as well as to take a more generalist pathway. Nurses in this specialty are often members of a multidisciplinary team working with other specialist nurses, consultants, general practitioners, physiotherapists, occupational therapists, pharmacists, and respiratory technicians (p.581). There are often many opportunities to direct and help the development of local services and care provision. Many nurses now cross the traditional boundaries of primary and secondary care working with patients wherever there is a perceived need.

For nurses working in the acute setting some hospitals have highly specialized respiratory units often providing regional services. However in the majority of units a large proportion of the workload combines acute respiratory and general medicine. It is generally recognized that respiratory conditions currently account for about a third of emergency admissions so the range of roles for nurses may encompass triage and front line assessment, care on respiratory or general wards, intensive or high- dependency care, and a range of specialist roles for immediate, early discharge and continuing care.

In the community nurses may work in walk-in centres, GP practices, health centres, and intermediate care settings or in the patients own home in a variety of roles. Some nurses will undertake their own respiratory clinics whilst others will incorporate their respiratory work into more generalist clinics.

Desirable qualities for a respiratory nurse

There are several personal qualities that are desirable for careers in respiratory nursing. Amongst these are:

- A good general medical knowledge and surgical knowledge if working with thoracic surgery patients
- A good knowledge of respiratory disorders
- Good communication skills
- The ability to work with other multidisciplinary team members
- The ability to work both within a team and often alone
- A willingness to explore new roles and boundaries
- An empathetic approach towards patients with chronic disorders, especially where therapeutic interventions are limited.

It is also essential that the nurse has a thorough understanding of the basic physiological and anatomical principles relating to the respiratory system, along with a fundamental knowledge of how different disease processes affect lung function (📖 p.13).

How do I become a respiratory nurse?

There are many ways in which a respiratory nursing post can be developed. These include undertaking relevant training courses and study days backed up by practical experience working with patients with respiratory problems. Joining the RCN respiratory nurse forum means that you will be kept informed of relevant respiratory matters by the newsletter 'Inspiration' and there are other respiratory publications available.

Opportunities exist for education and further training both locally and nationally.

Further training courses at all levels from diploma to MSc in respiratory are offered by:

Respiratory Education UK
University Hospital Aintree
Lower Lane
Liverpool
L9 7AL
Telephone: 0151 5292598
http://www.respiratoryeduk.com

Education for Health
The Atheneum
10 Church Street
Warwick
CV34 4AB
Telephone: 01926 493313
http://www.nrtc.org.uk

As well as the training centres many local universities and colleges run respiratory course and many respiratory nurses work as facilitators on these courses sharing their knowledge with others.

There are also many conferences specifically for respiratory disorders run through the RCN, BTS and also the training centres and pharmaceutical companies.

What are the current job prospects?

There are many opportunities for nurses with an interest in respiratory medicine and thoracic surgery to work in a variety of settings and in a variety of roles. Whilst some nurses are generalists many choose to have a subspecialty interest, such as asthma, chronic obstructive pulmonary disease (COPD), tuberculosis (TB), cystic fibrosis or lung cancer. Many nurses offer services such as smoking cessation, breathlessness management, counselling, and cognitive behavioural therapy (CBT) and many are involved in or run pulmonary rehabilitation schemes (📕 p.531).

A wide pathway of careers exist in respiratory nursing from Staff Nurse, Practice Nurse, Specialist Nurse, Nurse with a Specialist Interest, Nurse Practitioner, Lead Nurse to Consultant Nurse. Clearly respiratory nursing offers many opportunities for nurses seeking a challenging and fulfilling career.

The current job prospects are extremely good and there are often advertised vacancies within the nursing press. Pay scales vary enormously between jobs and between different areas of the country.

Useful addresses

Royal College of Nursing (RCN) Respiratory Nurses Forum
20 Cavendish Square
London
W1G 0RN

Association of Respiratory Nurse Specialists (ARNS)
17 Doughty Street
London
WC1N 2PL

British Lung Foundation (BLF)
73–75 Goswell Road
London EC1V 7ER
Telephone: 020 7688 5555

British Thoracic Society (BTS)
17 Doughty Street
London
WC1N 2PL

General Practice Airways Group (GPAIG)
http://www.gpiag.org.uk

Chapter 3

Anatomy and physiology

Introduction

This chapter covers some fundamental aspects of the respiratory tract, and will describe the structure and function of both the upper and lower airways, processes by which air is moved from the external environment to the gas exchange area of the lungs, and some of the aspects of the normal respiratory tract which are affected by the more common respiratory diseases.

Overall view of the respiratory tract

In its simplest form, the respiratory tract is a complicated infolding of tissue starting at the mouth and terminating at the areas of gas exchange, the alveoli. Its functions in terms of respiration are to facilitate the uptake of oxygen; eliminate carbon dioxide; and maintain the pH of the blood. Conventionally the tract is divided into upper and lower parts. The upper tract is composed of the mouth, nasal passages, and behind these a wide tube termed the pharynx. This receives inhaled air from the nose and mouth and accordingly is termed the naso- and oropharynx respectively.

Upper respiratory tract

The upper tract has a number of vital functions to perform; these are aimed at 'conditioning' inspired air. The specific function of the upper tract is to:
• Warm
• Humidify
• Cleanse inspired air.

The structure of the nasal cavities plays a part in this, particularly the cleansing of air, by altering the velocity of inspired air at different sites, and also altering turbulence in the airflow because of structures such as the conchae bones which project into the posterior nasal cavity. The conchae bones are also known as the turbinates. These alterations in velocity and turbulence help with removal of particulate matter from inspired air. In terms of humidification and warming of air, the conchae provide for an increased surface area, so allowing for maximum contact between inspired air and the tissue lining the upper tract, which is ciliated columnar epithelium. This has an abundant supply of mucus glands within it, and the rich blood supply of the mucosa, together with the mucus provide the warming and humidifying functions of the upper airways respectively. (see Figure 3.1)

The pharynx

The pharynx leads directly into the larynx, and this is an important area because of the proximity of the respiratory tract to the digestive tract, in particular the oesophagus. There is the potential for ingested matter to enter the trachea, where it may cause a number of problems. Normally, however, the epiglottis acts as a barrier to unwanted material entering the trachea.

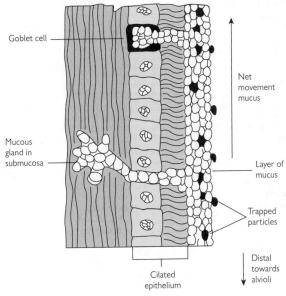

Fig. 3.1 Tissue structure in the upper respiratory tract
Reproduced with permission from Respiratory UK.

Lower respiratory tract

Trachea

This is the first structure in the lower respiratory tract. The trachea:

- Is the main air conducting passage
- It is approximately 13cms long in adults
- Divides to form two large airways, the bronchi (s. bronchus).

Bronchi

Each bronchus provides air entry to the left and right lungs. On entering the lungs, the bronchi divide into secondary and tertiary bronchi; these in turn continue to divide, eventually forming smaller airways called bronchioles. This continuing division of the airways once inside the lung is a key feature of respiratory anatomy, and helps explain how the large amounts of air needed on occasions can be delivered efficiently to the gas exchange area. As the airways continue to divide, they become narrower at each division. At the same time however the number of airways increases considerably.

To illustrate this concept, consider the following:

- We have one trachea
- This is approximately 2.5cm wide, and has a total cross-sectional surface area of 5cms
- At the end of the so-called conducting airways are the terminal respiratory bronchioles
- These number approximately 630, 000, and have an individual diameter of 0.45mm
- However, their total cross-sectional surface area is 1.71m^2. The total cross-sectional surface area of the conducting airways then could be likened to a trumpet, with a narrow top part and a flared end.

The conducting airways terminate in the alveolar ducts, and these lead into the alveoli. Alveoli are the structures involved in gaseous exchange, and as such could be viewed as 'what the lungs are all about'. However, from the preceding discussion it is apparent that all parts of the airway are important in each stage of respiration.

Airway structure

The main points re the upper respiratory tract have been described above. We will now consider some structural aspects of the lower tract, (many of which are depicted in Figure 3.2) starting with the trachea.

Trachea

As stated, this is approximately 13cm long in adults, and is approximately 2.5cm wide. This is sometimes described as a rigid tube, due to the presence of rings of cartilage surrounding it. However, these rings are incomplete, being described as C-shaped, with their opening facing posteriorly. A band of muscle joins the end of these rings, so while being very strongly supported, the trachea does have a degree of flexibility in that it can alter its diameter.

Bronchi

- The trachea divides at a particular cartilage called the carina to form the bronchi which supply each lung
- The first generations of the bronchi have complete rings of cartilage, but after this the cartilage becomes 'plates' which are attached to the airway wall
- As the airways continue to divide these plates of cartilage become smaller and thinner. They eventually peter out altogether at bronchiolar level
- Here the more predominant tissue is smooth muscle, and this has the role of regulating airflow in and out of the lungs. As demands for oxygen and production of carbon dioxide are variable, it can be appreciated that the ability to adapt to these variations is very important in maintaining respiratory health.

Tissue lining

In terms of lining tissue, the upper tract is very similar throughout, being pseudostratified ciliated columnar epithelium with mucus-secreting goblet cells. Mucus is also secreted by deeper lying bronchial glands. As described earlier this tissue type is important in conditioning and cleansing inspired air. Each epithelial cell has approximately 200 cilia on its surface, resulting in 1-2 billion cilia per cm^2 of mucosa. Below the mucosa is a supporting tissue, the lamina propria, and below this is a submucosa containing blood vessels and nerves.

- As with the cartilage, the epithelial cells change in nature as the airways divide and their walls become thinner
- The ciliated columnar cells seen in the upper respiratory tract gradually change to simple cuboidal epithelial epithelium which do not have cilia; in addition the number of mucus-secreting cells decreases
- At alveolar level the most significant change is the presence of squamous epithelial cells. Their structure enables them to meet their role which is to allow diffusion of respiratory gases from alveolar space to blood and vice versa.

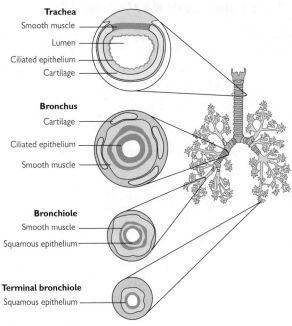

Fig. 3.2 Anatomy of the conducting airways
Reproduced with permission from Respiratory UK.

What happens during 'a breath'?

The main stimulus to breathing is in fact the pH of the blood, which in turn is driven by levels of carbon dioxide in the blood. This is constantly being produced as a result of cellular activity, and so has to be continually eliminated.

Carbon dioxide is important because following a set of well recognized chemical reactions hydrogen ions are formed. These tend to make the blood acidic. In basic terms, the acidity or alkalinity of the blood is measured on a scale called the pH scale. This runs from 1 (very acidic) to 14 (very alkaline), with blood having a normal range of 7.35–7.45. This narrow range illustrates how sensitively respiration is controlled and how important it is to maintain adequate respiratory function – to illustrate this point further, even a small drop in pH (down to approximately 6.9, which is less than one whole unit on the pH scale), is incompatible with life. The continual production of hydrogen ions, driven in turn by the continual production of carbon dioxide would, if not dealt with in some way, drive the pH down, i.e make the blood become more acidic. However, in normal circumstances the continued removal of carbon dioxide via expiration means that the pH of the blood is maintained within the normal homeostatic range. It is the hydrogen ions that are the major stimulus for breathing, as these activate the respiratory centres which control respiration.

A breath is achieved by:
- Structures called chemoreceptors in major blood vessels and in the brain detecting alterations in blood chemistry which are outside homeostatic limits
- They send messages to the respiratory centre in the brain, which initiates the sequence of events leading to inhalation/exhalation. The main muscle involved in breathing at rest is the diaphragm, with some input from the external and internal intercostal muscles situated between the ribs
- Nerve impulses arising from the respiratory centre stimulate these muscles, so causing them to contract
- Diaphragmatic contraction pulls the base of the lungs downwards, while costal muscle contraction pulls them upwards and outwards
- Impulses sent via the phrenic nerve stimulate the diaphragm to contract
- As it does it pulls the base of the lung downwards (via the visceral and parietal pleura; this in its simplest form is a double layer of tissue surrounding the lung)
- Pulling the lung downwards increases its overall volume and so decreases the pressure within it. The result is that there is a pressure gradient between the air inside the lung and the air in the external environment
- The very end result of this is that air moves down the concentration gradient, i.e. it flows from the environment in to lungs, and along the conducting airways, bringing oxygen as it does so
- Inspiration only lasts for a second or two, and a number of mechanisms are involved in the termination of inspiration

- At this point the diaphragm relaxes, and the base of the lung moves upwards. This returns the lungs to their 'original volume'
- However, they now have more air in them than at the start of the breath – so as they return to their original volume, the pressure in them starts to increase
- This pressure will eventually exceed the external pressure, so establishing a pressure gradient again – only this time the gradient is in the opposite direction
- Consequently the air now flows from inside the lungs to the external environment, taking carbon dioxide with it.

Many of these points plus some of the many influences on breathing are depicted in Figures 3.3 and 3.4.

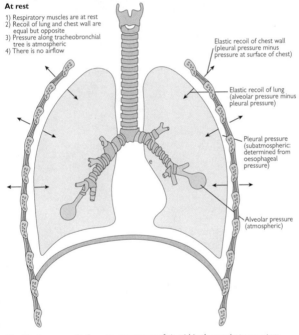

At rest
1) Respiratory muscles are at rest
2) Recoil of lung and chest wall are equal but opposite
3) Pressure along tracheobronchial tree is atmospheric
4) There is no airflow

Elastic recoil of chest wall (pleural pressure minus pressure at surface of chest)

Elastic recoil of lung (alveolar pressure minus pleural pressure)

Pleural pressure (subatmospheric: determined from oesophageal pressure)

Alveolar pressure (atmospheric)

Fig. 3.3 Pressures of influencing movement of air within the respiratory system
Reproduced with permission from Respiratory UK.

Regulation of airway calibre

As indicated previously, demands for oxygen and production of carbon dioxide which must be eliminated are variable. This is turn implies that the amount of air moved in and out of the lungs should also be variable in order to meet the increased/decreased demands. The two fundamental aspects of this process are increases in the rate and depth of respiration. The first of these processes is driven by changes in pH which directly influence the activity of the respiratory centre.

The second process, that of an increased depth of respiration, involves the movement of much larger amounts of air into and out of the lungs, and this in turn implies that the calibre of the airways must alter – this is indeed the case; this concept is important in both health and very common respiratory disorders such as asthma (📖 p.147) and chronic obstructive pulmonary disease (COPD) (📖 p.249).

Control of airway calibre

This is possible because of the presence of smooth muscle in the airways, referred to as airway smooth muscle (ASM). Smooth muscle in the upper airways is less prominent, and arranged in sheets. In the lower airways, notably from the bronchioles onwards, the muscle is arranged in rings which spiral around the airways. It is the contraction or relaxation of this smooth muscle which permits large variations in the amount of air entering the lungs.

Control of ASM and therefore airway calibre is performed by the autonomic nervous system. This has two divisions which have opposing actions.

Sympathetic division

The sympathetic division operates under the so called 'fight, fright or flight' mechanism. Sympathetic nerve endings are found in both the airways and in the adrenal glands. Under appropriate circumstances sympathetic nerves will:

- Stimulate the adrenal glands to secrete two hormones, adrenaline and noradrenaline
- Will directly secrete noradrenaline from sympathetic nerve endings which lie in close proximity to the ASM. Both of these hormones are in effect neurotransmitters, and will land on receptor sites situated on the plasma membrane of the ASM cells
- These receptors are termed β2 receptors. When adrenaline or noradrenaline bind to them a set of chemical reactions are initiated which eventually result in the ASM relaxing, and so increasing airway calibre.

Parasympathetic division

The opposite happens with the parasympathetic division. (Ninety percent of parasympathetic outflow occurs via the vagus nerve, and so many texts refer to the concept of vagal tone when discussing airways).

- Parasympathetic nerves tend to be trying to 'close the airways down' all of the time
- They achieve this by secreting a neurotransmitter called acetylcholine from their nerve endings
- This operates under the same principle as the sympathetic division in that the acetylcholine binds to a receptor (simply called a cholinergic receptor)
- This initiates a series of chemical reactions which ultimately result in ASM contracting, and so decreasing airway calibre. This system is overridden by the sympathetic division when more oxygen is required and we need to excrete more carbon dioxide.

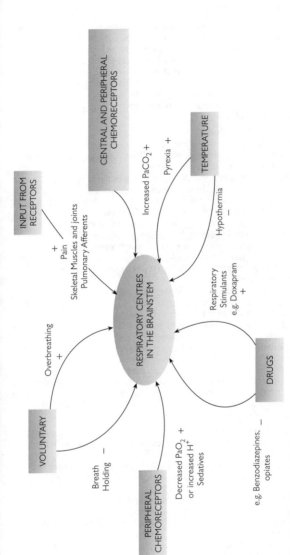

Fig. 3.4 Influences on respiration
Reproduced with permission from Respiratory UK.

Gaseous exchange

So far we have considered a number of aspects, viz the upper airways' role in conditioning inspired air; the structure and changing nature of the conducting airways and how their calibre can change; and something of the mechanisms underlying the whole process of getting air into and out of the lungs. The major function of respiration is however the uptake of oxygen by the blood, and the removal of the waste gas carbon dioxide from the body, and we need to consider here how gas exchange is achieved, and also the relationship between the lungs and the cardiovascular system (CVS).

External respiration

- The physiological principle underlying gas exchange is diffusion. By this process molecules move from areas of high concentration to low concentration until equilibrium is achieved
- The important points to bear in mind are that the areas of gas exchange, the alveoli, are surrounded by a dense network of capillaries
- These capillaries are derived from the pulmonary artery, which in turn is derived from the right side of the heart, and so contain blood which has a low oxygen and a high carbon dioxide content
- Separating this blood from the high oxygen low carbon dioxide environment of the alveolar space are the blood vessels and alveolar walls. Respiratory gases are highly lipid soluble; the implication of this is that these gases can easily pass through the cell membranes of both capillary and alveolar cells
- Because of this, diffusion of oxygen from alveolar space to blood, and of carbon dioxide from blood to alveolar space, happens very quickly (within seconds) so that by the time a capillary is leaving the alveolus it is maximally loaded with oxygen, and has offloaded much of the carbon dioxide it brought to the alveolus.

External respiration may seem a strange term for something which happens (or seems to happen) deep within the body. However, looking back at the start of this chapter, the term can be seen to be appropriate. As our airways divide they do become smaller and smaller, reaching the minute alveoli. Bear in mind however that on arrival at the alveolar membrane, no tissue has been breached, and while the space is small, it is still 'external' to the body-hence the use of the term external respiration.

Internal respiration

- The oxygen taken up by alveoli is bound to haemoglobin in red blood cells
- Blood leaves the lungs via increasingly large venuoles and veins, with two pulmonary veins leaving each lung and taking the oxygenated blood to the left side of the heart
- From there the blood is delivered to the body tissues, where diffusion again plays a part, only this time in reverse
- Oxygen diffuses from the blood (where it is in high concentration) to the tissues
- Conversely carbon dioxide diffuses from the tissues (where it is in high concentration) into the blood
- This process at tissue level is termed internal respiration

- Finally blood leaving body tissues does so via again increasingly large venuols and veins, with two large veins, the superior and inferior vena cava draining the now oxygen-poor, carbon dioxide-rich blood into the right side of the heart
- From there it will be pumped in to the lungs to continue the ongoing cycle so essential for life to continue.

The main points re respiratory anatomy and physiology have been covered here. The principles of the structure of the respiratory tree have been described, as have the important concept of our ability to adjust respiratory function in response to fluctuations in demand.

Respiration is vital not just to life per se, but also to quality of life. Normal respiratory function depends on a wide range of factors, not all of which have been covered in this brief overview. Alterations in normal respiratory physiology are seen in many common respiratory conditions, and hopefully this chapter will prepare the reader for the rest of this book.

Respiratory assessment

Introduction

Many nurses in both primary and secondary care are working as respiratory nurse specialists and nurse practitioners. These roles involve assessing and diagnosing many conditions, including common respiratory disorders. This chapter covers undertaking a respiratory assessment. It shows how making a diagnosis can be difficult because the principal symptoms of respiratory disease are common to many different conditions. The respiratory assessment also determines which investigations may be required to reach a diagnosis.

There is no substitute for experience: the nurses' practice improves the more respiratory patients seen. Respiratory assessments involve skilled communication with patients and carers and other medical professionals, along with an understanding of informed consent and the ethical implications of gaining consent.

The consultation

The consultation with a respiratory nurse gives the patient the opportunity to discuss healthcare issues that may involve physical, psychological or social issues. It is the nurse's responsibility to ensure that the consultation is properly and sensitively carried out. Sufficient time should be allocated so that the patient and their carers can freely describe details of their symptoms and discuss any underlying concerns. Open-ended and specific questions should be asked so that a full and detailed history is obtained.

Environment

The environment can greatly influence the history taking and assessment process. Lack of privacy may mean that patients feel inhibited about discussing their medical condition. Patients may be overheard, and confidentiality lost.

If relatives are present, ask the patient if they are comfortable for them to be present during the consultation.

Communication

Good communication with patients, carers and other members of the medical team is essential to any consultation. To help the patient feel in control of the interview, nurses should remember to involve the patient rather than talk at them.

Nurses working with respiratory patients need to be able to respond to emotions, and to help the patient vocalize how they are feeling. They may have to deal with conflict and anger, especially where bad news has been broken. The nurse should try to see the patient's point of view and always respect their autonomy. Table 4.1 shows the core communication skills required by nurses.

Table 4.1 Core communication skills

Skill	Nursing action
The right setting	You and the patient should be comfortably seated at the same level so you can face and observe one another
Non-verbal communication	Retain a friendly manner and be aware of your posture and gestures during the consultation
Introductions	Introduce yourself
	Establish the patient's identity
	Ask permission to take a history
Questioning	Make use of open questions to obtain a clear and precise history
	Use closed questions to clarify what the patient has said, or to obtain factual information that the patient may not have volunteered
	Avoid the use of medical jargon
Identifying and responding to patient perceptions and concerns	Help the patient feel in control of the consultation
	Deal with emotions before facts; put the emotions into words and offer them back to the patient
	Seek to understand the emotions. Be clear what the patient is feeling and identify the source of those feelings
	Show your empathy verbally and non-verbally
	Encourage the patient to elaborate on the background to their emotions
Summary	Summarize periodically and at the end of the consultation
	Give the patient a chance to add information or ask questions
Closure	Thank the patient for attending
	Arrange a follow-up appointment if necessary
	Provide any written information or equipment, such as peak flow meter and diary, management plan

History taking 1

The consultation begins with a comprehensive medical history. The story that the patient tells the nurse is vital when obtaining a history, before an appropriate physical examination is undertaken.

History taking has always been central to medicine, but with more nurses training to become nurse practitioners and nurse prescribers, it is now of increasing importance in nursing. The same core skills are required both by nurses and doctors. There must be a structure to history taking. The nurse needs to be skilled in ensuring that a consultation includes all the information required. The nurse must have sufficient knowledge to interpret and understand the relevant symptoms or situation described by the patient (see Table 4.2.)

Components of a medical history

When performing an assessment a framework of questions must be developed to help the nurse gather information in a systematic way. Patients must be allowed to tell their story, but this may be unstructured; it is up to the nurse to gather the information in a logical sequence. Some practitioners find it useful to have a template or an assessment form to follow, to ensure that all relevant facts are collected.

The key elements of a medical history include:
- Patient identification
- Presenting complaint
- History of presenting complaint
- Past medical history
- Current health and medications
- Family history
- Psychosocial history
- Review of systems.

Patient identification

The patient's name, age, date of birth, and computer or hospital number should be recorded. The date and time of the consultation should also be noted.

Presenting complaint

The patient should be encouraged to explain the problem in their own words. This should be summarized briefly in a few words, such as shortness of breath, cough.

Table 4.2 Core skill 3: applying knowledge while taking a history

Skill	Indices
Identify the main symptoms	These could include: • Cough • Wheeze • Shortness of breath • Lethargy • Weight loss/gain • Pain
Obtain information relevant to that symptom	• Timing of symptoms • Duration of symptoms • Precipitating factors • What may relieve the symptom • What may make the symptom worse
Think of the different causes of that particular symptom	In shortness of breath for example, this could include: • Asthma • COPD • Pneumothorax • Pulmonary embolism • Lung cancer • Pulmonary hypertension • Anaemia • Obesity • Lack of fitness
If a diagnosis seems likely, think of the risk factors predisposing to that disease	In asthma for example: • Strong family history of asthma • Evidence of atopy such as eczema, hay fever, allergies • Occupational exposure
Think also of other diseases that may complicate or be associated with the main problem	Using COPD as an example consider: • Cor pulmonale • Polycythaemia • Pulmonary hypertension • Osteoporosis
Think of possible effects of the disease on the patient	Using occupational asthma as an example: • Lost time from work • Loss of income • Ultimate job loss

History taking 2

History of present complaint

The patient should be encouraged to describe what they think has caused the problem, and what has led them to ask for help. They should be asked what impact the symptoms are having on their life. What provokes symptoms and what relieves them? For example, if the patient is complaining of breathlessness, they should be asked what exacerbates the breathlessness, and what treatment they may have tried either pharmacologically or non-pharmacologically to alleviate it.

Once the patient has given their account, the nurse can enquire about the presenting symptoms and illness. Patients with respiratory disease may have many chronic symptoms such as breathlessness or cough. The nurse must determine whether the patient is describing an acute worsening of their usual symptoms, and what has led them to seek medical attention. The timing and precipitants of the symptoms should be recorded as well as the impact on daily living.

Past medical history

Details of any previous or other current illnesses, operations or injuries should be recorded. For instance, a past history of tuberculosis is significant where the presenting complaint is haemoptysis and weight loss, particularly if treatment was inadequate or incomplete the first time.

Disease affecting other organs than the respiratory system is also significant. For example, a history of cardiac disease may be particularly relevant in an acutely breathless patient, as heart failure may be the cause of the symptoms, rather than respiratory disease.

Drug history

The patient should be asked to bring a list of any repeat prescriptions to the consultation, as many patients fail to remember drug names and dosages. The patient should also specifically be asked about:

- What medications they are currently taking, including 'over the counter' medication
- Any respiratory medications they may have been prescribed in the past, and why that medication had been stopped
- Whether they use nebulized drugs (🕮 p.440) or are on home oxygen therapy
- History of allergic reactions they may have had in the past, and what their symptoms were.

This last point is important, as many people confuse common side-effects such as nausea related to starting an antibiotic, for example, as an allergic drug reaction. This may result in the patient being denied drugs in the future that they may benefit from. Any true allergy should be clearly documented in the consultation notes.

Many drugs have pulmonary side effects. ACE inhibitors and beta blockers can cause cough for example. Aspirin, non-steroidal anti-inflammatories and beta blockers can all trigger asthma exacerbations.

Family history

Taking a family history will highlight conditions with genetic links which may be the cause of the patients' symptoms, such as cystic fibrosis (📖 p.298) or alpha one antitrypsin deficiency (📖 p.249). A strong family history of asthma, for example, may lead the nurse to consider this as a possible diagnosis in an individual presenting with nocturnal cough and breathlessness.

Social history

This is a crucial part of any respiratory assessment and should include:

Occupation

A detailed occupational history should be taken. This should include the nature, duration of the employment and what the job entailed. This is especially important for workers who were exposed to environmental hazards, such as passive smoking, silica, asbestos or coal dust (📖 p.541) (see Table 4.3). The nurse should enquire whether any respiratory or other protection was worn during the period of employment. If the patient is currently employed, then the nature and timing of the symptoms should be explored, especially if an occupational disease is suspected which is liable to compensation (📖 p.147). The patient should also be asked if any time has been taken off work because of respiratory illness.

Smoking and illicit drug use

Tobacco is a major cause of respiratory disease. The type and amount of tobacco smoked, along with the duration should be recorded and the individuals 'pack year' (📖 p.75) history documented.

Smoking pack years

It is important to quantify an individual's exposure to tobacco as accurately as possible. This is best done in terms of 'pack years'. Smoking 20 cigarettes a day (a pack) for a year equates to one pack year.

The formula to calculate this is:

$$\left[\frac{\text{Number smoked per day}}{20} \times \text{Number of years smoked} \right]$$

If a patient smoked 10 cigarettes a day from the age of 20 to 60 this equals

$$\left[\frac{10}{20} \times 40 = 15 \text{ pack years} \right]$$

If a patient smoked 25 cigarettes a day from the age of 18 to 75 this equals

$$\left[\frac{25}{20} \times 57 = 71 \text{ pack years} \right]$$

Not all patients buy ready-made cigarettes. The following are all equivalent of 20 cigarettes daily:
- 25g of rolling tobacco weekly
- 50g of pipe tobacco weekly
- 5 small cigars daily.

It is important to ask patients who are active smokers if they have ever stopped smoking, and if so, for how long. This period should then be deducted from the final calculation.

A significant smoking history is more than 15–20 pack years.

Details of the use of any illicit drugs should be obtained and the delivery route (injection, smoking) noted.

Social circumstances

The nurse should enquire whether the patient lives with someone, or has a carer, or whether they are the main carer for others (children, spouse, parents). The type of housing they are living in is important. A breathless person may struggle if the only toilet is upstairs. The condition of the home is also important. Damp may trigger asthma attacks. If the home is overcrowded, diseases such as tuberculosis may be considered in people presenting with cough and weight loss (p.541).

Ask the person what walking or household aids they may have, such as stair lifts or bathing aids. They should be asked about the distance they can walk before they develop breathlessness, and whether stairs or inclines make their breathing worse. They should be asked how they manage with shopping, cooking and cleaning, and who, if anyone helps them. All these factors are important when planning a patient's care, especially when organizing a safe discharge for a patient who is in hospital.

Travel history

Patients should be asked about any foreign or local travel where they may have been sitting still for long periods; this increases the risk of pulmonary embolism. If patients have visited areas where there are high levels of tuberculosis, HIV or malaria, this should be documented.

Ethnicity

The ethnic origin of the patient may be relevant. For example, the incidence of tuberculosis is higher in people from the Indian subcontinent.

Pets, hobbies and activities

Patients should be asked whether they currently or used to keep birds such as pigeons, parrots, or parakeets, as these can be the source of a respiratory condition such as bird-fancier's lung. Pets, such as dogs, cats and horses can worsen or trigger asthma exacerbations.

Systems review

The patient should also be asked about any non-respiratory or general symptoms. They may omit or forget to mention important symptoms that point to an underlying cause.

Ask the patient about:

- General symptoms, such as appetite, weight loss/gain, fevers, night sweats
- Gastrointestinal symptom, such as constipation, diarrhoea, reflux, heartburn
- Genitourinary symptoms, such as incontinence, prostate problems, polyuria, excessive thirst, period problems
- Cardiac symptoms, such as chest pain, palpitations, orthopnoea, paroxysmal nocturnal dyspnoea, oedema.

Summary

The nurse should briefly summarize the history in a few sentences. For example, '27-year-old single woman with a history of asthma presenting with a two-week history of nocturnal cough, increasing shortness of breath and wheeze'.

Table 4.3 Occupational causes of respiratory disease

Diesease	Examples of work area
Occupational asthma	Flour mills
	Bakeries
	Animal laboratories
	Spray paint shops
	Foundries
	Carpentry workshops
	Pharmaceutical plants
Asbestosis and malignant mesothelioma	Vehicle body workshops
	Demolition sites
	Shipbuilding yards
Pneumoconiosis	Coal mines
Silicosis	Mines
	Quarries
	Foundries
Farmer's lung	Farms where mouldy hay is stored

Symptoms of upper respiratory disease

Respiratory conditions can produce a wide variety of symptoms. The most common symptoms are cough, sputum production, chest pain and changes in breathing pattern or breathlessness. The most common symptoms will be discussed in depth and it will become evident how many of them overlap in different respiratory and non-respiratory conditions.

Upper airway symptoms in respiratory disease

Most respiratory diseases focus on the lower respiratory tract (trachea, bronchial tree, lung parenchyma and pulmonary vasculature) (p.13). The upper airways (nasal passages, larynx, vocal cords) are a continuum of the lower respiratory tract and should be considered collectively as the 'united airway'. Treating upper airway symptoms may also have a beneficial impact on the lower airways. This is especially important in asthma management.

Nasal symptoms

The commonest disorders of the upper respiratory tract are those that involve inflammation of the lining of the nose, particularly when associated with infection. Table 4.4 shows nasal symptoms and their causes.

Symptoms of the pharynx and larynx

The most common conditions to affect the pharynx and larynx are inflammatory conditions, or those that cause obstruction or restriction. Table 4.5 shows the common symptoms and the conditions that cause them.

Table 4.4 Nasal symptoms and causes

Symptom	Cause
Nasal obstruction	• Common cold • Influenza virus • Rhinitis • Polyps • Neoplasms
Rhinorrhoea (runny nose)	• Common cold • Influenza virus • Hay fever
Nasal discharge	• Acute sinusitis • Chronic sinusitis
Nose bleeds	• Acute sinusitis • Wegener's granulomatosis • Neoplasms
Sneezing	• Hay fever • Common cold

Table 4.5 Symptoms and causes of pharyngeal and laryngeal conditions

Symptom	Cause
Hoarse voice	• Laryngitis • Neoplasm • Croup • Inhaled steroids
Snoring	• Sleep apnoea • Enlarged adenoids or tonsils • Nasal deformities • Allergies, asthma, common cold • Alcohol or certain medications (anti-histamines, night sedation) • Smoking
Stridor	• Vocal cord dysfunction • Croup • Epiglottitis
Pain	• Laryngitis • Tonsillitis • Candidiasis

Non-specific and extra-pulmonary symptoms

During the consultation the nurse should encourage the patient to discuss any other symptoms they may have. Patients with lung cancer or tuberculosis, for example, could present with a history of fatigue, night sweats, anorexia and weight loss (>10% loss of body weight in the absence of dietary intervention), rather than cough or breathlessness.

Patients with respiratory failure (📖 p.494) may present with:
• Mood changes
• Depression
• Loss of appetite
• Lack of energy
• Sleep disturbance
• Morning headaches
• Ankle swelling.

Patients with decreased oxygen levels in the blood (hypoxaemia) may present with:
• Lethargy
• Tiredness
• Confusion
• Disorientation
• Seizures.

Patients with elevated levels of carbon dioxide in the blood (hypercapnia) may present with:
• Headaches
• Drowsiness
• Confusion
• Coma
• Flapping tremor
• Bounding pulse.

Lung cancer can present with:
• Finger clubbing
• Joint and muscular pain
• Limb weakness
• Confusion
• Hoarseness.

The nurse should also be aware that symptoms localized to other systems may be suggestive of respiratory disorders. For example, pneumonia often presents acutely in the elderly, with confusion and diarrhoea with sometimes very few respiratory symptoms.

Breathlessness 1

Breathlessness (dyspnoea) is defined as 'an unpleasant or uncomfortable awareness of breathing or need to breathe'. The overall experience includes the perception of difficult breathing and the physical, emotional and behavioural response to it.

A number of physiological factors underlie the sensation of breathlessness, and several mechanisms can coexist to cause it. Understanding the physiological basis of breathlessness is of limited help clinically. A good history is vital in determining the cause of the breathlessness.

The feeling and extent of breathlessness a person experiences will depend on the underlying disease responsible; there may be more than one disease causing the breathlessness. It may also be caused by lack of fitness or obesity (see Table 4.6).

Many patients complain of breathlessness on exertion. This may be a result of disturbances in the circulatory system or the respiratory system. Whatever the underlying cause, it is the sensation of breathlessness (and/or fatigue) which ultimately limits a person's ability to exercise.

Assessing the breathless patient

The nurse should aim to identify possible conditions by the patient's history of breathlessness, alongside other supporting evidence from the history and examination. Specific questions should be asked including:

- Whether the onset of breathlessness is sudden or gradual
- How long the breathlessness lasts
- How far the person can walk before becoming breathless
- What exacerbates the breathlessness
- What relieves it
- If their current level of breathlessness is normal for them
- Whether the individual becomes breathless when lying flat
- How many pillows they need to sleep on
- How it affects their daily life
- If their breathlessness becomes more pronounced if they feel anxious
- If there is a history of panic attacks.

Duration and onset of breathlessness

The duration of breathlessness can indicate what the underlying disease may be. A number of conditions can cause sudden acute shortness of breath that develops within minutes (see Table 4.6). Prompt recognition and treatment of such conditions could be life-saving so a good history is vital.

Other conditions may present with a more gradual onset or worsening breathlessness over days, weeks, months or years. The degree of breathlessness perceived by the individual can be assessed by means of tools such as the MRC or Borg scales (📖 p.75).

A patient may present when an acute event, such as a chest infection, worsens the underlying chronic condition, such as COPD or asthma. There may then be a worsening of their usual day to day breathlessness, for example, they may be breathless at rest, or after minimal exertion. It is important that the nurse documents the patient's usual exercise tolerance and compares it to their current tolerance. This is one of the factors that assist in deciding whether the patient may need to be admitted to hospital.

Appropriate hyperventilation

Some conditions cause an appropriate hyperventilation response. Examples are metabolic acidosis resulting from ketoacidosis, drug toxicity, and renal failure. In these conditions there is a build-up of acid (hydrogen ions) in the bloodstream (📖 p.75) which is then buffered by bicarbonate ions. This reaction produces CO_2 which is removed by the respiratory system increasing the respiratory rate leading to shallow and rapid breathing. Hyperventilation may also be a result of diseases such as pulmonary emboli.

Inappropriate hyperventilation

Inappropriate hyperventilation is known as idiopathic hyperventilation syndrome. The hyperventilation occurs in the absence of any cardio-respiratory conditions. Its cause is not completely understood, but it is thought to be induced by anxiety and panic.

Symptoms include:
- Breathlessness
- Dizziness
- Chest pain
- Tingling and parasthesia of the extremities.

Hyperventilation can coexist with other respiratory conditions.

Table 4.6 Causes of breathlessness

Cause	
Physiological	• Exercise • Altitude
Pathological	• Respiratory disorders, including asthma, COPD, pneumonia, pleural effusion, lung cancer, pulmonary fibrosis, pulmonary embolism • Cardiac disorders: chronic heart failure, left ventricular failure, arrhythmias • Obesity • Anaemia
Psychological	• Anxiety • Fear • Anger • Depression
Pharmacological	• Drug-induced respiratory disorders • Drug-induced cardiac disorders
Infection	• Bacterial • Fungal • Viral

Breathlessness 2

Other features of breathlessness

- Nocturnal breathlessness: can occur very rapidly and is seen in conditions such as left ventricular failure (LVF) and poorly controlled asthma
- Orthopnoea (breathlessness when lying flat): suggestive of LVF. This can also occur when the diaphragm muscles are weak or paralyzed due to any cause
- Breathlessness first thing in the morning, associated with a productive cough is suggestive of COPD
- 'Air hunger' is a real need to breathe and not being able to get enough air into the chest. It is seen in COPD and heart failure and is thought to relate to an increased respiratory drive
- Patients with pulmonary fibrosis may report a perception of increased effort in breathing at rest
- Patients with chest wall and neurological diseases causing respiratory muscle weakness may report a feeling of 'shallow' breathing.

Table 4.7 Onset of breathlessness

Onset	Common conditions responsible
Minutes to hours	• Pulmonary embolism • Acute left ventricular failure • Pneumothorax • Brittle asthma • Inhaled foreign body
Days to weeks	• Pneumonia • Lung cancer causing bronchial obstruction • Left ventricular failure • Exacerbations of COPD • Exacerbations of asthma • Pleural effusion
Months to years	• Lung cancer • COPD • Chronic heart failure • Pulmonary fibrosis

Cough

A cough is one of the commonest reasons for consulting a health profes-sional. Most coughs are caused by viral or bacterial infections of the upper and lower respiratory tract, they are easily identified and are self limiting.

Whilst some people have been coughing for years, the cause of the cough can be determined in at least 90% of cases. Therapies for cough have a success rate of at least 85%, and treatments should be aimed at the underlying cause, rather than medications that cover up the cough temporarily.

Coughing is a defence mechanism to protect the airway from inhaled foreign material as well as clearing secretions. It can be a voluntary action, but most coughs are involuntary responses to an irritant such as:
• Upper or lower respiratory tract infections
• Dust
• Cigarette smoke
• Danders (cat fur for example).

Anatomy and physiology of the cough reflex

Cough receptors are present in the larynx and tracheo-bronchial tree (📖 p.13). Stimulation of the receptors results in:
• Rapid deep inspiration
• Expiration against a closed glottis
• Sudden glottal opening
• Relaxation of expiratory muscles.

Acute and subacute cough

An acute cough is defined as one with a duration of less than three weeks. It usually results from respiratory infections; most frequently the common cold. Subacute cough has a duration of 3–8 weeks. Post-infectious cough due to irritation of cough receptors accounts for most of these. The most common causes of cough are listed in Table 4.8.

Chronic cough

A chronic cough is associated with a significant increase in morbidity, affecting quality of life. It can cause exhaustion, irritability, headaches, stress incontinence, sore throat, and embarrassment. In at least 25% of cases of a chronic cough, there are at least two medical conditions causing the person to cough.

Table 4.8 Causes of acute and chronic cough

Acute	Chronic
• Viral and bacterial respiratory infections including the 'common cold'	• COPD
	• Perennial rhinitis
• Acute sinusitis	• Asthma
• Pertussis (whooping cough)	• Cough variant asthma
• COPD exacerbations	• Gastro-oesophageal reflux
• Asthma exacerbations	• Post-viral cough
• Allergic rhinitis	• ACE inhibitors
• Pneumonia	• Chronic sinusitis
• Chronic heart failure	• Chronic aspiration
• Aspiration of foreign object	• Bronchiectasis
• Inhalation of cold air in people with reactive airways	• Tuberculosis
	• Interstitial lung disease
• Inhalation of noxious fumes	• Psychogenic cough
• Lung abscess	• Habit cough
• Pulmonary embolism	

Assessing the patient with cough

The patient should be asked:
- Whether the cough is acute (<3 weeks), subacute (3–8 weeks) or chronic (>8 weeks)
- If the cough is chronic in nature, has it changed recently and if so how?
- If the cough is productive (>30mls of sputum daily)
- The nature of the cough: barking, hard, painful, bubbling, tickling, wet, dry
- Timing of the cough: worse at night, worse first thing in the morning
- If any new medication, such as angiotensin-converting enzyme (ACE) inhibitors or beta blockers were prescribed
- What makes the cough better/worse
- If the cough is related to posture.

Management

Once a cause for the cough has been determined, the relevant treatment guidelines such as the British Thoracic Society asthma or COPD guidelines should be followed. If the patient fails to respond to the treatment, the diagnosis should be challenged. Patients should be referred to a respiratory physician if they have any of the following features:
- Haemoptysis
- Weight loss
- Night sweats
- Purulent foul-smelling sputum
- Difficult to control symptoms
- Difficulty in diagnosing cough.

Sputum

A healthy, non-smoking adult will produce approximately 100–150mls of mucus a day. This mucus will be transported up the airway's ciliary mucus escalator and swallowed. Expectorating this sputum is not a normal process. It is a sign that excess mucus has been generated. The excess mucus can be a result of irritation of the respiratory tract or from infection.

Sputum is classified as:
- Mucoid—clear, white or grey in colour
- Serous—watery or frothy
- Mucopurulent—yellow in colour
- Purulent—dark green or yellow in colour.

The type of sputum and the amount produced may indicate the underlying disease. Table 4.9 shows the characteristics of sputum and what the potential cause may be.

Assessing sputum production

Patients who produce sputum should be asked:
- How much sputum is produced on a daily basis
- At what time of the day the sputum is produced
- The colour and consistency of the sputum
- If sputum production is a chronic problem are there any changes?
- Has any blood been coughed up?
- Does the sputum have an offensive smell?
- Is it difficult to expectorate?

Management

If infection is suspected, a specimen of sputum should be obtained (🕮 p.75). If the patient has been diagnosed with pneumonia it may be necessary to start antibiotics whilst waiting for the sputum analysis. Sputum samples can be stained for acid-fast bacilli to diagnose tuberculosis and to identify cell type in lung cancer.

Table 4.9 Types of sputum

Characteristic of sputum	Potential cause
Large volumes produced	Bronchiectasis
Foul-tasting/smelling	Lung abcess Empyema
Thick, viscous, difficult to expectorate	Severe asthma *Aspergillosis* Chest infections
Pink and frothy	Pulmonary oedema
Yellow or green colour	Chest infections Eosinophil shedding in asthma
Rusty-brown colour	Pneumococcal pneumonia
Black colour	Cavitating lesions in coal miners
Blood-stained sputum	Carcinoma of lung Pulmonary infarction Bronchiectasis

Haemoptysis

Haemoptysis is coughing up blood. It is serious and can be alarming and frightening to the patient. It is important to ensure that the blood has come from the respiratory tract, and has not originated from the nasal or oral cavity. If the amount of haemoptysis is more than 200mls in 24 hours (massive haemoptysis), urgent medical treatment is required as the patient is at risk of severe haemorrhage.

There are many causes of haemoptysis which include:
• Pneumonia (particularly pneumococcal)
• Bronchial carcinoma
• Pulmonary emboli resulting in pulmonary infarction
• Tuberculosis
• Bronchiectasis
• Acute/chronic bronchitis
• Injury to the chest causing lung contusions
• Violent coughing.

Diagnosing haemoptysis

Haemoptysis is a symptom of disease, not a disease in itself. A detailed clinical history and physical examination is required to diagnose the underlying condition. Patients should be asked about any preceding events, such as history of deep vein thrombosis, recent chest infection, or travel to an area with a high incidence of tuberculosis.

Patients should be asked to describe the haemoptysis. For example:
• Frothy blood-tinged sputum may be a feature of LVF
• There is often a history of purulent sputum if the haemoptysis is caused by a chest infection
• Frank haemoptysis in a patient with a smoking history may be a sign of malignancy
• A long-standing history of haemoptysis with weight loss, loss of appetite, night sweats may suggest tuberculosis
• Streaks of haemoptysis in the presence of breathlessness may indicate pulmonary embolism.

Investigations required
• Chest X-ray
• Full blood count
• Sputum culture
• Bronchoscopy
• CT scan of chest and possible biopsy
• (📖 p.75).

Chest pain

Chest pain is a common feature of respiratory conditions. It can be difficult to determine if the pain is respiratory or cardiac in nature, but the patient's history can often distinguish the cause. Pain can originate from most parts of the chest and can be classified as central or lateral. It may be the presenting complaint for a number of potentially life-threatening diseases, and always requires a thorough history and investigation, including chest X-ray and electrocardiograph (ECG).

Common causes of chest pain

- Myocardial ischaemia
- Pleuritic pain
- Musculoskeletal
- Nerve root pain
- Gastric reflux.

Myocardial ischaemia

The chest pain associated with myocardial ischaemia is attributed to an imbalance between myocardial oxygen (O_2) supply and demand. Chest pain can be caused by conditions that increase myocardial O_2 demand (hypertension), or decrease O_2 delivery (anaemia, hypoxaemia). The following history would indicate cardiac chest pain:

- Central pain, usually with a sudden onset
- Pain described as dull, crushing, or a feeling of pressure
- Radiating pain to arm, jaw, or teeth
- Pain triggered by exertion, relieved by rest, or by taking medication such as glyceryl.

Pleuritic pain

The lung parenchyma and the visceral pleura are insensitive to most painful stimuli. Pain can arise from the parietal pleura, the major airways, the chest wall, the diaphragm, and mediastinal structures (🕮 p.13). The most common causes of pleuritic pain are inflammation (pleurisy).

Pleurisy itself is not a diagnosis, and the nurse needs to consider what is causing it. Pleuritic pain may be:

- Described as sharp or stabbing
- Worse when breathing, coughing or laughing
- Avoided by shallow breathing
- Referred to the shoulder tip if the diaphragmatic pleura is involved.

Pleurisy is commonly found in patients with a pulmonary embolism (PE), or a pneumothorax. The pain associated with a PE is thought to result from distention of the pulmonary arteries (🕮 p.471). Pain occurring later in the illness may be attributed to infarction of a peripheral segment of lung and inflammation of the adjacent pleura. In a patient with a pneumothorax, the pain is described as being of sudden onset, and unilateral.

Musculoskeletal and nerve root pain

Musculoskeletal pain is usually well localized, and can be described as sharp or dull. The patient may give a history of injury or trauma, such as a rib fracture. Rib fractures produce localized bony tenderness over the fracture site; pain is also produced by pressing on the same rib, away from the fracture. Inflammation of the costochondral cartilage of the rib is common and is known as 'Tietze's syndrome'.

Viruses, such as *Varicella* (shingles) may cause chest wall pain. The pain is often the first symptom of the condition. Nurses must always be aware that lung tumours may be the cause of chest wall pain. This may be because the tumour has invaded the nerve roots, the chest wall or the mediastinum, giving rise to a dull constant ache in the chest.

Gastric reflux

The chest pain from gastric reflux is caused by acid irritation of the oesophageal mucosa. Gastric reflux can be confused with myocardial ischaemia. If the nurse is any doubt, the pain should be treated as cardiac until proven otherwise. Patients with gastric reflux may describe pain that is:

- Worse on lying flat or bending forward
- Relieved by sitting up or taking antacids
- A central dull ache, occasionally radiating to the throat, neck or left arm
- Related to eating or drinking alcohol
- Coexistent dyspepsia (indigestion)
- Rarely associated with exertion.

Assessing chest pain

As with any type of pain, the nurse should enquire about the:

- Site of pain
- Mode of onset
- Characteristics of the pain (sharp, stabbing, burning, aching)
- Radiation, and if so where to
- Intensity
- Precipitating, aggravating, or relieving factors
- Response to any analgesics taken
- Relationship of the pain to breathing, coughing or movement.

Respiratory examination

The nurse should adopt a routine in the examination of the respiratory system. They should first introduce themselves, if this has not already been done, and gain informed consent.

There are exceptions. For example, if the patient is admitted 'in extremis', and is too unwell to give consent. In this situation it is felt that a physical assessment may be life-saving and is in the best interest of the patient. If the patient does not have the mental capacity to give consent, the carer or family can be asked to give consent for the examination.

The nurse should ensure that the surroundings are appropriate for a physical examination. The dignity and comfort of the patient should be ensured, remembering that they may need to remove their upper-body clothing. The room should be warm and well lit, with enough space to conduct the examination.

Patients should be asked whether they would like a chaperone present throughout the examination. The name of any chaperone should be recorded in the documentation.

Before the examination, the patient should be asked whether they are in any pain or discomfort, and if so where the pain is situated, so that extra care can be taken not to cause further pain during the examination process.

The patient should be asked to remove their upper garments, seated in a comfortable position, ideally at an angle of 45° with their hands down by their sides. Their head may be supported by pillows, if this makes them more comfortable.

A physical examination of the respiratory system follows four steps:
- Inspection
- Palpation
- Percussion
- Auscultation.

General inspection

A general inspection of the patient should be the starting point for the respiratory examination. Ideally the practitioner should stand in front of the patient and ask themselves the following questions:

- Does the patient appear comfortable at rest? Patients will appear uncomfortable if they are in pain or are breathless.
- Is the patient using their accessory muscles to help them breathe?
- Does the patient look unwell or distressed?
- Does the patient look pale or flushed?
- Does the patient have any obvious abnormalities such as scarring, rashes, disfigurements?
- Does the patient look alert or appear confused or sleepy?
- Is the patient overweight or thin?
- Do the veins in the neck appear engorged?
- What is the general state of the skin?

Table 4.10 shows the potential respiratory causes of these visual signs.

Breathing pattern

The practitioner should look closely at how the patient is breathing. This includes counting the amount of times the patient breathes in one minute (respiratory rate). The normal respiratory rate for an adult is between 12–15 breaths per minute. A rate higher than this is known as tachypnoea. Causes of tachypnoea include:

- Anxiety
- Pain
- Infection
- Pneumothorax
- Pulmonary embolism.

A respiratory rate of <12 breaths per minute is known as bradypnoea. Causes of bradypnoea include:

- Respiratory depression secondary to neurological lesions or drug overdoses
- Morbid obesity causing hypoventilation.

Along with the rate, the depth of breathing should also be noted. For example, patients with deep sighing respirations could have an acute massive pulmonary embolism.

Other areas to be noted include whether the patient is using their accessory muscles, for example, the sternomastoids, to help them breathe. Posture is also important. Some patients 'fix' their upper body by leaning forward, supporting their arms on a chair or table in an effort to maximize the use of accessory muscles. Some patients with COPD adopt a 'pursed lip' breathing technique to prevent the collapse of small airways due to airflow limitation and to increase the time spent on expiration.

Any noise that the patient makes when breathing (wheeze, stridor) should be noted.

Table 4.10 Visual signs observed and the diagnostic inference

Test performed	Signs observed	Diagnostic inference
Observation of the skin	Thin, shiny skin with excessive bruising	Steroidal skin caused by prolonged use of corticosteroids. Found in: • COPD • Asthma • Fibrosing alveolitis
	Generalized dryness and scaling of the skin	• Eczema • Sarcoidosis
	Pale skin	• Anaemia • Shock
Observation of body weight: Cachexia	Generalized muscle wasting and lack of body fat. Dry and wasted skin.	• Malignant lung disease • Tuberculosis • Severe COPD
Morbid obesity	Very high body mass index (>40)	Obesity hypoventilation syndrome (Pickwickian syndrome)
Observation of thoracic scarring	Scars present from previous operations	Surgical intervention for: • Lung cancer • Pneumothorax • Tuberculosis
Observation of the chest wall	Depression in pectus excavatum (funnel chest)	Benign condition, no treatment required
	Prominence in pectus excavatum (Pigeon chest)	May be secondary to severe childhood asthma
	Barrel chest	Hyperinflation seen in asthma and COPD
	Increased lateralcurvature of spine (scoliosis) and increased forward curvature of the spine (kyphosis)	Structural abnormalities resulting in reduced lung capacities

Examination of the hands and limbs

Hands

The nurse should examine the patients' hands, looking for tar staining on the fingers, an indication that the patient is or has been a heavy smoker.

The hands should also be examined for signs of rheumatoid disease. This may affect the lung, producing pulmonary nodules or pulmonary effusion. The temperature of the hands should also be noted. Abnormally warm and cyanosed hands are a sign of carbon dioxide (CO_2) retention.

The most common sign in relation to the respiratory system is finger clubbing. Finger clubbing is a painless enlargement of the finger tips. It is accompanied by softening of the nail bed and loss of the nail bed angle (see Figure 4.1).

The causes of finger clubbing include:
- Carcinoma of the lung
- Mesothelioma
- Idiopathic pulmonary fibrosis
- Asbestosis
- Bronchiectasis
- Lung abcess
- Empyema
- Cystic fibrosis
- Hypertrophic pulmonary osteoarthropathy.

The nurse should remember that the clubbing may be a congenital phenomenon, and ask the patient how long the clubbing has been present. Other non-respiratory causes of clubbing include chronic liver disease, inflammatory bowel disease, and congenital heart disease.

Examination of the pulse

The normal resting pulse is between 60-100 beats per minute. A pulse rate >100 is known as tachycardia, a pulse rate <60 is known as bradycardia. The pulse should be counted for a minimum of 15s and the rate multiplied by four to give the rate per minute. Causes of tachycardia include:
- Pain
- Shock
- Infection
- Sarcoidosis
- Pulmonary embolism
- Drugs such as salbutamol (📖 p.391).

The pulse rate should be regular. An irregular pulse could be a sign of cardiac arrhythmias such as atrial fibrillation. A bounding pulse is a sign of CO_2 retention, anaemia, and fever.

Tremor

The patient should be asked to hold out their hands in front of them. The nurse should observe hands at eye level. A fine tremor may be easier to observe if a piece of paper is placed on the hand over the fingers. If a fine tremor is noticed, it may be caused by bronchodilator drugs, such as salbutamol, stimulating β-receptors (📖 p.391).

The patient should then be asked to hold their arms outstretched in front of them, with the palms facing downwards. They should then fully flex their hands upwards. The nurse should wait 30 s and then observe the hands for a flapping tremor, from the wrist. The flap tends to be irregular in nature and is a sign of CO_2 retention. It can also be a sign of liver failure.

Examination of the limbs

The patients' ankles should be checked for oedema by applying pressure with the fingers and thumb for a few seconds. Pitting in the skin will be seen if oedema is present. Bilateral pitting oedema is seen in patients with cor pulmonale (p.249).

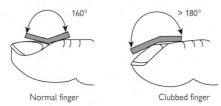

Normal finger   Clubbed finger

Fig. 4.1 Illustration of finger clubbing

Inspection of the head and neck

Eyes

The patient should be asked to look up, the lower eyelid should be gently lowered and the colour of the mucous membrane noted. A pale mucous membrane may indicate anaemia, which may be the cause of breathlessness. Anaemia can only be conclusively diagnosed by measuring haemoglobin levels.

Tongue

The patient should be asked to open their mouth and put out their tongue. The nurse should observe the colour of the underneath of the tongue. It should be pink; if it appears blue, this may be a sign of central cyanosis.

Neck

The jugular venous pressure should be measured. The jugular venous pressure (JVP) and characteristics of the waveform gives the nurse important information about the fluid balance of the body (central venous pressure), as well as indicating the pressure in the right atrium of the heart.

To measure the JVP the patient should be positioned at an angle of 45° with the head turned to the left and fully supported. The patient should try to relax, as it is impossible to assess JVP if the sternomastoid muscles are tensed. The nurse should look for the internal jugular venous waveform, and once this is located, determine whether or not it is abnormal or the venous pressure is elevated. The venous pulsation should not be higher than 4cm when measured with a ruler extending vertically above the sternal angle (see Figure 4.2). If the JVP cannot be visualized when the patient is lying flat, lower than normal volumes of blood circulating in the body (hypovolaemia) is suggested. The JVP may be easily visible if raised to the level of the earlobes. This is commonly caused by any condition causing an increase in right atrial pressure, fluid overload, or congestive cardiac failure. Table 4.11 lists causes of a raised JVP.

The neck should be palpated for lymphadenopathy. The patient should be asked to sit upright. The nurse should position themselves behind the patient and using both hands feel for enlarged lymph nodes, taking care not to cause the patient any discomfort.

Table 4.11 Causes of raised JVP

Sign observed	Common cause
Elevated JVP	Tension pneumothorax
	Severe hyperinflation in asthma or COPD
Elevated non-pulsatile JVP	Superior vena cava obstruction usually caused by malignant enlargement of the right bronchus
Elevated pulsatile JVP	Cor pulmonale
	Paratracheal lymph nodes
Depressed JVP	Shock
	Dehydration
	Severe infection

The area to palpate includes:
• Pre- and post-auricular (ears)
• Under the chin
• Submandibular
• Cervical chain
• Supraclavicular.
The presence of lymphadenopathy could indicate:
• Infection
• Carcinoma
• Tuberculosis
• Sarcoidosis.

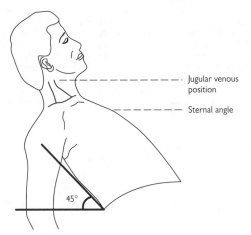

Jugular venous position

Sternal angle

45°

Fig. 4.2 Position of the jugular vein

Palpation

Chest expansion

The main purpose of palpation in the respiratory examination is to determine the degree of expansion of the lungs. This may be affected unilaterally or bilaterally by disease.

Palpation is performed anterioraly and posterioraly. The nurse should place their hands symmetrically on either side of the upper sternum with the thumbs in the midline. The thumbs should be slightly lifted off the chest so that they are free to move with respiration (see Figure 4.3). The patient should be asked to inhale and exhale deeply. The relative movement of the two hands and the separation of the thumbs reflect the overall movement of the chest and any asymmetry between the two sides (see Figure 4.3).

When assessing for expansion, the nurse should also feel for the rise and movement of their own hands on the chest wall, as well as judging the distance moved by the thumbs. If any abnormality is detected, the nurse should determine whether the expansion is reduced symmetrically or unilaterally, and the degree of reduced expansion present. Reduced expansion is indicated by an expansion of <1½ cm when the patient inhales.

Chronic respiratory conditions that cause a pattern of symmetrically reduced expansion include:

- COPD
- Pulmonary fibrosis
- Neuromuscular disease.

Localized respiratory conditions that cause a pattern of unilateral or asymmetric expansion include:

- Pleural effusion
- Pneumothorax
- Collapse of one or more lobes of a lung secondary to tumour, foreign body or sputum plug.

Tactile vocal fremitus

Tactile vocal fremitus refers to the ability to palpate vibrations set up by the voice in the large airways and transmit these to the chest wall. This involves the practitioner placing the edge of their hand in a systematic manner on the chest wall and asking the patient to say '99'. The vibration felt by the examiner is the key to interpreting the physical sign. The vibration is decreased or absent in cases where there is a greater distance for the sound waves to travel to reach the examiner's hand. An example of this would be if the pleural space is filled with air or fluid, as in a pneumothorax or pleural effusion. Other causes of decreased vocal fremitus include pulmonary fibrosis and pneumonia.

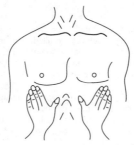

Chest expansion on inspiration: the thumbs
move apart.

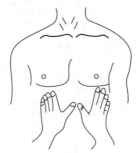

Chest expansion on expiration: the thumbs
move back.

Fig. 4.3 Assessment of chest expansion

Percussion

Percussion is the technique of tapping the chest to produce sounds which indicate if the underlying structures are filled with air, fluid, or are solid. There are four common types of percussion note that may be heard:

- *Resonant*: the note obtained when percussing a normal air-filled lung
- *Dull*: abnormal dullness found over areas of lung consolidation (pneumonia)
- *Stony dull*: the note obtained when a significant quantity of fluid, pus or blood is in the pleural cavity (pleural effusion, empyema, haemothorax)
- *Hyper-resonant*: a large air-filled space such as a pneumothorax, or emphysema (🔖 p.249), may produce a hyper-resonant note.

Percussion technique

- Place the non-dominant hand on the chest wall
- Separate the fingers and press the middle finger down firmly
- With the tip of the middle finger of the dominant hand, strike the middle finger of the non-dominant hand at the level of the middle phalanx
- The movement should come from the wrist of the dominant hand, not the elbow or upper arm.

The nurse should percuss the anterior and the posterior chest wall in a number of areas in a symmetrical manner (see Figure 4.4). The areas to percuss include the apices of the lungs, the axillae and the lung bases. All areas should be percussed, paying particular attention to comparison between the two sides. In healthy lungs there should be a symmetrical distribution of sounds.

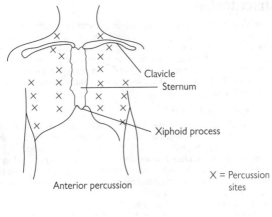

Clavicle
Sternum
Xiphoid process

Anterior percussion

X = Percussion sites

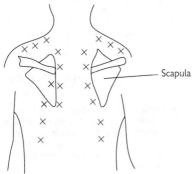

Scapula

Posterior percussion

Fig. 4.4 Key areas of the chest for lung percussion

Auscultation

Auscultation is the process of listening to the sounds of breathing via a stethoscope. The stethoscope contains a diaphragm and a bell. The bell of the stethoscope should be used during auscultation, as it is more sensitive to sounds of lower frequencies which characterize most breath sounds. The ear-tips of the stethoscope should closely fit the ear canal, and incline towards the nose, matching the angle of the ear canal, to block out external noise.

Auscultation technique

It is important to auscultate the chest in a quiet room, as some breath sounds have frequencies which are hard for the human ear to hear. It also helps to listen with the eyes closed, to focus attention on the sound. The stethoscope should be placed on the chest wall in the same positions used in percussion (Figure 4.4). Each location is matched symmetrically with the same location on the opposite side. Before commencing the examination:

- Explain the technique to the patient
- Warm the end of the stethoscope
- Ask the patient to take deep breaths in and out of their mouth
- Listen to a full inspiration and expiration at each position in both lungs
- If the breath sounds are faint, ask the patient to breath more deeply
- Note the pitch, intensity and duration of inspiratory and expiratory sounds
- Ensure that the stethoscope tubing does not touch any clothing or extra sounds may be heard
- Do not listen through clothing as the breath sounds will be muffled.

Vocal resonance

Vocal resonance is the auscultatory equivalent of tactile vocal fremitus and has largely replaced it. The practioner again listens with the stethoscope in the same area, but asks the patient to say '99'. Transmission is increased over the presence of consolidated lung (solid conducts sound better than liquid or air), and decreased if the pleural space is occupied by fluid (pleural effusion) or air (pneumothorax).

Abnormal breath sounds

Normal lung sounds are categorized as tracheal, bronchial, bronchovesicular and vesicular. As air moves through the bronchi, it creates sound waves that travel to the chest wall. The sounds produced by breathing change as air moves from large airways to smaller airways. Sounds also change as the air passes through fluid, mucus, and through narrow obstructed airways. The properties of breath sounds (loudness, frequency, pitch) are modified according to any disease which alters the lungs and airways. Certain conditions will therefore cause changes in the breath sounds heard with the stethoscope.

Wheeze

A wheeze is a musical sound heard mainly on expiration. It is caused by air forcing its way through narrowed airways, causing it to vibrate, producing the characteristic high-pitched sound. Wheezes are classified as being monophonic (just one note) or polyphonic (of many different notes). A monophonic wheeze indicates that a single airway is partially obstructed; a polyphonic wheeze is often heard in patients with widespread airflow obstruction. Conditions causing wheeze are:
• Asthma
• COPD
• Infection
• Heart failure
• Tumour
• Foreign body.
Patients should be asked when they wheeze. If the wheeze is worse first thing in the morning, the cause may be COPD. If the wheeze is worse during the night or when exercising, the cause may be asthma.

Stridor

Stridor is an audible, high-pitched noise heard on inspiration. It is an indicator of partial obstruction of the upper, larger airways, such as the larynx, trachea, and main bronchus. Conditions causing stridor are:
• Tumour
• Inhalation of a foreign body
• Laryngeal spasm.
Any patient with stridor requires urgent investigation so that the cause is identified.

Crackles

Crackles are intermittent, non-musical sounds. The crackling sound is caused by collapsed or fluid-filled alveoli popping open. Crackles are classified as either fine or coarse.

Fine crackles
Fine crackles are distinguished by:
• Occuring when the patient stops inhaling
• Usually heard at the base of the lungs
• Sound like Velcro™ being pulled apart.
Fine crackles tend to occur in diseases such as:
• Diffuse parenchymal lung disease

- Asbestosis
- Silicosis
- Atelectasis
- Heart failure
- Pneumonia.

Coarse crackles

Coarse crackles are distinguished by:
- Occuring when the patient starts to inhale and sometimes present when the patient exhales
- Being heard through the lungs and at the mouth
- Sounding like bubbling or gurgling, as air moves through secretions in large airways.

Coarse crackles tend to occur in diseases such as:
- COPD
- Bronchiectasis
- Pulmonary oedema
- Severely ill patients who cannot cough.

Pleural rub

A pleural rub is caused by the two surfaces of the pleura (visceral and parietal) making contact. The sound produced resembles leather rubbing against leather. It is caused by the surfaces becoming abnormally inflamed. A pleural rub is heard on both inspiration and expiration and does not alter on coughing. It may be caused by any condition which causes inflammation of the pleural surfaces. These include:
- Pulmonary embolism
- Pneumonia
- Connective tissue disease.

Completing the respiratory assessment

After completing the history and the physical examination the nurse should finish the assessment by checking any basic observation or peak flow charts, inspect any sputum produced by the patient, and check if any investigations such as blood tests, chest X-ray or arterial blood tests have already been performed. The nurse should then integrate the findings of the history and examination and reach a potential diagnosis. All findings should be documented in the patient's records.

Experienced clinicians rarely view the respiratory system in isolation during the physical examination, even when there is a strong suspicion that a lung disease is present. A good understanding of general medicine is required to achieve competency in respiratory assessments. This assessment includes a thorough history, a respiratory and general systems examination, before proceeding to investigations which, in a large number of cases, will only confirm the nurse's suspicions.

Respiratory investigations

Introduction

There are many investigations in respiratory medicine, ranging from basic tests to more invasive procedures. Respiratory investigations are the final pieces in the jigsaw to help respiratory nurses and nurse practitioners reach a diagnosis.

Many nurses do not work in specialized respiratory units and will not have access to the most sophisticated investigations. However, all respiratory nurses should understand what tests are available, be aware of how the tests are performed, and of any preparation required before and after the test, so they can explain these procedures to their patients.

Peak expiratory flow rate (PEFR)

PEFR is the maximum flow of air that a patient can expel from their lungs from a full inspiration. The PEFR is achieved after a tenth of a second and is measured using a peak flow meter. Peak flow meters provide a cheap method of measuring airflow obstruction and are available on prescription. A peak flow meter can be used by most adults, and by children over 6 years of age. Children under 6 years of age are not usually prescribed peak flow meters because they might confuse the blowing out for a peak flow reading with the sucking in of their inhaled medication.

The patient blows into the meter as forcibly as possible and the flow of air is measured in litres per minute. PEFR is most commonly used to:
- Diagnose asthma
- Assess the severity or stability of asthma
- Measure ongoing response to asthma therapies.

The maximal flow rate that the patient can attain depends on:
- The resistance to flow through the bronchi
- Patient effort
- Patient motivation
- Correct technique
- Any restrictions of the chest wall.

Maximal PEFR also depends on the patients' age, gender, height and ethnic origin—a set of predicted values have been produced (see Figure 5.1). Peak flow readings vary from person to person, so it is difficult to say exactly what a person's predicted peak flow should be. It is important to ask the patient what their 'best' peak flow measurement has been, as this can be more meaningful than looking at predicted values alone.

Patients' should be provided with their own meter. There are several different types of meter available. Patients should be advised to bring their own meter to clinic appointments so that comparable blows are measured.

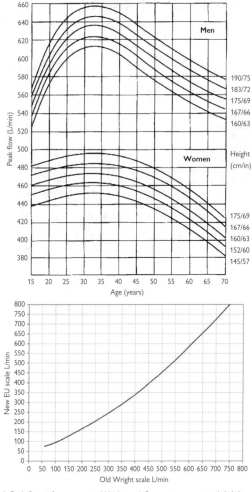

Fig. 5.1 Peak flow reference ranges Wright peak flow meters over-read slightly (approx. 50 l/min) in the midrange (approx. 300 l/min), compared to gold-standard-measurements. From October 2004, new peak flow meters will have a corrected scale (in yellow to identify them). This will introduce some confusion if old and new meters are mixed indiscriminately. The following page is a conversion chart to be used when rewriting a management plan, based on peak flow measurements, and the patient is converting from an old to a new meter.

Reproduced from Chapman, S, Robinson, G, Stradling, J, and West, S, Oxford Handbook of Respiratory Medicine Ranges, 2005. Appendix 1, Peak Flow Reference Ranges, 712, with permission from Oxford University Press.

Performing the PEFR test

PEFR is a quick and simple test to perform. It is also easy to perform the test incorrectly.

The patient should:
- Ensure that the pointer on the meter is set at zero
- Stand or sit in an upright position and always repeat recordings in the same position
- Take a deep breath in to full inspiration
- Place the lips around the mouthpiece to make a good seal
- Hold the peak flow horizontally
- Blow out as hard and as fast as possible (the blow should not last longer than one second)
- Note the reading on the meter and return the pointer to zero
- Repeat and note the blow two more times
- Note down the highest of the three readings.

There may be significant variability in PEFR. This is called 'diurnal variation'. In normal health there is an increase of 5% in PEFR at midday compared with midnight. Asthma is a variable disease (p.145) and this variation is small when the patient is well controlled, but there may be a difference of >10% in the morning and evening values.

The BTS/SIGN asthma guidelines (see below) suggest that a diurnal variation of >20% for three or more days per week on two consecutive weeks is diagnostic of asthma.

Further information

http://www.peakflow.com

British Thoracic Society/Scottish Intercollegiate Guidelines Network (2003) British Guideline on the management of asthma. *Thorax*, 58: S1–94.

http://www.sign.uk/gu/published/numlist.html.

BTS ISBN 978 1905813 285

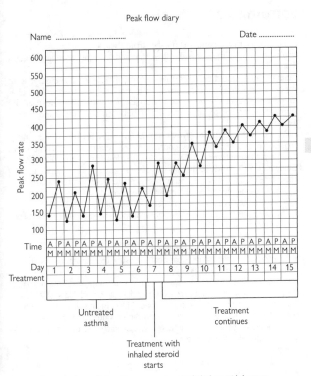

Fig. 5.2 Example of a peak flow diary pre and post inhaled steroid therapy

Spirometry

Spirometry is a method of assessing lung function by measuring the volume of air that a patient can expel from their lungs following maximal inspiration. It also measures the flow rate and gives far more information than PEFR alone.

Spirometry should be undertaken if lung disease is suspected. It is an important tool in assisting diagnosis, and in monitoring patients with respiratory disease, especially when used in conjunction with other investigations. Spirometry can identify and differentiate between obstructive and restrictive lung disorders.

People with persistent symptoms of wheeze, breathlessness and a productive cough should be considered for referral for spirometry, as these are all symptoms of COPD (📖 p.249). In addition, the NICE COPD Guidelines[1] (2004) advise that people over 35 years of age who are lifelong heavy smokers should have a spirometry test to identify early disease.

Other reasons for referral for spirometry are:

• To assess the severity or progression of a respiratory disease
• To assess the therapeutic effect of respiratory medication such as bronchodilators or steroids
• To assess the risk of surgery
• To assess the response to allergens
• To assess the effect of occupational exposure to respiratory irritants such as dust and fumes (📖 p.145).

The indices most commonly measured in spirometry are Vital Capacity (VC), both as a relaxed blow (RVC) and as a forced blow (FVC), and Forced Expiratory Volume in one second (FEV_1). Most spirometers contain computer software to calculate the predicted values and the percentage of predicted that the patient achieves. The predicted value is based on the following patient characteristics:

• Age
• Height
• Gender
• Ethnic origin.

Readings that are 20% either side of the predicted values are considered to be within the normal range, and healthy individuals should achieve at least 80% of the FEV_1 and FVC values predicted for them.

References

1. Chronic obstructive pulmonary disease–management of chronic obstructive pulmonary disease in adults in primary and secondary care. http://www.nice.org.uk

Spirometry measurements

The Vital Capacity (VC) is the maximum volume of air that can be breathed out of the lungs following a maximal inhalation. It is a measure of the size of the lungs and can be measured in two ways:

- Relaxed Vital Capacity (RVC) or Slow Vital Capacity (SVC). The air is exhaled in a relaxed or slow manner. Because air is exhaled slowly, there are fewer limitations on the flow from narrow airways or damaged lungs
- Forced Vital Capacity (FVC) is where the air is exhaled rapidly from full inspiration to full expiration. As the air is being blown forcibly out of the lungs, the positive pressure inside the chest can cause premature closure of the smaller airways. This can cause air to 'trap' in the alveoli. This will be seen if the FVC measures less than the SVC.

In healthy people, the SVC and the FVC are normally within 200mls of each other, but in people with obstructive lung diseases, such as asthma and COPD, premature closure of the airways may lead to greater differences. It is recommended that both are measured if there is a suspected obstructive lung disease.

FEV_1

This is the volume of air exhaled in the first second of a forced exhalation from maximum inhalation, using maximum effort. Several factors influence the FEV_1, including the elastic properties of the lung, the size of the lungs and the caliber and collapsibility of the airway.

FEV_1 and VC are expressed in absolute values, in litres per minute and as a percentage of the predicted value.

FEV_1 ratio

This is the ratio between the volumes exhaled in one second (FEV_1) to the total of air exhaled, either the SVC or FVC, whichever is greatest. It is an excellent measure of airflow limitation and allows differentiation between obstructive and restrictive lung disease.

It is calculated by:

$$\frac{FEV_1 \times 100}{FVC \text{ or } VC} = FEV_1/VC \text{ ratio}$$

The FEV_1/VC ratio measurement ranges from 0.75–0.85 in a normal adult. Anything below 0.7 may indicate obstructive disorders as it takes longer to exhale the air. The FEV_1/VC ratio is normal or high in restrictive disorders as the flow of air is not reduced (see Table 5.1).

The volume of air exhaled is plotted on a volume/time curve (see Figure 5.3). Volume in litres is plotted on the y axis and time in seconds on the x axis. In Figure 5.3 it can be seen that most of the air is expelled from the lungs in the first second (FEV_1). This is because there is no obstruction present in the individual's airways and the air is exhaled at a normal rate.

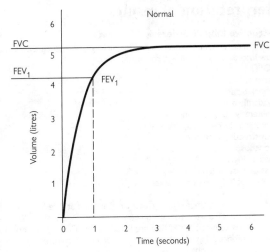

Fig. 5.3 Normal volume-time graph

Interpretation of results

Obstructive lung disorders

Anything that reduces the diameter of the airways will reduce the rate of airflow into or out of the lungs. For example:
- COPD
- Asthma
- Bronchiectasis
- Cystic fibrosis
- Obliterative bronchiolitis
- Tumour or foreign body in the airways.

The obstruction is caused by:
- Bronchospasm
- Mucus plugging
- Loss of elastic recoil
- Release of inflammatory markers
- Scarring.

A reduced airway diameter means that air is exhaled at a reduced speed. The definition of obstructive spirometry is a FEV_1/FVC ratio <0.7. The FEV_1 is usually reduced at <80% of predicted but the FVC may be normal, or slightly reduced. Figure 5.4 shows the volume/time spirometry tracing for a patient with an obstructive picture.

Restrictive lung disorders

- Fibrosing lung diseases such as idiopathic fibrosing alveolitis (📖 p.311), sarcoidosis and pneumoconiosis
- Skeletal deformity such as kyphosis or scoliosis
- Pulmonary oedema (📖 p.137)
- Neuromuscular disorders such as muscular dystrophy
- Previous surgery, such as pneumonectomy or lobectomy
- Malignancy
- Obesity.

Reduced lung volumes are a result of the inability of the lungs to expand and relax at the rate and completeness the diaphragm and intercostal muscles demand. Figure 5.5 shows the volume/time spirometry tracing for a patient with a restrictive picture. Restrictive spirometry is indicated by a reduced VC, both slow and forced at <80% of predicted. The FEV_1 is also reduced, not because there is any obstruction present, but because predicted values for FEV_1 are based on normal volumes of air being present. However, the FEV_1/FVC ratio is normal or high.

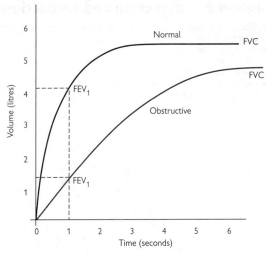

Fig. 5.4 Volume/time graph showing obstruction

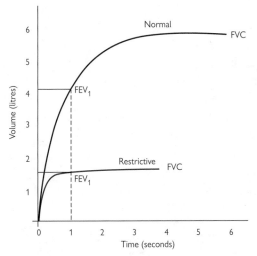

Fig. 5.5 Volume/time graph showing restriction

Combined obstruction and restriction

Conditions that produce a combined obstructive and restrictive pattern of spirometry include:
- Severe airflow obstruction in advanced COPD
- Cystic fibrosis
- Severe bronchiectasis.

This results in reduced VC, especially the FVC, reduced FEV_1 and reduced FEV_1/FVC ratio. The volume/time spirogram seen in Figure 5.6 illustrates this.

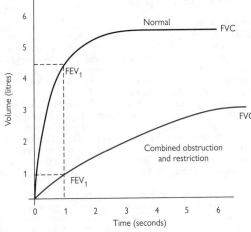

Fig. 5.6 Volume/time graph showing a combined picture

Flow volume graphs

Flow volume curve

Apart from volume/time graphs, most spirometers also produce a graph of flow rate against volume. This is known as a flow volume curve. The graph produced represents the flow of air in and out of the lungs—plotted on the y axis—against the volume of air along the x axis from maximal inspiration to maximal expiration. The flow volume curve can provide information about the nature of airway obstruction.

At the beginning of expiration following a full breath in, the expiratory muscles are at their strongest, the lungs at their biggest and the airways at their most open. This means that the highest flow rates are possible at the beginning of the blow; the point at which the gradient of the curve is at its steepest, and reaches a peak in about a tenth of a second in the PEF rate. The flow then declines linearly until the lung is empty. If the measurement is continued into subsequent full inspiration, a full flow-volume loop is produced.

Extra readings can be taken from the curves, such as mid expiratory flow (MEF 25–75). This is a measurement of what flow is like during the middle of a forced breath. Although it is often said to be a measurement of small airways obstruction, the MEF 25–75 is fairly non-specific and reductions can be seen with a number of non-obstructive diseases. An isolated reduction in the MEF 25–75 serves as an important clue to mild obstructive lung disease when the FEV_1/FVC ratio is normal. For example, this occurs in early COPD and in asthmatics when they are relatively symptom-free.

Flow volume loop

The flow volume loop can plot inspiratory and expiratory flow against lung volume during a maximal expiratory and inspiratory manoeuvre. As with the flow volume curve, the patient starts from full inspiration to full expiration as above, then they inspire maximally again. Although the inspiratory muscles are at their strongest, the airways are at their smallest so the flow rates start low and increase as the airways open up. As this happens, the inspiratory muscles are weakening. This means the flow rates fall again and give the rounded appearance seen on the inspiratory limb of the flow volume loop (see Figure 5.7).

The greatest value of the flow volume loop is to assess for upper airway obstruction (for example, a laryngeal cancer). If there is a fixed upper airway narrowing, (for example from a tracheal tumour), then the size of the airway at this point becomes so narrow that it limits maximal flow.

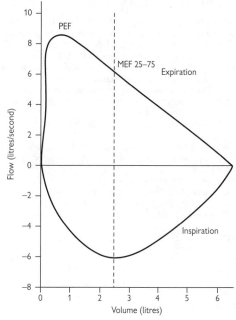

Fig. 5.7 Flow volume loop

Table 5.1 Interpretation of spirometry

FEV$_1$%	FVC%	FEV$_1$/FVC ratio	Interpretation
>80	>80	>0.7	Normal
<80	>80	<0.7	Obstruction
<80	<80	>0.7	Restriction
<80	<80	<0.7	Combination of obstruction and restriction

Reversibility testing

Spirometry alone will not diagnose disease. If the baseline test shows the presence of airflow obstruction, this could indicate either asthma or COPD. The obstruction is either fixed or irreversible, as in COPD, or reversible, as in asthma. Reversibility testing has traditionally been used to differentiate between the two. However the NICE COPD[1] guidelines no longer advocate reversibility testing because:

• Repeated FEV_1 measurements can show small spontaneous fluctuations
• The results of a reversibility test performed on different occasions can be inconsistent and not reproducible
• Over-reliance on a single test may be misleading unless the change in FEV_1 is greater than 400 ml
• Long-term symptomatic response to bronchodilators cannot be determined by the response to a dose of bronchodilator given during a reversibility test.

To help resolve cases where the diagnosis is in doubt, a reversibility test can be undertaken. Reversibility can be assessed using short-acting bronchodilators such as salbutamol, terbutaline or ipratropium bromide (📖 p.391), or over a period of weeks using oral or inhaled steroids.
   Tests should be performed when:

• The patient is clinically stable and free of infection
• The patient should not have taken any short-acting bronchodilators in the past 4 h, long-acting beta2-agonists in the past 12 h, long-acting anticholinergics or theophyllines in the past 24 h
• If any bronchodilators have been taken prior to the test, this should be documented
• The patient should not have smoked in the past 24 h.

Bronchodilator reversibility

If short-acting bronchodilators are used to assess reversibility, high doses need to be given. The most convenient way to deliver high doses is to use a nebulized bronchodilator. High doses may be given from a metered dose inhaler and spacer device (📖 p.391). Suitable doses would be:

• Salbutamol 2.5–5mg nebulized or 400mcg inhaled
• Terbutaline 5–10mg nebulized or 2000mcg inhaled
• Ipratropium bromide 500mcg nebulized or 80 mcg inhaled
• Or any combination of salbutamol and ipratropium bromide.

Repeat spirometry should be undertaken 15 min post salbutamol and terbutaline, and 30 min post ipratropium bromide.

Corticosteroid reversibility

The NICE COPD guidelines recommend that prednisolone 30 mg is given daily for 7–14 days. The GOLD guidelines suggest a 6–12 week trial of high-dose inhaled steroids (beclometasone 1000mcg daily or equivalent) (📖 p.391) which may be a more reliable and safer option. Response to corticosteroids does not predict responses to inhaled corticosteroids.

   A positive reversibility test is when there is at least 400mls increase in FEV_1 from baseline or if the FEV_1 returns to normal predicted values for the individual patient.

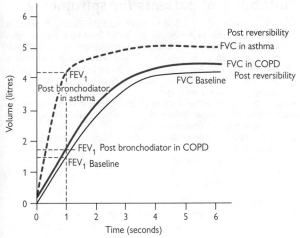

Fig. 5.8 Volume/time graph pre and post reversibility

Suitability of patients for spirometry

Spirometry involves a great deal of effort from the patient. Poor effort can affect the validity of the results. The effort involved can cause light-headedness in some people, and can cause some people to cough. Certain conditions could affect the reliability of spirometry measurements. Also, FVC manoeuvres may aggravate these conditions and the test should be postponed until the condition has resolved. These conditions are:

- Haemoptysis of unknown origin
- Pneumothorax (or within 2 weeks of resolved pneumothorax)
- Unstable cardiovascular status such as recent myocardial infarction, unstable angina or pulmonary embolus
- Thoracic, abdominal or cerebral aneurysms (danger of rupture due to increased thoracic pressure)
- Recent eye surgery (cataract)
- Recent thoracic or abdominal surgery
- Nausea and vomiting.

Test procedure

Before a spirometry test the patient's height (barefoot) and weight (indoor clothing) should be accurately measured. If the patient is unable to stand to be measured, or has marked kyphoscoliosis, they can be asked to stretch their arms and hands out to their sides as far as possible, and a fingertip to fingertip measurement can then be taken. This gives a very close estimation of their overall height. The patient's ethnic origin and age should also be noted. The time and dose of any bronchodilator medication taken should be recorded.

Prior to the test the patient should avoid:

- Wearing tight clothing—or anything that might restrict the chest
- Vigorous exercise—for at least 30 minutes
- Alcohol—for at least four hours and a large meal for at least two hours
- Bronchodilators—if reversibility test is to be performed
- Tobacco for 24 hours.

Quality assurance

As spirometry relies on patient cooperation and effort, it is essential that the technician is trained not only on the use and maintenance of the equipment used, but also on how to encourage the patient to perform to their maximum potential.

To achieve this, careful explanation of the procedure before the test, and encouragement of the patient during the test will be required.

The patient should be advised:
• To empty their bladder before the test
• To remove loose-fitting dentures. Well-fitting dentures should remain *in situ* so that a better seal can be formed around the mouthpiece
• To sit upright, in a chair with arms
• To place feet flat on the floor.

Measuring a relaxed vital capacity (RVC)

The patient should be instructed to:
• To keep the head up and shoulders back
• Inhale as deeply as possible
• Place lips tightly around the mouthpiece
• Blow the air out steadily and as completely as possible
• Verbal encouragement to keep blowing should be given.

Measuring a forced vital capacity (FVC)

As for the RVC, except the patient should be asked to blow the air out as hard and fast as possible.

Testing errors

Common faults when testing are:
• Failure to achieve full inspiration and incomplete exhalation, resulting in a reduced vital capacity
• Leakage of air from the patient's nose or mouth. A nose clip or a smaller mouthpiece may be required
• A delay in the start of the blow, resulting in a reduced FEV_1
• Obstruction of the mouthpiece by the teeth or tongue
• Coughing during expiration (Fig 5.9).

If any of these errors occur, the test should be rejected, the patient's technique corrected, and the test repeated until at least three technically satisfactory tests have been achieved; of which the best two are within 100ml, or 5% of each other. No more than eight blows should be attempted.

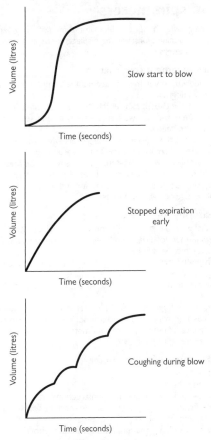

Fig. 5.9 Technical faults seen on volume/time graphs

Types of spirometers

There are many different spirometers on the market. They vary in price, but there are two main types: volume displacement spirometers and flow measuring spirometers.

Volume displacement spirometers

The most widely used volume displacement spirometer is the dry wedge bellows (e.g. Vitalograph)

- In this system, the patient exhales into bellows contained in a metal box
- The expansion of the bellows is recorded by a pen fixed to a plate resting over the bellows
- The pen records the movement onto a chart which moves horizontally at a fixed rate, recording a volume/time measurement
- This device only allows an expiratory manoeuvre to be measured.

This type of device is most commonly used in secondary care settings where they do not need to be moved around. Figure 5.10 illustrates a Vitalograph wedge bellows spirometer.

Flow measuring spirometers

Measures airflow and electronically converts the values into volumes.

- This measurement of airflow (in litres/second) can then be integrated to give a volume measurement
- Usually have the facility to enter age, height, gender and race, and will then automatically calculate predicted values
- This type of spirometer can also measure flow volume curves and loops
- An example of a flow measuring spirometer is a rotating vane spirometer such as a MicroMedical's microlab spirometer (see Figure 5.11).

The performance of both types of spirometer is the same as long as the equipment is used appropriately.

Essential features of a spirometer

- Easy to use
- Reliable and robust
- Easy to clean (follow manufacturers instructions)
- Meets the British Thoracic Society and Association for Respiratory Technology and Physiology (1994) criteria
- Supplied by a company that provides technical support and assistance.

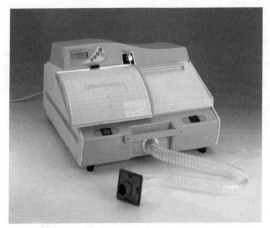

Fig. 5.10 Wedge bellows spirometer
Reproduced with permission from Vitalograph.

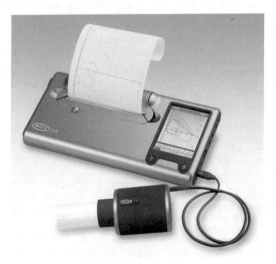

Fig. 5.11 Rotating vane spirometer Digital Volume Transducer Spirometer or Turbine Type
Reproduced with permission from Cardinal Health.

Standardization

It is important that whenever a patient's lung function is measured, the results obtained are of the highest possible accuracy and reliability. It is not unusual for spirometry to be repeated over a period of time, for example before and after a steroid trial. It is important to know if any change in FEV_1 and FVC during this time is due to the treatment given, rather than poor spirometry technique. The most important feature in obtaining reliable data is the competence of the technician.

The following are important for achieving standardized results:

- Equipment performance—the machine should be capable of measuring at least eight litres, and have a graphical display which can be easily viewed
- Equipment quality control—the equipment should be calibrated, cleaned and serviced as instructed by the manufacturer
- Patient input—spirometry is effort dependent and requires careful instructions, understanding, coordination and cooperation
- Measurement procedures—all health practitioners measuring spirometry should have local protocols based on recognized national guidelines such as those written by the Association for Respiratory Technicians and Physiologists
- Acceptability—the FVC needs to be checked by looking at the volume/time and flow volume graphs. The volume/time graph should curve smoothly upwards to a plateau and the flow volume trace should rise almost vertically to a peak. Inadequate blows should be rejected
- Reproducibility—a minimum of three forced manouveres should be recorded and the best two readings of FVC and FEV_1 should be within 5% and 100 ml of each other
- Accurate results—the best FEV_1 and FVC from any of the traces should be reported as the patient's values. The ratio between FEV_1 and the vital capacity should be calculated from either the relaxed VC or FVC, whichever value is greater.

Resources

Training in spirometry and its interpretation is available from the following organizations:

Association for Respiratory Technicians and
Physiologists (http://www.artp.org.uk)
Respiratory Education UK (http://www.respiratoryeduk.com)
Education for Health (http://www.educationforhealth.org.uk)
Indications for performing spirometry are available from the American Lung Association (http://www.thoracic.org.ca.html)
Spirometer equipment is available from:
http://www.micromedical.co.uk
http://www.vitalograph.co.uk

Respiratory function tests

In secondary care, a systematic combination of lung function tests are carried out in lung function laboratories. The two tests of lung function that are often carried out routinely, in addition to spirometry, are the measurement of lung volumes and diffusing capacity. The gas held by the lungs is thought of in terms of subdivisions, or specific lung volumes. A definition and description of the specific tests measured can be seen in Table 5.2.

Lung volume measurements

- One important lung volume, residual volume (RV), cannot be measured using simple spirometry because gas remains in the lungs at the end of each breath
- If no air was left in the lungs at the end of expiration, the lungs would collapse
- The RV needs to be measured so that the functional residual capacity (FRC) and total lung capacity (TLC) can be calculated
- In healthy subjects RV is approximately 30% of TLC
- In obstructive lung diseases the lungs are hyperinflated with 'air trapping' so that RV is greatly increased and the ratio of RV to TLC is also increased.

There are three methods of measuring RV: nitrogen washout, helium dilution and plethysmography.

Nitrogen washout

- This test measures FRC which can be used in combination with plethysmography to determine the amount of trapped gas in the lungs
- This technique is based on the assumption that the concentration of nitrogen (N_2) in the lungs is 75–80%
- It consists of a rapid response gas analyser in conjunction with a spirometer, to provide breath-by-breath analysis
- The patient breathes 100% O_2 for several minutes
- After this time N_2 is gradually washed out of the lungs
- There is a residual N_2 remaining which is why the test is continued until alveolar concentrations of N_2 reach 1% (approximately 7 minutes)
- In the presence of airflow obstruction and air trapping, the test may be extended to increase accuracy.

Helium dilution

- Helium is an inert gas that can be used to indirectly calculate FRC
- A dry rolling seal spirometer is filled with a known concentration of helium (approximately 10%) room air and O_2
- Measurements of the exact concentrations are recorded prior to testing, the patient then re-breathes the gas concentration until equilibrium is reached within the lungs and the re-breathe circuit
- It is essential to control for the levels of CO_2 during this procedure
- Lung divisions such as RV, TLC, ERV and IC are derived from a relaxed VC manoeuvre.

Plethysmography

- Determines changes in lung volumes by recording changes in pressure
- The patient sits in a large airtight box and breathes through a mouthpiece
- At the end of a normal expiration, a shutter closes the mouthpiece and the patient is asked to make respiratory efforts
- As the patient tries to inhale, box pressure increases
- This method measures all intrathoracic gas including cysts and bullae.

Table 5.2 Subdivisions of the lung

Subdivision	Abbreviations	Definition
Tidal volume	TV	Volume of air breathed in and out in a single breath (approximately 0.5L)
Inspiratory reserve volume	IRV	Volume of air breathed in by a maximum inspiration at the end of a normal inspiration (approximately 3.3L)
Expiratory reserve volume	ERV	Volume of air breathed out by a maximum expiration at the end of a normal expiration (approximately 1.0 L)
Residual volume	RV	Volume of air that remains in the lungs at end of maximum expiration (approximately 1.2 L)
Inspiratory capacity	IC	Volume of air breathed in by a maximum inspiration at the end of a normal expiration (TV+IRV)
Functional residual capacity	FRC	Volume of air remaining in lungs at the end of a normal expiration (ERV+RV)
Total lung capacity	TLC	Total volume of lungs when maximally inflated

How to interpret respiratory function tests

- Multiple FRC measurements by gas dilution should be made
- Results should be interpreted with at least two trials agreeing within 10% of the mean
- ERV measurements should agree within 5% or 60ml of the mean, whichever is the larger
- Variable measurements should be documented as not achieving the reproducibility criteria
- FRC varies with body size, change in posture, diurnal variation and racial or ethnic background
- FRC> 120% predicted is suggestive of air trapping
- Increased RV demonstrates that the lungs contain an abnormally increased volume
- Elevated RV may occur in acute asthmatic exacerbation but this is usually reversible
- Fixed obstructive lung diseases, especially emphysema (☐ p.249) result in an increase in RV and RV:TLC ratio caused by chronic air trapping
- As RV increases greater ventilation is required and the work of breathing increases for adequate gas exchange
- This correlates with an increase in either TV or breathing frequency or a combination of both
- Increased RV is also associated with type I or type II respiratory failure (☐ p.494)
- In severe emphysema the TLC can show a marked increase
- Restrictive lung disease is associated with a decrease in FRC, RV and TLC.

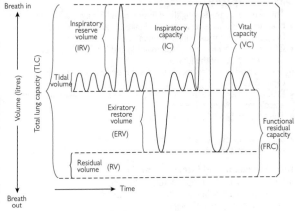

Fig. 5.12 Scheme of lung volumes

Diffusing capacity test

- This is used for measuring the diffusion membrane capacity of the lungs
- It is carried out by estimating the uptake of carbon monoxide (CO) by the pulmonary gas exchange mechanism
- CO readily combines with haemoglobin and is a fast way of deriving diffusing capacities of the lung
- The method most commonly used is the single-breath CO diffusing capacity (DLCO)
- DLCO measures the milliliters of CO diffused per minute across the alveolocapillary membrane
- The test can help identify impairment in both obstructive and restrictive lung disease
- Diffusing capacity tests can involve the patient holding their breath for ten seconds; this may be problematic in the very breathless patient.

Indications for and interpretation of the test

- Evaluation and follow-up of interstitial lung disease such as idiopathic fibrosing alveolitis. In interstitial lung disease (📖 p.311) the DLCO is impaired due to loss of lung capillaries
- Evaluation of patients with emphysema, which is characterized by the destruction of the alveolar membrane. The capacity for gas exchange is compromised and the DLCO will be decreased (📖 p.249)
- Evaluation of other diseases associated with dust inhalation such as asbestosis, which results in a low DLCO as the airborne asbestos particles cause diffuse fibrosis
- Drug related reactions such as cardiac drugs (amiodarone) and rheumatoid drugs
- Evaluation of patients with arterial desaturation on exercise. This is found in some patients with obstructive lung disease, but is more profound in those with restrictive disease. A DLCO < 50% is usually accompanied by a clinically significant fall in oxygen
- Following inhalation of toxic gas or organic agents. This may cause inflammation (alveolitis) which causes a reduction in diffusion which may be due to a related loss in lung volume
- Assessment of disability.

Further information
AARC Clinical Practice Guidelines. *Respiratory Care* 1999: 44 (5).

Exercise testing

One of the main symptoms of respiratory disease is breathlessness, especially on exertion. When assessing a patient, testing exercise capacity will:

- Determine the level of impairment in disability
- Enable a safe and effective exercise programme to be prescribed
- Test the effects of therapy such as pulmonary rehabilitation on exercise capacity
- Assess the extent of lung disease, by stressing the system
- Assist in the diagnosis of unexplained breathlessness on exertion.

Six minute walk test (6MWT)

For this test:

- The patient is encouraged to walk as far as possible at his or her own pace for 6 min
- Standardized encouragement is given, but there is a learning effect and two or three practice runs need to be done
- The total distance walked is measured
- The patient is fitted with a pulse oximeter and oxygen saturations are measured throughout
- The distance covered correlates well with lung function and diffusing capacity but not with oxygen saturations during the walk
- A typical COPD patient with an FEV_1 of about 1 litre or 40% of predicted, would walk about 400 metres
- There is a lot of intersubject variability, which depends on motivation, emotional state, and expectations.

Shuttle walk test (SWT)

For this test:

- The patient walks around two markers, 10 metres apart
- The pace of walking is set by an audio signal which increases in frequency
- The patient continues the shuttle until they cannot keep up, and the distance walked is expressed in metres
- The SWT is a reproducible test of maximal capacity; the 6MWT is less reproducible, but is closer to real life activity.

Nursing considerations for 6MWT and SWT

- Testing should be performed in a location where a rapid, appropriate response to an emergency is possible
- Absolute contraindications are unstable angina and myocardial infarction during the previous month
- There should be oxygen, sublingual nitroglycerine and salbutamol available (metered dose inhaler or nebulizer) (📖 p.391)
- A telephone or other means should be available to enable a call for help
- If a patient is on domiciliary oxygen therapy, oxygen should be given at their normal rate.

Cardiorespiratory exercise test

This test assesses the ability of the respiratory and cardiac systems to cope with an increase in work, particularly the increase in oxygen delivery and carbon dioxide removal. Patients with unexplained breathlessness, normal lung function and those with symptoms of exercise- induced asthma are often referred for this test.

For this test:

- The patient exercises on a treadmill or cycles on an exercise bike
- A mouthpiece with sensors is inserted to measure the rate and volume of respiration
- The oxygen levels of the blood are measured using pulse oximetry and the CO_2 levels are measured in the exhaled air
- Cardiac function is measured by recording the heart rate, blood pressure, and by using an electrocardiogram.

Nursing considerations

- The patient needs to know why the test is being performed
- They need to be reassured that they will be monitored extensively; an explanation of all the monitoring equipment may need to be given
- The patient should be warned that they will be exercised until they experience a considerable degree of breathlessness
- This exertion may put a strain on the heart and cause angina (if they have coronary artery disease); a glycerol trinitrate spray should be available.

Table 5.3 Contraindications to cardio-respiratory exercise test

Absolute	Relative
Recent acute cardiac event or unstable angina	Electrolyte or metabolic disturbance
Uncontrolled cardiac failure	Ventricular aneurysm
Complete heart block	Cardiomyopathy
Severe aortic stenosis	Chronic infective illness
Recent pulmonary embolism	Neuromuscular or musculoskeletal problems
Acute infection	Pregnancy

Breathlessness rating

Breathlessness is a subjective term; it is important to determine how the breathlessness affects the individual. There are several scales for assessing it subjectively. Those most commonly used are:
- The Medical Research Council (MRC) dyspnoea scale
- The 'oxygen cost' diagram
- The Borg scale[1].

Table 5.4 Dyspnoea assessment tools

Test	Description
MRC dyspnoea scale	Patients grade themselves on a scale of 0–5 according to the activity that induces breathlessness
Oxygen cost diagram	This diagram lists activities along a 10cm line and the patient marks a line at the point above which they would become breathless. The score is the distance along the line
Borg scale	This scale is used to measure short-term changes in the intensity of breathlessness during a particular task. For correct usage of the scale the exact design and instructions given by Borg must be followed[1]

Table 5.5 MRC dyspnoea score

Grade	Degree of breathlessness related to activities
1	Not troubled by breathlessness except on strenuous exercise
2	Short of breath when hurrying or walking up a slight hill
3	Walks slower than contemporaries on the level because of breathlessness, or has to stop for breath when walking at own pace
4	Stops for breath after walking about 100m or after a few minutes on the flat
5	Too breathless to leave the house, or breathless when dressing or undressing

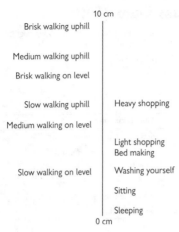

Fig. 5.13 'Oxygen cost' diagram

1. *The Borg CR Scales® Folder. Methods for measuring intensity of experience.* Hasselby, Sweden. borgperception@telia.com.

Body mass index (BMI)

The simplest measure of nutritional status is body weight, from which BMI can be calculated. The formula to calculate an individual's BMI is:

$$BMI = \frac{\text{Weight (in kg)}}{\text{Height}^2 \text{ (in metres)}}$$

Table 5.6 BMI scale

BMI	Nutritional status
<16	Severe malnourishment
16–18.5	Moderate malnourishment
18.5–20	At risk
20–25	Ideal
25–30	Moderate obesity
>30	Severe obesity

- The normal range for BMI is 20–25
- A low BMI (<20) is a poor prognostic feature in respiratory patients and increases the risk of death in COPD
- Patients with a low BMI have an increased risk of lean muscle mass loss
- This leads to peripheral muscle weakness and makes exercising more difficult
- Breathlessness can make eating difficult. Practical advice, such as eating small, frequent high-calorie meals can help reverse the weight loss
- Patients with a low BMI who do not respond to simple advice should be referred for dietetic advice and be encouraged to exercise
- Patients with a high BMI are likely to have greater impairment of activity and more breathlessness than patients with a normal BMI
- This in turn can lead to the patient having even less exercise and a worsening quality of life
- Patients should be given advice on how to lose weight.

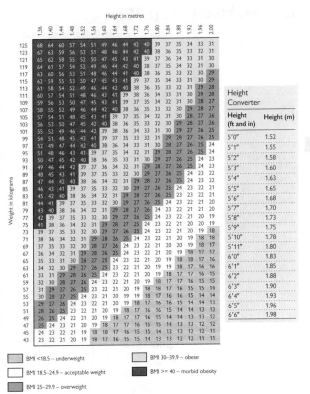

Fig. 5.14 BMI calculator and height converter

Reproduced from Chapman, S, Robinson, G, Stradling, J, and West, S, Oxford Handbook of Respiratory Medicine, 2005, Appendix 5, BMI Calculator and Height Converter, 737–8, with permission from Oxford University Press.

Arterial blood gas (ABG)

ABG analysis evaluates gas exchange in the lungs by measuring the acidity or alkalinity of the blood (pH), respiratory function (oxygen and carbon dioxide) and metabolic measures (bicarbonate and base excess). The respiratory and metabolic systems work together to keep the body's acid-base balance within normal limits.

Indications for ABG analysis include:
- To diagnose and establish the severity of respiratory failure
- To evaluate the need for long-term oxygen therapy (📖 p.359)
- Manage patients in a critical care setting
- Monitor the patients receiving non-invasive ventilation
- Assess patients' condition following cardiac/respiratory arrest
- Establish a baseline prior to surgery
- Monitor patients during cardiorespiratory exercise tests and sleep studies.

The parameters measured are:
- pH—an indication of hydrogen ion (H+) concentration in the blood, pH shows the blood's acidity or alkalinity
- Partial pressure of arterial oxygen (PaO_2)—PaO_2 reflects the body's ability to pick up oxygen from the lungs
- Partial pressure of arterial carbon dioxide ($PaCO_2$)—$PaCO_2$ reflects the adequacy of lung ventilation and carbon dioxide elimination
- Bicarbonate (HCO_3)—known as the metabolic parameter it reflects the ability of the kidneys to retain and excrete HCO_3 (📖 p.494)
- Base excess—a mathematically calculated figure that reflects the amount of acid or base needed to change one litre of blood to a pH of 7.4.

Table 5.7 Normal values of arterial blood gases

Parameter	Normal values
pH	7.35–7.45
PaO_2	11.5–13.0kPa
$PaCO_2$	4.7–6.0kPa
HCO_3	22–26mmol/L
Base excess/deficit	–2 to +2mmol/L
SaO_2	> 93%

A systematic approach should be followed when interpreting ABG tests, and the results should be considered in the context of the patient's history. The results can be misleading if there are mixed respiratory and non-respiratory factors.

Table 5.8 ABG definitions and meanings

Parameter	Definition	Normal values
pH	pH <7.35 indicates acidosis pH >7.5 indicates alkalosis	A normal pH means either the blood gas is normal, in which case so will the $PaCO_2$ and the HCO_3, or full compensation is present in which case the $PaCO_2$ and HCO_3 will be outside normal values as one parameter is compensating for the other. It is possible for the PaO_2 to be low without affecting the pH
PaO_2	PaO_2 <11.5kPa indicates insufficient oxygen in blood (hypoxaemia) PaO_2 >13kPa indicates more oxygen in blood than necessary	Assess whether the value is normal, high or low. This should be considered in the light of any supplementary oxygen the patient may be receiving
$PaCO_2$	$PaCO_2$ <4.7kPa indicates alkalosis $PaCO_2$ >6.0kPa indicates acidosis	$PaCO_2$ assesses the respiratory component. If the $PaCO_2$ is deranged it is important to check whether it follows the same direction (acidosis or alkalosis) as the pH. If so this is the primary disorder
HCO_3	<22 mmol/L indicates acidosis >26 mmol/L indicates alkalosis	HCO_3 assesses the metabolic component. If the HCO_3 value is abnormal check whether it follows the same direction (acidosis or alkalosis) as the pH. If so this is the primary disorder
Base excess	>+2mmol/L indicates a base excess in the blood <−2mmols/L indicates a base deficit in the blood	A base excess is defined as the amount of acid required to restore 1L of blood to a normal pH of 7.4 A base deficit is defined as the amount of alkali required to restore 1L of blood to a normal pH of 7.4

Compensation

This is the body's attempt to maintain a normal pH level. The body uses the respiratory and metabolic systems to oppose each other to maintain a normal pH. Three types of compensation are possible:

- Uncompensated
- Partially compensated
- Fully compensated.

Uncompensated

The pH is abnormal and either the $PaCO_2$ or HCO_3 is abnormal. There is nothing in the results to indicate that the opposite system has tried to correct for the other. This is often seen when a patient is acutely unwell. An example of uncompensated respiratory acidosis would be:

pH	7.17	This is low (acid)
PaO_2	6.6kPa	This is low (hypoxic respiratory failure)
$PaCO_2$	9.4kPa	This is high which explains why the pH is acid
HCO_3	25	This is normal so no evidence of compensation

Partially compensated

The pH is again abnormal and both the $PaCO_2$ and the HCO_3 are also abnormal. One of the parameters will follow the same direction as the pH. This will indicate the primary problem (respiratory or metabolic). The third parameter will be moving in the opposite direction in order to compensate for the primary disorder but will not have changed enough to normalize the pH. An example of partially compensated respiratory acidosis would be:

pH	7.3	This is low (acid)
PaO_2	6.8kPa	This is low (hypoxic respiratory failure)
$PaCO_2$	8.6kPa	This is high which explains why the pH is acid
HCO_3	30	This is high, so evidence that compensation is starting to take place

Fully compensated

The pH is normal but may be at the upper or lower range of normal. The $PaCO_2$ and HCO_3 will be abnormal and moving in opposite directions, one compensating for the other

pH	7.37	This is just within normal limits but slightly acid
PaO_2	6.9kPa	This is low (hypoxic respiratory failure)
$PaCO_2$	7.3kPa	This is high which explains why the pH is slightly acid, so the problem is respiratory in origin
HCO_3	29.8	This is high, the kidneys have produced bicarbonate which explains why pH is in normal limits despite a high CO_2

Table 5.9 Causes, signs, and symptoms of deranged ABGs

Disorder and ABG finding	Possible causes	Signs and symptoms
Respiratory acidosis	Mechanisms that reduce ventilation such as: • COPD/asthma • blocked airway by tumour or foreign body • spontaneous lung collapse • chest wall injury Central nervous system depression from: • drugs (morphine, barbiturates) Hypoventilation from: • pulmonary, cardiac, musculoskeletal or neuromuscular diseases	• Headache • Tachycardia • Confusion • Restlessness • Sweating • Fatigue • Twitching
Respiratory alkalosis	Hyperventilation from: • anxiety • pain • infection causing fever • brainstem damage • drugs (aspirin) Increased ventilation–caused by hypoxic drive: • pneumonia • diffuse interstitial lung disease • high altitude	• Rapid respirations • Numbness • Light-headedness • Twitching • Anxiety • Fear
Metabolic acidosis	• HCO_3 depletion from diarrhoea • Liver, renal and endocrine disease • Drug intoxication	• Deep respirations • Fatigue • Headache • Drowsiness • Nausea/vomiting • Abdominal pain • Coma (if severe)
Metabolic alkalosis	• Loss of hydrochloric acid from prolonged vomiting • Loss of potassium from diuretics or steroids • Excessive alkali ingestion	• Slow, shallow respirations • Restlessness • Twitching • Confusion • Irritability • Coma (if severe)

Arterial blood sample

Arterial sample

Arterial blood samples can be obtained by an arterial puncture or 'stab', or they can be taken from an indwelling arterial cannula. If frequent samples need to be taken, an indwelling cannula enables blood to be taken painlessly. For one-off samples, the most commonly used arterial sampling sites are the radial, brachial, and femoral arteries. Of these three sites the radial artery (lying in the wrist area beside the thumb) is the preferred site because:

- It is easy to access
- It is a superficial artery that is easy to palpate, stabilize, and puncture
- It has a collateral blood supply from the ulnar artery.

A modified Allen's test should be performed prior to taking the sample. This is a test to check the integrity of the radial and ulnar arteries at the wrist.

- The examiner compresses the patient's radial and ulnar arteries at the wrist
- The patient is then asked to open and close the hand rapidly until the palm appears white
- The examiner then releases either the radial or the ulnar artery and looks for return of pink colour and circulation to the hand
- The test is then repeated releasing the other artery
- The hand should return to its pink colour within six seconds if circulation through that artery is adequate (see Figure 5.15).

Taking the sample

- An arterial stab is performed with a 21 gauge needle attached to a syringe that is pre-filled with heparin (0.1–0.2ml of 1000iu heparin/ml)
- The heparin prevents the sample from clotting
- The needle is inserted at an angle of 45° and the amount of blood drawn ranges from 0.5ml (children) to 3ml, depending on local policy and the blood gas analyser available
- Pressure needs to be applied to the puncture site for 5 mins, longer if the patient is on anticoagulant therapy or has a bleeding disorder
- Once the sample is obtained, care should be taken to eliminate visible gas bubbles, as these bubbles can dissolve into the sample and cause inaccurate results
- The sealed syringe should be taken to a blood gas analyser immediately
- If the sample cannot be analysed immediately it should be kept on ice to slow down metabolic processes that may cause inaccuracy
- The machine aspirates this blood from the syringe and measures the pH and the partial pressures of oxygen, carbon dioxide and the bicarbonate concentration, as well as the oxygen saturations of haemaglobin
- The results are usually available within 5 mins, and are then ready for interpretation
- It is important to record whether the patient is breathing air or receiving oxygen when the sample is taken. If the patient is on oxygen, the percentage of oxygen inspired should be recorded.

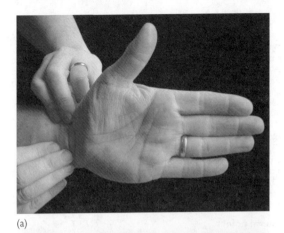

(a)

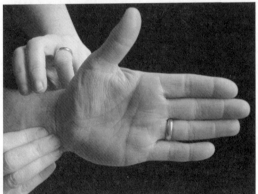

(b)

Fig. 5.15 Modified Allen's test. (a) Radial and ulnar artery occluded; (b) ulnar artery released

Capillary blood samples

Blood can also be taken from the earlobe or a digit for occasional ABG samples; this technique is considered less invasive and painful than an arterial stab.

- A capillary tube is required to collect the sample
- If the earlobe is used it needs to be warmed and a vasodilator cream applied
- This ensures a rapid flow of blood through the capillary
- If a digit is used, vasodilator cream does not need to be applied
- A small nick with a pointed scalpel or lancet will cause a large spot of blood to ooze out, which can be collected in the tube
- The tube is then sealed and taken immediately to the blood gas analyser
- Care is needed to ensure that air bubbles are not present in the sample
- The $PaCO_2$ corresponds well with those obtained from arterial samples, but the accuracy of the PaO_2 depends on good technique in arterialization of the earlobe or digit.

General points

- The procedure should be explained to the patient; they should be warned that it may be painful
- The patient should be advised to breathe normally throughout the test; if the patient is hyperventilating the results may be inaccurate
- Certain conditions may interfere with the test results, for example, venous blood in the sample may lower PaO_2 and elevate $PaCO_2$ levels
- Air bubbles in the sample result in gas equilibration between the air and the arterial blood, lowering the $PaCO_2$ and increasing the $PaCO_2$
- Wait at least 20 mins before drawing blood for an ABG after initiating, changing or discontinuing oxygen therapy
- Document the amount of oxygen the patient is receiving when the sample is drawn
- If the patient is pyrexial when the sample is drawn, the blood gas analyser may need to be adjusted, as most are set to analyse samples at 37° C
- The puncture site should be observed for signs of bleeding, or circulatory impairment, such as numbness, pain, tingling or swelling.

Pulse oximetry

Arterial oxygenation can be easily measured, and provides an estimate of the level of oxygenation of the blood arterial oxygen saturation (SaO_2). It is measured with a pulse oximeter placed either on a finger or an earlobe. The oximeter uses a red and infrared light to detect the absorbed characteristics of oxygenated and deoxygenated haemoglobin. The results are expressed as a percentage of haemoglobin saturated with oxygen. Normal oxygen saturation is usually around 95–98% when breathing room air.

Pulse oximetry is accurate to within + or −3 to 5% but the measurement is unreliable at saturations below 70%. It can be inaccurate if the patient has poor circulation, such as peripheral vascular disease or Raynaud's disease.

An SpO_2 of 90% would be equivalent to a PaO_2 of approximately 8kPa. If the SpO_2 is <92% on air, arterial blood gases should be taken to check CO_2 levels.

General considerations

- Explain to the patient that the test assesses the oxygen content of their haemaglobin
- Patients should remove nail polish prior to the test
- If false nails are *in situ* an ear probe should be used
- Place the probe or clip over the finger or ear lobe, so that the light beams and sensors are opposite each other
- Protect the transducer from strong light
- If the probe is to be kept *in situ* for long periods, check the site frequently and rotate at least every four hours to avoid skin irritation.

Blood tests

Many routine blood tests are performed when a patient has either an acute or a chronic respiratory disease. Some blood tests are done specifically to monitor drug levels (e.g. theophylline) (🔲 p.391)or to confirm a diagnosis (e.g. specific IgE levels in inhalant allergy) (🔲 p.145), but most are indicators of a disease process such as infection. The more common tests and the associated lung diseases are listed in Table 5.10.

Table 5.10 Common blood tests and associated diseases

Blood test	Disease
White blood cell count (WBC)	Elevated in infections such as pneumonia
Haemaglobin (Hb)	Anaemia (low Hb) is often present in chronic pulmonary abscesses
	Erythrocytosis (high red blood cell (RBC)) is sometimes seen in COPD and may indicate hypoxaemia
C-reactive protein (CRP)	An inflammatory index, which can be raised in adults with bacterial pneumonia, pulmonary abcess, infective exacerbations of COPD and asthma. Can be raised in idiopathic pulmonary fibrosis
Erythrocyte sedimentation rate (ESR)	Another inflammatory index, increased during infection. Can be raised in idiopathic pulmonary fibrosis
Blood cultures	Important to obtain during lung or other respiratory infection, prior to starting antibiotics
Serum IgE	Total serum IgE and specific IgE levels rise in allergic bronchopulmonary aspergillosis.
	In asthma, specific IgE antibodies (radioallergosorbent tes [RAST] tests) are measured to confirm diagnosis of inhalant allergies.
	Total IgE shows a positive correlation with prevalence of asthma, but is not diagnostic
Serum $\alpha_1$antitrypsin levels	Should be measured in younger patients with emphysema. If level is low, the phenotype or genotype should also be identified
Serum immunoglobulins and IgG subclasses	These tests should be performed in patients suspected of having bronchiactasis: as immunoglobulin deficiency is a relatively common cause
D-dimer	This test is an indirect, but suggestive marker of intravascular thrombosis. It has a low specificity and can be positive not only when there is pulmonary embolism or deep vein thrombosis, also in the presence of malignancy and after trauma

Radiological investigations

Chest X-ray

A chest X-ray is the basic screening test for patients with respiratory symptoms. It is regarded as standard for patients presenting with chronic problems or acute potentially serious symptoms. It allows visualization of conditions affecting the lung such as:

- Pneumothorax—the accumulation of air in the pleural space
- Lung mass—such as carcinoma (📖 p.344)
- Collapse (atelectasis)—a loss of volume of a lung, lobe or segment for any cause. The most common cause is obstruction of a major bronchus by a tumour, foreign body or mucus plug
- Tuberculosis
- Fibrosis
- Over-inflation in airways disease such as asthma and COPD
- Consolidation—seen as an area of white lung it represents fluid or cellular matter, where there would normally be air. Most commonly seen in infection such as pneumonia or pulmonary oedema (📖 p.455).

Nursing considerations

What the patient needs to know:

- There will be no discomfort during the test and there is very little risk involved
- In women of reproductive age, an X-ray should be performed within 10 days of their last menstruation, unless it is an acute situation
- They will need to remove any metal objects and jewellery from their neck and chest
- They will be asked to stand in front of a photographic plate, with the X-ray beam positioned two metres behind them
- They will be asked to inhale fully, and to hold their breath
- The X-ray beam fires a short beam of X-rays through the patient onto the photographic plate
- These X-ray beams scatter as they pass through the chest structures
- This distortion influences the pattern of X-rays hitting the plate, allowing the structures in the chest to be identified
- Patients who are too ill or too breathless to stand for an X-ray in the radiology department can have a portable X-ray
- The film obtained by portable X-ray may be inferior to the standard X-ray obtained in the radiology department.

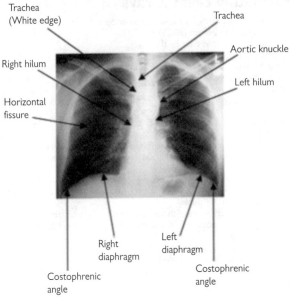

Fig. 5.16 Normal chest radiograph

Evaluating chest X-rays

- Always view an X-ray on a viewing box or on a Picture Archiving and Communication System (PACS)
- Check the name and date on the X-ray
- Note that the radiograph contains right or left-side markers
- You should be able to count six ribs anterior to the diaphragm if there was sufficient inspiration
- Make sure the whole lung field is included
- Divide the lungs into zones—upper, middle and lower and compare like with like
- Examine the area around the rib cage for masses, swelling, air or foreign objects
- Observe the diaphragm—normally the right side looks higher than the left. The diaphragm normally curves downward (costophrenic angle) with clear delineated margins
- Examine the bony structures, looking for unusual densities or fractures
- Look at the heart and check it is of normal shape and size and that the cardiac borders are visible
- Look at the trachea, which should be central—if the trachea has shifted this suggests a problem within the mediastinum or pathology within one of the lungs
- Compare the lung fields looking for adequate lung expansion, and similar areas of density in both lungs
- You generally cannot see the pleura unless they are abnormally thickened.

Computerized tomography (CT) scan

Availability of CT scans has greatly enhanced imaging of the chest, and it is now a routine test in specialist clinical practice. It allows a detailed examination of the lung fields and the central chest. It also allows very high quality images of the chest and the contents of the thoracic cavity, by having many X-rays of the same area performed at different angles. These are collected and processed by a computer into a single image (see Figure 5.17).

Nursing considerations

What the patient needs to know:
• Why the test needs to be performed
• That the test involves exposure to a moderately large dose of X-ray material, approximately 100 times that of a standard chest X-ray
• They may be given intravenous contrast
• That the test involves lying flat and motionless, often difficult for a patient who is breathless, on a bed inside a tube for approximately 15 mins
• They will need to be able to hold their breath for a period of up to 10 s
• The scanner takes the images quickly and silently
• The pictures are then transferred to a computer that processes the information.

What the CT scan identifies

• Pulmonary nodules
• Mediastinal masses
• Carcinoma of the lung
• Pleural lesions
• Vascular lesions.

High-resolution CT scan (HRCT)

HRCT is used in imaging diffuse lung diseases as it looks at thin sections of 1–2mm, which show greater lung detail.
   This scan identifies:
• Bronchiectasis
• Interstitial lung disease such as sarcoidosis, occupational lung disease, and interstitial pneumonia
• Atypical infections, where HRCT is used to provide earlier diagnosis, monitoring disease and response to treatment, and evidence of disease activity and destruction.

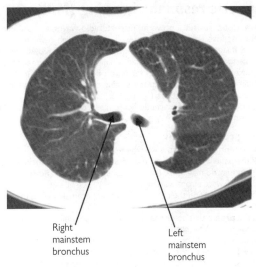

Right
mainstem
bronchus

Left
mainstem
bronchus

Fig. 5.17 Normal CT scan

Magnetic resonant imaging (MRI)

MRI is a test that uses a powerful magnet, radio waves, and a computer to help diagnose respiratory diseases. It provides high-resolution, cross-sectional images of lung structures and traces blood flow. An MRI scan can be of additional value to a CT in examining spinal and some soft tissue pathologies. Although a CT scan tends to offer similar detail to MRI, the MRI scan can be very helpful in the staging of lung cancer as it looks for spinal and cerebral metastases (📖 p.323).

Because of the use of magnetic fields, metal objects cannot be placed in the scanner.

Nursing considerations

- The patient needs to know why the test needs to be done
- Ask the patient to remove all jewellery and empty their pockets. The magnet may de-magnetize the magnetic strip on debit and credit cards, and stop a watch from working
- Inform the doctor if the patient has a heart pacemaker or orthopaedic pins or disks
- Tell the patient that he or she will have to lie on a table that slides into a tunnel inside the magnet
- The patient should be advised to breathe normally, but not to talk or move during the test to avoid distorting the results
- The test can take up to 45 minutes with the patient lying flat throughout, this can be difficult if they are very breathless
- Warn the patient that the machinery is very noisy, with sounds ranging from a constant ping to loud bangs. Provide ear plugs or play music of the patient's choice
- Some patients may feel claustrophobic and sedation may need to be offered.

Bronchoscopy

Bronchoscopy is the direct inspection of the trachea and larger bronchi. It can be used to sample lung tissue via brushings, lavage or biopsy. There are two types of bronchoscopes used: flexible fibreoptic bronchoscopes and rigid bronchoscopes.

Flexible bronchoscopy is the most common type as patients only need to be lightly sedated. This reduces anxiety and suppresses the cough mechanism. Topical anaesthetic, such as lignocaine, is used to anaesthetize the pharynx and the vocal cords.

Rigid bronchoscopy is relatively unusual and is sometimes performed as part of other procedures, such as cryotherapy or laser therapy, where better control of the airway is needed with respect to bleeding. Rigid bronchoscopy needs to be performed under a general anaesthetic.

The main indications for bronchoscopy are:
- Diagnosis of lung cancer following an abnormal chest X-ray or haemoptysis
- Staging of lung cancer
- Diagnosis of diffuse lung disease
- Diagnosis of infection
- Removing foreign bodies, mucus plugs, or excessive secretions.

Nursing considerations
- Explain to the patient what the examination entails and why it is being performed
- Advise the patient not to eat or drink for 4–6 h before the test
- Advise the patient that a sedative will be given before the test and that a topical anaesthetic will be administered
- Advise the patient that they will need to lie on a couch and the bronchoscope will be inserted through their nose or mouth
- Advise the patient that a pulse oximeter will be used to continuously monitor their oxygen levels, and that supplementary oxygen will be given if indicated
- Report any increase in wheeze, breathlessness, chest pain or haemoptysis to the doctor immediately
- Withhold food, fluid, and oral drugs until the gag reflex returns.

Skin-prick testing

A skin-prick test can help to identify whether someone is allergic to a compound. The primary function of the test is to confirm a diagnosis of atopy (📖 p.145), to confirm the clinical history and to allow for correct advice and treatment to be given. It is used most frequently in patients with a history of asthma and allergic rhinitis.

Skin-prick testing is a simple, quick and inexpensive test, which can be performed using a wide range of allergens, and results can be available within 15 min. The principle of the test is that if the patient is allergic to a compound they will have produced specific immunoglobulin (IgE) to that compound. This immunoglobulin will recognize the compound when it is administered.

Skin-prick testing should relate to the clinical history of the patient, which should indicate the allergens selected. In the test, a small amount of the allergen is placed under the skin. If the patient is allergic to the allergen, the IgE that sits on top of the mast cells will recognize the allergen and cause the mast cells to degranulate. Mast cell degranulation causes increased blood flow to the area, causing it to become red, hot and swollen.

How the test is performed

- The test is generally carried out on the skin of the inner forearm
- The arm is labelled in advance with numbers indicating specific allergens, together with a positive control (histamine) and negative control (saline) (see Figure 5.18)
- A drop of allergen is placed on the skin beside the appropriate label and pricked gently into the epidermis using a lancet
- A new lancet should be used for each allergen
- After two minutes the area can be blotted with a clean tissue
- The test sites are read at 15 mins for the presence of erythema (redness) and weal
- The size of the weal is measured and a weal 3mm> the negative control is considered positive
- Large weals at all sites or failure of all tests including the positive control site suggest the need for an alternative test such as specific IgE.

Nursing considerations

- The patient should be advised not to take antihistamines before the test as the result will be unreliable
- Patients should not be on high-dose oral steroids at the time as the test results will be unreliable
- It is safer to avoid skin-prick testing in patients with a past history of anaphylaxis, or with moderate to severe eczema
- The patient should be warned that a positive response to the allergen may be uncomfortable as the skin swells and gets warm
- Very rarely, a patient may develop a severe reaction such as an anaphylactic response to the allergen
- Because of this risk, resuscitation equipment and trained personnel should always be available when skin tests are being performed.

Major allergens tested for:
- House dust mite
- Cat
- Dog
- Grass pollen
- Tree pollen
- Feathers.

Food allergens are less reliable, as false positives to food occur in up to 5% of patients. The test may also cause anaphylaxis and is therefore avoided. Specific RAST tests can be done instead.

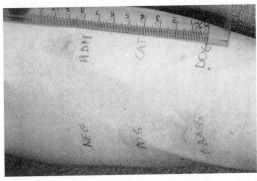

Fig. 5.18 Illustration of skin-prick test site

Reproduced with permission of ALK-Abello.

Sputum tests

Sputum is the material expectorated from the lungs and bronchi during coughing. Analysis of a sputum sample helps diagnose respiratory disease, determine the cause of respiratory infection, and identify abnormal lung cells.

A sputum specimen is examined under a microscope and, depending on the patient's condition, sometimes cultured. Culture and sensitivity testing identifies a specific microorganism, and which antibiotic it is sensitive to. A negative culture does not always rule out infection, as it may be that an infection is viral in nature. The most commonly found organisms and the therapy indicated are listed in Table 5.11.

Sputum can be obtained in three ways: expectoration, tracheal suctioning, or bronchoscopy.

Nursing considerations for obtaining sputum sample

- Explain to the patient why the test is being performed
- Encourage the patient to produce the sputum sample in the morning when sputum production is greatest
- To prevent contamination of the sample, ask the patient not to eat, clean his teeth or use a mouthwash before expectorating
- When the patient is ready to expectorate, encourage him to take three deep breaths and force a deep cough
- If the patient has difficulties expectorating, nebulized saline may be given which loosens the sputum. Alternatively, a physiotherapist may be required to assist the patient to expectorate
- A sterile specimen pot should be used to transport the sample
- Before sending the sample, ensure that the specimen is sputum, not saliva. Saliva has a thinner consistency and more froth or bubbles than sputum
- Include on the laboratory request slip the patients details, date and time of specimen, the original diagnosis, any medication the patient may be taking, and any known drug allergies
- The sample should be sent to the laboratory as soon after it is collected as possible.

Table 5.11 Common microorganisms and antimicrobials indicated

Bacterium	First-line antimicrobials	Second line antimicrobials
Streptcoccus pneumoniae	Amoxycillin Benzylpenicillin	Erythromycin Clarithromycin Cefuroxime Cefotaxime
Haemophilus influenzae	Amoxycillin (co-amoxyclav for ß-lactamase producing strains)	Cefuroxime Cefotaxime Ciprofloxacin Levofloxacin
Legionella pneumophila	Clarithromycin + rifampicin	Ciprofloxacin Levofloxacin
Chlamydia pneumoniae *Mycoplasma pneumoniae*	Erythromycin Clarithromycin	Tetracycline Ciprofloxacin Levofloxacin
Moraxella catarrhalis	Co-amoxiclav	Erythromycin Tetracycline

Table provided by Professor K Kerr Consultant Microbiologist/Honorary Clinical Professor of Microbiology, Harrogate District Foundation Trust.

Chapter 6

Acute respiratory distress syndrome

Definition

Acute Respiratory Distress Syndrome (ARDS) is not a single entity but represents the severe end of a spectrum of acute lung injury resulting in a non-cardiogenic pulmonary capillary permeability which allows fluid and protein to leak into the alveolar spaces with pulmonary infiltrates. It is characterized by rapid progressive hypoxaemia, due to shunt from ventilation/perfusion (VQ) mismatch, and reduced lung compliance increasing the work of breathing.

ARDS is the severe form of the respiratory component of the Systemic Inflammatory Response Syndrome (SIRS). The reader is encouraged to read more widely about SIRS, sepsis and multiple organ failure.

ARDS is the severe form of acute lung injury (ALI) and is characterized by:

PaO_2/FiO_2 ratio <200 (mmHg) or 27kPa

- PaO_2 = partial pressure of oxygen in arterial blood, obtained from blood gas analysis and may be measured in mmHg or kPa. FiO_2 is the fraction of inspired oxygen (e.g. 40% oxygen is an FiO_2 of 0.40). The ratio is an indication of oxygen dependence (e.g. a patient with a PaO_2/FiO_2 ratio of less than 200 mmHg or 27kPa will need an inspired oxygen concentration of 40% to achieve a PaO_2 of 10.8kPa)
- Bilateral central batwing infiltrates on chest radiograph, (not usually limited to the basal regions as with pulmonary oedema) and due to the fibrotic stage. This is often accompanied by a normal heart shadow on the cxr
- No evidence of left atrial hypertension, Pulmonary capillary wedge pressure (PCWP) <18 mmHg (excluding hydrostatic pulmonary oedema as seen in cardiac failure).

The above criteria apply to patients with a defined risk factor for ARDS and the absence of severe chronic lung disease.

The scenario of the patient with ARDS and underlying cardiac dysfunction, or post cardiopulmonary bypass ARDS is a challenging clinical entity both for diagnosis, management and care.

ALI is characterized by:
- PaO_2/FiO_2 <300 mmHg or 40kPa
- Bilateral infiltrates on chest radiograph
- No evidence of left atrial hypertension
- ARDS may predominate the clinical picture, or may be of lesser importance than failure of other organ systems.

Incidence

The incidence of ARDS is approximately 25–45% in critically ill patients.

Aetiology

ARDS forms part of an exaggerated inflammatory response which may be either:

- *Direct*, as in the case of lung contusion, lung infections, inhalation injury etc, or
- *Indirect*, as in the case of sepsis, pancreatitis, burns, severe tissue injury etc.

The most common cause is sepsis. Approximately 40% of patients with sepsis exhibit ARDS.

Onset occurs within 24 h of the predisposing cause in 80% of cases and within 72 h in 95% of cases.

Pathophysiology

Histology shows activation and aggregation of neutrophils and platelets, patchy alveolar infiltrates caused by proteinaceous exudate, and elements of fibrosis from an early stage of the pathophysiological process of ARDS. The development of ARDS includes dysfunction of both the respiratory capillary endothelium and the pulmonary pneumocytes. Inflammatory mediators (interleukins, tumour necrosis factor [TNF], prostaglandins, nitric oxide, endothelins etc.) and inflammatory cellular elements (leucocytes, platelets, fibroblasts etc.) all play a variable part in the pathophysiology.

ARDS is classically divided into an early exudative phase due to increased capillary permeability, activation and aggregation of neutrophils and platelets, and patchy alveolar exudate, followed by a fibroproliferative phase showing varying degrees of resolution, organization and fibrosis.

Treatment and general management

- Remove the cause wherever possible. Surgical drainage of infection or debridement of infected or necrotic tissue, fixation of long bone fracture, early effective antibiotic therapy etc
- Oxygen or non-invasive continuous positive airway pressure (CPAP) are the first line of ventilation therapy. Intubation and mechanical ventilation with appropriate sedation offer a more controlled support. For more unstable patients, appropriate paralysing agents may be considered
- Haemodynamic monitoring and appropriate therapy to maintain oxygen delivery to tissues
- Support of other organ function. The *Surviving Sepsis Guidelines* published by the European Critical Care Society provides common general treatment principles for other forms of acute critical illness (see Further reading at the end of this chapter).

Respiratory support

Initially oxygen saturation should be supported with appropriate increases in administered oxygen by face mask in the spontaneously breathing patient (📖 p.359). Patients requiring higher than 40–60% oxygen should receive high-flow humidified oxygen. High-flow oxygen is delivered via a high-flow generator at flows of above 4L per minute. It can cause drying of the mucosa and of secretions, and should always be warmed and humidified.

The addition of CPAP may be considered to maximally recruit those alveoli without capillary shunt.

An intensive care unit referral with intubation and invasive ventilation may be necessary if the patient is unable to sustain oxygenation or the work of breathing with non-invasive therapy.

Ventilation needs for the patient will be:

- Increased inspiratory to expiratory (I:E) ratio ventilation
- Tidal volume (Vt) should be limited to 6–8 ml/kg predicted body mass and plateau pressures limited to <30–35 cmH2O where achievable to prevent ventilator associated lung injury (VALI). Where higher pressures need to be used, increased positive end expiratory pressure (PEEP) (up to 20cmH2O) helps protect the lungs from further damage.

Complications of mechanical ventilation are common and include ventilator associated pneumonia (VAP), and pneumothorax necessitating the placement of often multiple chest drains.

Serial chest radiographs and CT scan as indicated will confirm correct positioning of tubes and monitor lung changes (📖 p.75).

Blood gas values should be aimed at survival and not necessarily the achievement of normal values. Permissive hypercapnia may be indicated and reductions of SaO2 to 80% may be tolerated provided that organ function is maintained.

Position changes

Rotation or prone positioning may improve oxygenation by improved ventilation/perfusion matching, but has not been shown to improve outcome and may carry practical risks such as injury, access limitation and risk of line/tube displacement. A 30–45° head-up position reduces the incidence of aspiration and nosocomial pneumonia.

Other treatments

Inhaled nitric oxide (NO) or nebulized epoprostenol (PGI2) (2–10ng/kg/min) have shown improvements in oxygenation in up to 60% of patients, but have not shown outcome benefit. There is no benefit to be derived from the use of surfactant.

Steroids do not prevent ARDS. Steroids on days 7–10 may improve gas exchange in 50–60% of patients but their use is debated and may be detrimental in the presence of concurrent infection.

In severe ARDS an ICU may consider referral to a specialist centre for $ECCO_2R$ (extra corporeal CO_2 removal) or ECMO (extra corporeal membrane oxygenation) where the patient's blood is pumped outside the body through a membrane oxygenator, though these treatment modalities remain controversial with trials ongoing.

Other treatments, with varying uptake and benefit, include independent lung ventilation, tracheal gas insufflation, partial liquid ventilation (experimental) and high-frequency oscillation or jet ventilation. None of these are proven to improve outcome.

Prognosis

Prognosis is dependent on the:

- Nature of the primary insult—ARDS associated with certain underlying precipitating causes may carry a good prognosis and reverse rapidly (fat embolism—90% survival), while other causes (sepsis)—may be more severe in all aspects of the condition
- The extent of such insult
- Age and health of the patient
- Presence and extent of other organ dysfunction
- The mortality rate has fallen over the past decade from 60–70% to around 35%
- 80% of deaths in patients with ARDS are from sepsis and/or multi-organ failure and not from respiratory failure
- The majority of survivors have residual mild to moderate respiratory impairment, a small percentage are severely impaired and some return to normal function but may still have some deficit on lung function testing.

Nursing care

Nursing care in a general ward area is aimed at identification of early deterioration in respiratory function and prompt management of signs and symptoms. Regular observations of basic physiological parameters such as heart rate, blood pressure and respiratory rate must be recorded (📖 p.31).

Accurate recording of fluid balance with running totals will be key when managing hypotension and pulmonary oedema. The use of a track and trigger or early warning scoring system will also aid the identification of deterioration for the more junior staff member.

Optimization of oxygen delivery and commencing high-flow oxygen and humidification will give some symptomatic relief. Consideration of reducing oxygen demand by timing and planning nursing interventions will aid symptomatic relief.

Patient positioning and reassurance will support breathlessness. Oral intake may be reduced and oral care should be offered. Monitoring of nutritional intake needs to be carried out and dietician referral made. IV fluids will often be needed.

Early referral to a higher level of care should be considered.

Care within the critical care unit will be aimed at preserving organ function and will include invasive ventilation, haemofiltration, inotropes and other system support. The reader is advised to select a specialist intensive care book for further reading on this area.

The nursing care of the patient with ARDS will be the best supportive care provided in an appropriate setting. The impact of the severity of the illness on the patients' family and of the high mortality will need careful handling.

Further reading

Acute Respiratory Distress Syndrome Network. Ventilation with lower tidal volumes as compared with traditional tidal volumes for acute lung injury and the acute respiratory distress syndrome. *N Engl J Med* 342: 1301–1307, 2000.

Artigas A, Bernard GR *et al.* The American-European consensus conference on ARDS. Part 2: Ventilatory, pharmacologic, supportive therapy, study design strategies, and issues related to recovery and remodelling. *Am J Respir Crit Care Med* 157: 818–824, 1998.

Bernard GR, Artigas A, Brigham K *et al.* The American European consensus conference on ARDS: Definitions, mechanisms, relevant outcomes and clinical trial coordination. *Am J Respir Crit Care Med* 149: 818–824, 1994.

Dellinger RP, Carlet JM, *et al.* Surviving Sepsis Campaign Guidelines for management of severe sepsis and septic shock. *Intensive Care Medicine* 30: 536–555, 2004.

Gattinoni L, Tognoni G *et al.* Effects of prone positioning on the survival of patients with acute respiratory distress syndrome. *N Engl J Med* 345: 568–573, 2001.

Herringe MS, Cheung AM *et al.* One-year outcome in survivors of the acute respiratory distress syndrome. *N Engl J Med* 348: 683–693, 2003.

Jantz MA, Sahn SA. Corticosteroids in acute respiratory failure. *Am J Respir Crit Care Med* 160: 1079–1100, 1999.

McIntyre RC Jr, Pulido EJ *et al.* Thirty years of clinical trials in acute respiratory distress syndrome. *Cri Care Med* 28: 3314–3330, 2000.

Ware BL, Matthay MA. The acute respiratory distress syndrome. *N Engl J Med* 342: 1334–1338, 2000.

Wyncoll DLA, Evans TW. The acute respiratory distress syndrome. *Lancet* 354: 497–501, 1999.

Asthma and allergies

Introduction

Asthma is a significant problem in the UK affecting approximately 5.2 million people; occuring in 21% of children and 15% of adults. Whilst there is no cure for asthma, current medications can effectively abolish symptoms in most people. Despite this, there is still considerable morbidity amongst people with asthma, with over half experiencing symptoms that regularly wake them at night and two-thirds reporting difficulty in running for a bus or taking part in exercise.

Allergy is an important component of asthma, and most people with asthma are sensitive to one or more common aeroallergens. Approximately 80% of people with asthma also have rhinitis (essentially a runny, blocked nose), which is associated with a significant impact on quality of life.

Key components for improved asthma and rhinitis control are: accurate diagnosis, appropriate use of the therapeutic options available, regular review, and effective patient education. Identification of allergic triggers may be useful where avoidance measures have been shown to be both effective and feasible. It is essential that patients and their families or carers are involved in decisions about their treatment and that health professionals work in partnership with them to enable them to better manage their own condition.

To improve asthma control and reduce the impact of symptoms on an individual's quality of life, it is essential that all health professionals who come into contact with people with asthma (and rhinitis) are familiar with the most up to date methods of treating both conditions, and are fully conversant with current clinical guidelines.

Asthma: a definition

For many years experts have struggled to find a simple definition for asthma. There is considerable debate as to whether asthma should be considered as a single disease entity, or whether it should be considered a dynamic heterogenous clinical syndrome which has a number of different patterns. There is agreement, however, that it is characterized by the following features:

- Chronic airway inflammation
- Increased airway responsiveness
- Widespread variable airflow obstruction
- Reversible airflow obstruction.

The definition used in the current British Guidelines on the Management of Asthma is that of the International consensus report 1992 which describes asthma as:

> a chronic inflammatory disorder of the airways…in susceptible individuals, inflammatory symptoms are usually associated with widespread but variable airflow obstruction and an increase in airway response to a variety of stimuli. Obstruction is often reversible, either spontaneously or with treatment.

This is similar to the National Institutes of Health Global Initiative for Asthma(GINA) guidelines definition of 1998:

> chronic inflammatory disorder of the airways. In susceptible individuals this inflammation causes recurrent episodes of wheezing, coughing, chest tightness and difficulty in breathing. Inflammation causes airway sensitivity to stimuli such as allergen and irritants.

Common features of the definitions are asthma is a chronic inflammatory condition with onset, symptom severity and response to stimuli as variable.

Pathophysiology

Everyone's airways react to inhaled irritants, for example, on entering a fume-filled room or inhaling a crumb, most people will cough. Although they are not aware of it, their bronchial smooth muscle contracts and mucus production increases as part of the body's normal protective mechanisms.

In asthma this reaction becomes exaggerated and the airways of people with asthma react much more readily to lower levels of provocation and to triggers that might not bother other people. This exaggerated response is known as bronchial hyperreactivity (BHR). Whilst characteristic of asthma, BHR is not exclusive to it. Long-term smokers may develop BHR and sometimes an acute respiratory infection such as bronchitis or influenza can lead to a temporary rise in BHR.

Exposure to a trigger then sets off a chain of events causing an inflammatory response. In *atopic* or *extrinsic* asthma this is an immunoglobulin E- (IgE) mediated series of events but in *non-atopic* or *intrinsic* asthma the mechanisms leading to inflammation are less clear.

It is the underlying inflammation that causes narrowing of the bronchioles through three main mechanisms:

Bronchospasm

Bronchospasm is the sharp contraction of bronchial smooth muscle which narrows the bronchioles and distorts the epithelium and sub-mucosa. Attention is often given to bronchospasm because it is readily perceived by the person with asthma who is experiencing symptoms and it can easily be reversed by β_2 agonist drugs such as salbutamol and terbutaline (📖 p.391).

It is important to remember that bronchoconstriction is caused by other mechanisms and that unless these are appropriately treated symptoms will return quickly and may become persistent.

Frequent or prolonged bronchospasm can result in smooth muscle growth (hypertrophy) causing thickening of the muscle and permanent reduction in airway size. This may be one of the reasons why people with poorly controlled asthma can go on to develop an element of irreversible airway obstruction.

Epithelial damage and oedema

The capillaries in the submucosa dilate and become leaky, causing the epithelium and submucosa to become swollen with watery fluid. Epithelial cells are shed causing the submucosa and the vagal nerve endings of the basement membrane to become exposed. The basement membrane can also become thickened and persistent inflammation can result in permanent changes.

Mucus production

Mucus glands enlarge and mucus-secreting cells multiply resulting in the over-production of sticky yellowish mucus. In severe attacks it is possible for mucus plugs to be coughed up, cast in the shape of smaller airways, containing shed epithelial calls, inflammatory cells and plasma exudates.

Epithelial damage, oedema and excess mucus production do not respond to bronchodilators, and treatment with systemic or inhaled corticosteroids (depending on the severity of presentation) is required to control them.

Allergen exposure: early and late phase responses

As mentioned previously, a large proportion of people with asthma are allergic to one or more allergens. This can be demonstrated by their tendency to produce IgE in response to these allergens (measured by skin-prick or blood tests) (📖 p.75). However, much of the damage to the lungs of an asthmatic person is not caused directly by IgE-mediated mechanisms. When someone is exposed to an allergen to which they are sensitized, the allergen binds to the IgE on the mast cells and basophils causing these cells to release their inflammatory mediators. One of these is histamine, which causes many of the symptoms of allergies, such as in rhinitis. In asthma, however, although histamine will cause an immediate bronchoconstriction in the lungs, it is the influx of other inflammatory cells (in response to not only histamine but other mediators and cytokines released by mast cells and T cells) that is behind the main changes in the lungs in asthma, and which induce the so-called late asthmatic response following allergen challenge.

Early asthmatic response

Following sensitization to a particular allergen, re-exposure to that allergen results in rapid bronchoconstriction, starting within minutes, peaking at 15 min, and disappearing within about 3 h. This is known as the early asthmatic response. The most important mediators that are released in the early response are histamine, prostaglandins and leukotrienes. (Fig. 7.1).

Late asthmatic response

Approximately 50% of allergic adults and over 70% of asthmatic children will go on to develop a late asthmatic response several hours after exposure to the allergen. The late response lasts for up to 18–24 h. However, even after the peak expiratory flow rate (PEFR) has returned to normal, bronchial hyperreactivity may persist for up to 3 weeks after a single allergen exposure. This late response is caused by the recruitment (by mediators released during the early phase) of inflammatory cells such as eosinophils, neutrophils and lymphocytes into the area. The mediators released from these cells are more toxic and longer-lasting than the mediators released from mast cells. They lead not only to sustained bronchospasm but also to further plasma exudation from the capillaries along with increased bronchial hyper-responsiveness and inflammation. (Fig. 7.1).

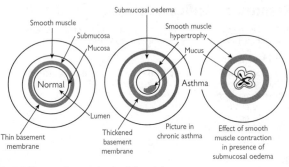

Fig. 7.1 Diagram of a normal and an inflamed airway

Reproduced with permission from Education for Health
http://www.educationforhealth.org.uk.

Asthma classification

Asthma can be classified in different ways but it is important to remember that patients rarely fit neatly into specific categories.

Extrinsic asthma

Now more commonly referred to as atopic asthma, it is characterized by:
- Childhood onset
- Intermittent symptoms
- Positive skin tests
- Clearly identifiable triggers
- Family history of allergy
- Good prognosis.

Intrinsic asthma

Now more commonly referred to as non-atopic asthma, it is characterized by:
- Adult onset
- Persistent symptoms
- Negative skin tests
- Trigger factors not clear
- Possible family history of asthma
- Fair prognosis.

Patterns of asthma

Another way of classifying asthma is to consider the pattern in which symptoms occur. Asthma can then be divided into three broad groups:

Episodic

Occasional well-defined attacks, lasting hours or days. In between attacks symptoms completely resolve.

Frequent episodic

More frequent exacerbations lasting longer, sometimes days or weeks.

Persistent

Acute exacerbations on a background of some continuous symptoms even when 'well'. These persistent symptoms between more severe attacks are sometimes referred to as interval symptoms.

Occupational asthma

The exact incidence of occupational asthma is difficult to ascertain, but it is estimated that occupational causes may account for about 9–15% of adult onset asthma. It is now the commonest industrial lung disease in the world with over 400 reported causes. Occupational asthma can have significant impact, with many people having to change jobs to avoid contact with the substance which caused their asthma, or in more severe cases causing major disablement resulting in early retirement.

Work-aggravated asthma

Pre-existing asthma (or co-incidental new onset asthma) made worse by non-specific factors such as dust or fumes in the workplace.

Occupational asthma

Asthma caused by sensitization to a specific agent in the workplace. Occupational asthma can be subdivided into two groups:

Irritant-induced occupational asthma

Symptoms typically occur within a few hours of exposure to a high concentration of an irritant gas, fume or vapour at work. This type of occupational asthma is sometimes termed reactive airway dysfunction syndrome (RADS).

Allergic occupational asthma

About 90% of all occupational asthma is caused through an allergic response and this is what is generally meant when referring to occupational asthma. In this allergic response the exposure to a respiratory sensitizer at work is followed by a latency period before development of symptoms. Agents that induce workplace asthma through an allergic mechanism can be broadly divided into those of low- or high-molecular weight. Those of high-molecular weight are usually proteins and appear to act through a type 1, IgE-associated hypersensitivity. Whilst some low-molecular weight agents also act through IgE-mediated mechanisms, the action of the majority is less clear.

The diagnosis of allergic occupational asthma should be suspected in all adults with symptoms of airflow obstruction. It should be positively searched for in those working in high-risk occupations or with high-risk substances because early removal from the causative agent has an improved prognosis with the best chance of complete recovery. Workers who remain in the same employment; and with the same exposure after diagnosis, are unlikely to improve and symptoms may worsen. The chance of improvement or resolution of symptoms is greatest in those who have no further exposure to the causative agent. This may have significant employment and financial implications for the worker and for this reason early referral to a specialist occupational chest physician is recommended.

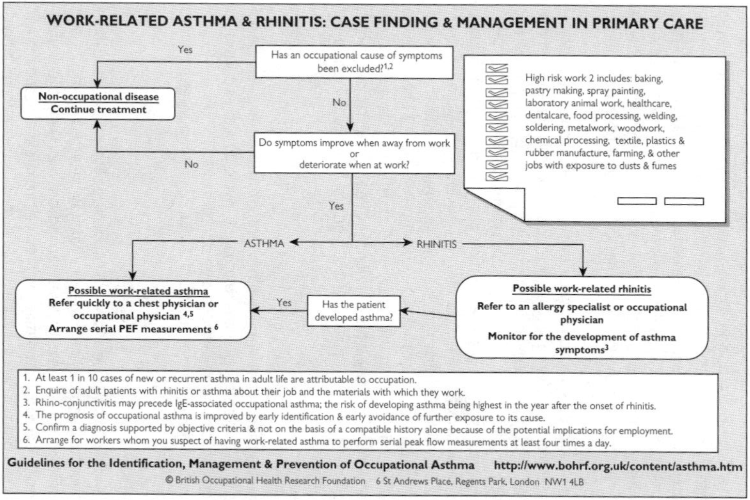
WORK-RELATED ASTHMA & RHINITIS: CASE FINDING & MANAGEMENT IN PRIMARY CARE
Has an occupational cause of symptoms been excluded?1,2
Yes
No
Non-occupational disease
Continue treatment
Do symptoms improve when away from work or deteriorate when at work?
No
Yes
High risk work 2 includes: baking, pastry making, spray painting, laboratory animal work, healthcare, dentalcare, food processing, welding, soldering, metalwork, woodwork, chemical processing, textile, plastics & rubber manufacture, farming, & other jobs with exposure to dusts & fumes
ASTHMA
RHINITIS
Possible work-related asthma
Refer quickly to a chest physician or occupational physician 4,5
Arrange serial PEF measurements 6
Yes
Has the patient developed asthma?
Possible work-related rhinitis
Refer to an allergy specialist or occupational physician
Monitor for the development of asthma symptoms3
1. At least 1 in 10 cases of new or recurrent asthma in adult life are attributable to occupation.
2. Enquire of adult patients with rhinitis or asthma about their job and the materials with which they work.
3. Rhino-conjunctivitis may precede IgE-associated occupational asthma; the risk of developing asthma being highest in the year after the onset of rhinitis.
4. The prognosis of occupational asthma is improved by early identification & early avoidance of further exposure to its cause.
5. Confirm a diagnosis supported by objective criteria & not on the basis of a compatible history alone because of the potential implications for employment.
6. Arrange for workers whom you suspect of having work-related asthma to perform serial peak flow measurements at least four times a day.
Guidelines for the Identification, Management & Prevention of Occupational Asthma http://www.bohrf.org.uk/content/asthma.htm
© British Occupational Health Research Foundation 6 St Andrews Place, Regents Park, London NW1 4LB

Fig. 7.2 Work-related asthma and rhinitis: case finding and management in primary care (Algorithm).

Reproduced with permission from Newman Taylor AJ, Nicholson PJ. (eds). Guidelines for the prevention, identification and management of occupational asthma: Evidence review and recommendations. British Occupational Health Research Foundation. London 2004

Risk factors for the development of asthma 1

No single cause for asthma has been identified, but there are several different factors that may be implicated in the development of asthma.

Genetic influences

There is no doubt that asthma does tend to run in families and is associated with a genetic predisposition to atopy but it can occur in individuals in whom there is no family history of either asthma or atopy.

It is estimated that a child with first-degree relatives with asthma or atopy is two to three times more likely to develop asthma than one without a close family history. There is a slightly higher risk from maternal asthma than paternal asthma and the risk is further increased if both parents are affected.

Whilst a genetic predisposition may be part of the reason for the development of asthma, it is clear that a more complex interaction of other environmental factors is involved in the development of symptoms. For example when children from areas with low asthma prevalence have been relocated to areas of higher prevalence they have been found to develop asthma at a similar prevalence to that of their new location. Although many factors may be involved, studies like this have generally shown that a move to a more modern, urban, economically developed society seems to be associated with an increase in the occurrence of asthma. This is seen with the reunification of Germany, where lower prevalence rates amongst children in East Germany caught up with West German rates over a period of around ten years.

Gender

Male sex is a risk factor for the development of asthma in prepubertal children with male infants being approximately twice as likely to develop asthma in early childhood as their female counterparts.

Female sex is a risk factor for the persistence of childhood asthma into adulthood.

Pollution

Whilst it is evident that high levels of atmospheric pollution can contribute to exacerbations of asthma the evidence that it is linked to an increase in new presentations is less clear. Studies carried out following the unification of Germany demonstrated that the lifetime prevalence of asthma and sensitization to common aeroallergens was higher in those from Munich in the west compared to Leipzig in the East. This study suggests that 'classical' air pollution from sulphur dioxide and particulates is unlikely to be a contributory factor to the development of asthma, as those from Leipzig had been exposed to much higher levels of these due to poorly regulated heavy industry and high domestic use of coal.

Some recent studies have, however, suggested that ambient air pollution, particularly prolonged exposure to diesel fumes, may act as an adjuvant for the sensitization to common aeroallergens. This type of exposure might possibly be considered to have a causal relationship to asthma.

Indoor pollutants such as nitrogen dioxide fumes from gas cookers or fires have also been implicated in some studies as contributing to the development of asthma (📖 p.541).

Allergen exposure

There has been much interest in the role that early exposure to potential allergens might play in the atopic person developing asthma. It has been thought that the amount of exposure (allergen load), the type of allergen and the timing of exposure are all factors that might have a role to play in the development of asthma.

It is likely that with the advent of modern living with central heating, double glazing and fitted carpets we have increased exposure to allergens such as house dust mite. Some studies have suggested that reducing exposure to these types of allergens during pregnancy and early life may be protective for wheezing at one year of age for children with a high genetic risk. Unfortunately studies have often failed to be conclusive and in fact are often contradictory. Some studies demonstrate that early exposure to high levels of allergens such as cat or dog, may be protective whilst others link early exposure to higher levels of sensitization. So it is difficult to say whether early allergen exposure is causative in asthma.

Maternal smoking

Many studies demonstrate a link between maternal smoking in pregnancy or exposure to passive smoking in early life increasing the risk of wheezing illness in the first few years of a child's life. Children exposed to cigarette smoke in this way are twice as likely to suffer a serious respiratory illness such as bronchiolitis, pneumonia or bronchitis requiring hospital admission or medical treatment.

The evidence for parental smoking as a causative factor for childhood asthma is less clearly defined although in children with established asthma parental smoking is associated with more severe disease.

Exposure to infection (hygiene hypothesis)

There is some evidence to demonstrate that a reduction in environmental bacterial load might in some way be connected to an increase in allergen sensitization. Some have suggested that exposure to some infections could even be protective for the development of asthma.

The 'hygiene hypothesis' is based on the idea that the immature immune system is biased towards the production of cytokines that are also associated with allergy. The exposure to infection focuses the maturing immune system towards the type of response that is not related to allergy and so sensitization and allergic response is less predominant.

In contrast there is evidence that some viral infections such as respiratory syncytial virus (RSV), *Chlamydia pneumonia* or varicella may be linked to the development of asthma. It is possible that certain infections like these trigger an immune response which in turn affects the way in which the immune system reacts to allergens with or without sensitization.

Dietary factors

The evidence surrounding the links between diet and the development of asthma is limited. It has been suggested that too much sodium and omega-6 fatty acids and too little antioxidant and omega-3 fatty acids may be responsible. There is limited evidence that a diet high in fish oil may be protective against the development of childhood asthma.

Breastfeeding

The evidence in relation to the development of asthma and breastfeeding is contradictory. Some studies have shown protective effects against the development of asthma and other atopic illness with a significant reduction in serum IgE levels in those who have been breastfed. Others, whilst showing protection against early childhood wheezing, have failed to show any benefit with regard to the later development of asthma.

Given the other health benefits of breastfeeding it should always be recommended when possible.

Inhaled allergens as triggers for asthma

The airway hyper-responsiveness associated with asthma results in an exaggerated reaction to a variety of inhaled allergens and also following exposure to irritants, cold air, and exercise or in response to hyperventilation.

Most people with asthma will have more than one trigger factor for their asthma symptoms. Not all people with asthma have the same trigger factors, thus what provokes asthma symptoms in one person may not present a problem to another.

Trigger factors can be either allergens where the specific IgE-mediated response is seen (Type 1 hypersensitivity) or irritants which are non-specific but still cause asthma exacerbations.

Inhaled allergens including pollens, animal dander, house dust mite

In allergic asthma and rhinitis, allergen triggers are generally those that are airborne, although occasionally food allergy can induce asthma and/or rhinitis symptoms. The most important of the aeroallergens are those that are found indoors. This is because most people spend around 90% of their time indoors. With the increase in carpets and soft furnishings and the reduction in ventilation in modern houses, the concentration of airborne allergens indoors is much higher than it was around 30 years ago. Asthma and rhinitis symptoms can have both allergic and non-allergic triggers.

Causes of seasonal allergic asthma and rhinitis
- Grass pollens (e.g. Timothy grass, rye grass)
- Tree pollens (e.g. birch, cedar, London plane)
- Weed pollens (e.g. mugwort)
- Moulds (e.g. *Aspergillus Fumigatus, Cladosporium*).

Seasonal symptoms commonly occur in February/March (trees), May/July (grasses) and August (weeds). The diagnosis is usually straightforward and based on a clear history of typical seasonal symptoms of itch/sneeze, watery discharge (rhinorrhea) and associated allergic conjunctivitis. The peak for seasonal symptoms varies from the south to the north of the UK, with the latter tending to be later.

Causes of perennial allergic asthma and rhinitis
- House dust mites (Dermatophagoides Pteronyssinus)
- Cat dander (from saliva, urine or skin scales)
- Dog dander.

Perennial symptoms are more difficult to attribute to allergen exposure due to the persistent nature of indoor allergens. Predominant symptoms include nasal blockage and watery rhinorrhea.

Differences between seasonal and perennial rhinitis symptoms

It is likely that the primary differences between seasonal (sneezing, itching, rhinorrhea) and perennial (nasal blockage) symptoms are the result of intermittent versus persistent allergen exposure. Pollen counts rise and fall during the pollen season, giving repeated but not necessarily persistent exposure to allergen, whilst constant levels of house dust mite or a cat in the home lead to prolonged exposure. For effective management, it is important that both immediate (intermittent) and persistent symptoms are recognized and treated appropriately.

Allergen avoidance

House dust mite

Single house dust mite avoidance measures (e.g. mattress encasings) have not been shown to have any effect in reducing asthma or rhinitis symptoms in adults. There is some evidence that both single and multifaceted interventions based on individual sensitization in children are associated with a meaningful and sustained improvement in asthma control.

Animal allergens

There is little evidence that reducing cat allergen in the home whilst continuing to live with a cat is either possible or effective. Removal of the animal from the home is probably the only effective option, although prolonged and vigorous cleaning is required to eradicate allergen effectively. Evidence to support the use of pet avoidance in early life to prevent subsequent sensitization or symptoms is contradictory.

Pollens

Grass pollen is light, easily carried on the wind over large distances and is therefore ubiquitous in the summer months in urban and rural areas. There is no evidence that pollen avoidance measures are effective in reducing symptoms. Tree pollens are larger, heavier and tend to fall to the ground more quickly; because of this they often cause problems in some areas more than others and are theoretically more avoidable.

Moulds

Mould spores (rather than the mould itself) can cause allergic symptoms. Mould spores are often released when there is a change in the environment, when moist conditions suddenly become warm or when the central heating first goes on in a damp house. Outdoor mould spores are often more prolific in late summer and autumn, during the harvest time and as fallen leaves collect on the ground.

Other triggers for asthma

Respiratory infections

Viral respiratory infections are the most common trigger for asthma symptoms causing 50–80% of wheezing illness and asthma exacerbations. Young infants tend to be more affected, possibly because of their small airways. There is increasing evidence that there is a synergy between viral-induced inflammation and allergen-induced inflammation. It has also been suggested that altered cytokine responses to the viral infection allow allergens to enter the bloodstream via the respiratory tract more readily, thus triggering an exacerbation.

Exercise

Many people with asthma suffer from bronchoconstriction after exercise. This is different from the normal breathlessness that anyone might experience during exercise. If the exercise is the only trigger for symptoms then the condition is termed 'exercise-induced asthma'. It has been suggested, however, that because changes in airway inflammation or hyper-responsiveness are not always involved, the term 'exercise-induced bronchospasm' might be more appropriate.

It is thought that it is the drying and cooling effect of rapidly inhaled air during exercise that may be the cause of the bronchospasm. There seem to be fewer problems in the presence of warmer more moist air which may be the reason why some activities may be less problematic than others.

For many people with asthma, exercise will not be their only trigger and the presence of exercise-induced symptoms is often considered to be a marker of suboptimal asthma control.

Environmental triggers

Pollution

Several different indoor and outdoor pollutants can trigger asthma exacerbations. These include:

- ozone (even at low levels)
- sulphur dioxide
- nitrogen dioxide
- cigarette smoke
- fumes from gas cookers/fires (probably nitrogen dioxide)
- vehicle emissions.

Cold air

Sudden decreases in temperature such as breathing in cold air or exposing the face to cold air can precipitate bronchoconstriction in both asthmatic and non-asthmatic subjects. For people with asthma simply going out of the house on a cold day or possibly eating a cold ice cream on a hot summer's day can cause asthma symptoms.

Thunderstorms

Although infrequent it is not uncommon for asthma epidemics to occur as the result of thunderstorms, when a set of complex pre-conditions exist.

It is thought to be the result of pollen grains or mould spores being picked up by the rising air and then bursting due to the high humidity in the base of the cloud.

Characteristics of those most likely to be affected include:
- Hayfever with previous chest symptoms
- Allergy to the pollen or fungal spores present
- Possibly no previous asthma diagnosis.

Environmental factors involved include:
- High levels of pollen or fungal spores
- High temperatures for at least 7 days
- Humidity in correct range (80–90%)
- Ozone (possibly)
- Mesoscale thunderstorm (large-scale, low-level convergence of air).

Food and drink

Foods are rarely the cause of asthma attacks, although wheezing and bronchoconstriction may occur secondary to skin symptoms during anaphylaxis.

Food causing allergic reactions:
- Cows' milk
- Eggs
- Nuts (particularly peanuts)
- Fish/seafood.

Only about 2.5% of people with asthma will show a bronchoconstriction reaction to challenge with food, yet up to 60% consider that certain foods are a trigger factor for their asthma.

Foods causing non-allergic (irritant) reactions:
- Tartrazine
- Alcohol
- Sulphur dioxide
- Sodium metabisulphate.

Food allergy is more common and more life-threatening in children although many children appear to lose or grow out of their food reaction around the age of 7.

Food-induced rhinitis

Rhinitis may (rarely) occur after consuming certain foods or drinks. This may occur via neural mechanisms, nasal vasodilatation, food allergy and/or other undefined mechanisms. Food allergy is rarely the cause of rhinitis unless the patient also has gastrointestinal, skin or systemic symptoms. The syndrome of copious watery rhinorrhea occurring immediately after eating foods, particularly hot and spicy foods, has been termed 'gustatory rhinitis' and is mediated via the vagus nerve. Intranasal anti-cholinergic agents are of particular value in treatment of gustatory rhinitis.

Alcohol is a common cause of nasal blockage (as well as local flushing or non-itchy urticaria) due to its vasodilator effects. This is not an allergic reaction and should not be interpreted as a precursor to anaphylaxis.

Pregnancy and menstruation

The hormonal changes during pregnancy and menstruation can affect asthma symptoms. The links between hormonal influences and asthma are not clearly understood, but for some women there is a definite association between asthma symptoms and the different phases of their menstrual cycle and reproductive life.

In pregnancy approximately:

- One-third of women experience an improvement in symptoms
- One-third of women find symptoms get worse
- One-third of women find symptoms are unchanged.

A small subgroup of women experience increased asthma symptoms pre-menstrually, possibly related to the amounts of circulating oestrogen. These asthma attacks are most likely to appear either:

- Three days before menstruation
- Four days into menstruation.

The menopause is another time in a woman's reproductive life cycle when there is significant fluctuation in hormone levels and again it can be associated with changes in asthma symptoms. For the majority of women with pre-existing asthma there is no change in symptoms but some women do present with asthma for the first time at menopause.

Psychological stress

For some people stress or other strong psychological factors can trigger asthma symptoms. For young children the excitement of a birthday or Christmas can be enough to trigger symptoms and later the stress of exams, job interviews or pressures at work may all trigger or aggravate asthma symptoms.

Stress may also induce panic attacks with hyperventilation which may then go on to trigger asthma symptoms. In these cases it can sometimes be difficult to distinguish between a panic attack with hyperventilation and a true asthma attack.

Drugs

Certain medications can trigger asthma symptoms.

Beta blockers

If stimulating beta receptors causes bronchodilatation then it is clear that blocking these same receptor sites could cause bronchoconstriction. It is important that people with asthma are not given beta blockers because even locally acting ones such as eyedrops for the treatment of glaucoma can produce significant symptoms.

In the case of people with asthma who have had myocardial infarction the risk–benefit of using beta blockers must be considered and it may be possible to use a more cardioselective beta blocker.

Aspirin and non-steroidal anti-inflammatory drugs (NSAIDs)

About 10% of adults with asthma are sensitive to aspirin. In addition to asthma symptoms aspirin and other NSAIDs can also cause hay-fever like symptoms, urticaria and angioedema. As these drugs are all available as over the counter preparations it is important to caution patients with asthma about the potential risks and for them to use other medications.

Occupation

Some of the most commonly reported and at risk occupations include:

- Paint sprayers
- Bakers and pastry makers

- Nurses
- Chemical workers
- Animal handlers
- Welders and metal workers
- Plastics and rubber workers
- Food processing workers
- Electronic production workers
- Timber workers
- Painters
- Cleaners
- Farm workers
- Dental workers
- Laboratory technicians
- Waiters
- Textile workers.

Common causative agents

Many hundreds of causative agents have been reported and new causes are regularly being documented. The most frequently reported causes include:

- Isocynates
- Flour and grain dust
- Colophony and fluxes
- Latex
- Animals
- Aldehydes
- Wood dust.

Incidence and epidemiology of asthma

The prevalence of a condition is defined as the number of the population suffering from it at any one time. It is difficult to be completely certain about the actual percentages or numbers of people with asthma because asthma symptoms are variable, may be self-reported or may be tolerated without a specific diagnosis. The prevalence of asthma will obviously depend on the definition of the condition used, and where a history of wheeze is used as a marker of disease the prevalence may be higher than in studies that look for regular wheeze or objective evidence of variable airflow obstruction. The diagnosis may also be incorrectly applied to other respiratory conditions such as chronic obstructive pulmonary disease (COPD) (📖 p.249) or hyperventilation syndrome which share the same symptoms.

Current data from Asthma UK suggests that:
- 5.2 million people in the UK have asthma
- 4.1 million adults are affected
- 1.1 million children are affected
- 1 in 12 adults over 16 have asthma
- 1 in 10 children aged 2–15 have asthma.

Other studies, however, report higher levels of asthma and the British Thoracic Society in 2006 gave the incidence of doctor diagnosed asthma as:
- 21% in children
- 15% in adults.

The incidence of asthma is defined as the number of new episodes that occur during a defined time period. Current measures of incidence do not always separate the first diagnosis of asthma from new episodes of asthma or acute attacks. The number of first or new presentations of asthma in general practice has risen steadily over the last 25 years although it does now appear to have reached a plateau. It is unclear whether this is due to a reduction in the incidence of asthma itself or to better more proactive management of the condition resulting in less need for acute intervention.

It is currently estimated that there are approximately 4.1 million GP consultations for asthma every year.

Asthma tends to be more common in developed parts of the world such as the USA, Scandinavia and western Europe and prevalence in the UK is thought to be broadly in line with these areas at 4–8% of the population overall.

Natural history of asthma

The commonest age of onset is in childhood with another smaller peak later on in the 30s age group. The important thing to remember is that asthma can begin at any age.

For some children asthma symptoms tend to 'disappear' as they get older, but for about half these they will experience symptoms again in later life. If there is no evidence of atopy and the asthma symptoms are only related to viral infections then the prognosis is better. The more frequent and the more severe the asthma then the more likely it is to persist into later life. It is impossible to say, however, whether an individual child will grow out of asthma and even if they do appear to then there is a good chance that symptoms may re occur in adulthood.

Adult asthma may:
- Be a continuation of childhood asthma
- Be reactivation of quiescent childhood asthma
- Occur for the first time in adult life.

It is estimated that about a third to two-thirds of adults with asthma develop it for the first time during their working lives, and it is important to remember that about 9–15% of adult-onset asthma may be attributable to occupational causes.

Asthma in the elderly may be under diagnosed and although some elderly people with asthma will have had symptoms since childhood, it is thought that for about 80%, symptoms will have started in adult life. True numbers are difficult to ascertain but it is thought that there may be slightly more elderly men with asthma than women. Reversible airflow obstruction in the elderly may be poorly perceived, poorly recognized by healthcare professionals and suboptimally treated. The biggest challenge in older people is often to distinguish between COPD, pulmonary oedema and asthma, all of which can result in symptoms of shortness of breath, wheeze and cough and may coexist (📖 p.31).

Economic impact of asthma

Financial costs occur as a result of direct medical costs such as medicines and the use of NHS resources and indirect costs such as the loss of productivity and payment of benefits. Analysis of these costs has shown that the greatest proportion is related to the care of people with poor asthma control. Suboptimal asthma control means that people are unable to perform many of the tasks of normal daily living, including paid work, and result in much more intensive use of NHS services including admissions and increased consultations.

It is estimated that asthma is costing the UK over £2.3 billion per year and that costs in 2001 were broken down as follows:
- Prescriptions—£659 million
- Dispensing—£117 million
- Hospital admissions—£49 million
- GP consultations—£63 million
- Work days lost—£1200 million
- Benefits—£260 million.

It is likely then that improved asthma control could not only improve an individuals' quality of life but also significantly reduce the financial impact on society as a whole.

Morbidity and mortality

Asthma morbidity

Despite significant advances in asthma management in recent years considerable morbidity still exists. Someone with poorly controlled asthma may:

- Have time off school or work
- Be unable to perform to their full potential due to disturbed sleep
- Be unable to take part in sport or leisure activities
- Experience anxiety and disruption to their normal lifestyle.

In a report by Asthma UK in 2004 they found that of people with asthma:

- 49% reported more than one attack per week
- 1 in 6 stated that they experienced one attack a week severe enough to cause difficulty in speaking
- 44% reported that asthma significantly affected their social lives
- 66% reported difficulty in running for a bus or taking exercise
- 50% reported waking at night with symptoms.

Many people with asthma may accept symptoms as a normal part of life. They may have low expectations of treatment outcomes and accept significant limitations to their lifestyle. The Asthma in Real Life study found that:

- 79% of people with asthma reported it as well or completely controlled
- Almost three-quarters of the 79% had used reliever medication twice or more on the previous day
- A third of those reporting good asthma control actually had symptoms at least once a week.

The reasons for continued morbidity from asthma despite advances in treatments are likely to be related to:

- Inappropriate diagnosis
- Under treatment
- Lack of follow-up
- Poor understanding of the disease and treatments by health professionals and patients
- Lack of patient education.

Asthma mortality

On average an individual healthcare professional can expect to see one asthma death in their whole career.

In the UK:

- There are around 1400 asthma deaths each year
- One person dies from asthma approximately every 7 hours
- More than two-thirds of asthma deaths are in those over 65
- Most asthma deaths occur before the patient reaches hospital.

In comparison to respiratory diseases such as COPD, which causes 30,000 deaths, and lung cancer which causes 38,000 deaths, asthma mortality may appear small. Its significance, however, lies in the fact that:

- Most asthma deaths are thought to be preventable by better use of existing management techniques
- Preventable asthma deaths are evidence of poorly controlled and suboptimally managed asthma.

Important factors that are associated with a higher risk of asthma mortality have been identified as:

- Severe asthma as defined by previous admission for asthma
- Previous ventilation
- Repeated Emergency department (ED) attendance
- Brittle asthma usually defined as type 1 where patients have wide peak flow variability despite appropriate therapy and type 2 where there are sudden severe attacks set against a background of apparently good control
- Using three or more classes of asthma medication
- Heavy use of short-acting beta agonists
- Adverse psychosocial factors
- Domestic stress (including abuse)
- Homeless or living alone
- Unemployed or other work stress
- Extreme poverty
- Separated or single parent
- Alcohol or drug abuse
- Depression or psychosis
- History of self-harm
- Learning disability
- Non-compliance with treatment
- Failure to attend appointments
- Self-discharge from hospital.

Assessment of the asthma patient

The diagnosis of asthma is essentially a clinical one as there are no definitive confirmatory diagnostic tests. Diagnosis relies largely on detailed history taking and where possible the demonstration of variable airway obstruction, using lung function tests such as PEFR or spirometry (📖 p.75).

Symptoms

People with asthma can suffer a variety of symptoms none of which are specific to asthma. Common symptoms include:
- Wheeze
- Shortness of breath
- Chest tightness
- Cough.

The hallmark of asthma is that these symptoms tend to be:
- Variable
- Intermittent
- Worse at night
- Provoked by triggers including exercise.

Asthma symptoms can vary within and between patients and not all people with asthma will experience all of the symptoms.

Signs

Commonly none.

People with chronic asthma may sometimes have signs of:
- Hyperinflation
- Wheeze.

During acute episodes there may be:
- Reduced lung function
- Wheeze which is
  - Diffuse
  - Polyphonic
  - Bilateral
  - Predominately expiratory.

Other indicators

There may an increased likelihood of asthma if there is:
- Personal or family history of atopic conditions such as
  - Eczema
  - Rhinitis
  - Asthma
- Worsening of symptoms in association with triggers such as:
  - Pollens or spores
  - Viral infections
  - Exercise
  - Animals
  - Chemical agents
  - Smoking
  - Aspirin or other non-steroidal anti-inflammatory medication or beta blocker agents including eyedrops.

Key questions to ask when taking a history

Current symptoms

- Specific symptoms of cough, wheeze, shortness of breath, chest tightness and nasal symptoms of running or blocking
- Severity of symptoms—how do they affect normal activity, do they cause time off school or work?
- Frequency of symptoms—how often, daily, weekly or less frequent?
- Variability of symptoms—seasonal or diurnal variation, particularly looking out for nocturnal symptoms
- When did the symptoms start?
- What makes symptoms worse—any specific triggers?
- What makes symptoms better?
- Have these symptoms ever occurred before?
- Non respiratory symptoms such as tiredness, lethargy, irritability, weight loss or in children failure to thrive or not meeting developmental milestones.

Past medical history

- Any previous chest problems
- Any hospital admission with respiratory symptoms
- Cardiac disease—shortness of breath or cough can be cardiac in origin
- Congenital abnormalities
- Rhinitis, eczema or other allergic disease.

Family history—ask about any immediate family with the following:

- Asthma
- Eczema
- Rhinitis
- Any respiratory or cardiac disease.

Social history and lifestyle—ask about the following:

- Contact with pets or other animals
- Hobbies—consider potential triggers e.g. glues; solder; paints
- Exercise—are symptoms triggered by exercise or limiting ability to exercise
- Living conditions—moulds and damp conditions or paint fumes
- Smoking—active or passive can be a trigger for asthma and is associated with a higher risk of developing COPD
- Recreational drug use—can trigger asthma or result in other respiratory problems.

Occupation

- Past and present to look for at risk occupations and exposure.

Medication

Consider over the counter, complementary medicines and prescribed medications particularly
- Oral and topical beta blockers
- Aspirin and NSAIDs.

Asthma severity

The type, frequency and severity of respiratory symptoms experienced in asthma varies over time. In the British Guidelines asthma severity is not formally categorized into levels of severity but is linked to the potential treatment that the patient requires. The important thing to recognize is that asthma severity is dynamic: it should be treated as appropriate to the presentation and severity of symptoms at the current time. At any level of asthma severity any asthma patient may experience an acute episode severe enough to require hospital admission.

Asthma can be broadly classified as:

Mild asthma

Occasional (episodic), short attacks lasting a few hours with complete remission in between.

Moderate asthma

The presence of continuous or persistent mild symptoms with occasional more severe exacerbations that can last days or weeks.

Brittle and severe asthma

Severe asthma is usually considered to consist of the presence of continuous symptoms with frequent severe exacerbations. The spectrum of severe or difficult to manage asthma includes the disease entity of 'brittle asthma' which is thought to affect about 0.05% of people with asthma. Brittle asthma has been classified into two categories:

Type 1

Asthma that consistently shows wide PEFR variability (greater than 40% diurnal variability for at least 50% of days), despite maximal medical therapy including at least 1500mcg inhaled beclometasone or equivalent (📖 p.391). There is an increased frequency of this type of brittle asthma in women aged between 15 and 55 years.

Type 2

Asthma appears to be well controlled between attacks. Attacks are sudden in onset (often occurring within minutes) and are associated with loss of or disturbance in consciousness on at least one occasion. Type 2 brittle asthma appears to be equal in prevalence in men and women.

Brittle asthma is associated with considerable morbidity, frequent attendances at ED departments, hospital admissions and using considerable amounts of medication. Patients with type 1 brittle asthma are likely to be taking maintenance oral corticosteroids (📖 p.391) and will be at significant risk of side effects such as osteoporosis, weight gain, diabetes and gastro-oesophageal disturbances. People with brittle asthma are more likely to have increased psychosocial morbidity and may be more likely to delay in seeking help, preferring to continue self-administering β_2 agonists. Although people with brittle asthma are more likely to experience the factors associated with asthma deaths as given previously it is not known what proportion of people with brittle asthma die from their condition.

Treatment and management of chronic asthma

The British guidelines for the management of asthma provide the clinical framework for the diagnosis and treatment of asthma. Useful BTS/SIGN algorithms for the management of chronic asthma in both adults and children are available at the end of this chapter. The mainstay of asthma therapy for all but the mildest intermittent symptoms is regular anti-inflammatory treatment. The overall aim is to minimize symptoms and maximize lung function. Whilst it is important to step up treatment when asthma is poorly controlled, it is equally important to step down treatment once control is established. The overall aim is to use the minimum medication whilst maintaining good asthma control. Due to the variable nature of asthma it is a question of constant titration of medication to suit the needs of the moment, which is why it is so important that patients should be able to monitor their condition and adjust treatment appropriately.

Stepping up treatment

The guidelines adopt a stepwise approach to the pharmacological management of chronic asthma. For those with very mild and infrequent symptoms (less than three times a week) it is possible to treat symptomatically with the use of intermittent bronchodilators alone. The majority of people with asthma, however, will require the use of regular inhaled corticosteroids (preventers) to control airway inflammation and the intermittent use of bronchodilators (relievers) to control breakthrough symptoms. In cases of poor control on low doses of inhaled corticosteroids then diagnosis, inhaler technique and compliance should all be checked before increasing therapy. Only if they are found to be satisfactory should treatment be stepped up by the addition of other agents. To control symptoms in severe disease, higher dose inhaled steroids may be required along with the addition of multiple other agents and possibly regular oral steroids. At any step of the current guidelines a short course of oral steroids may be required to treat an acute exacerbation and regain control.

Stepping down therapy

Stepping down treatment once asthma is well controlled is an important but often overlooked part of asthma management. Considerable use of unnecessary high dose treatment occurs although clearly for many patients the dose of inhaled corticosteroid could be reduced without loss of control. When stepping down therapy it is not always clear which is the best drug to reduce first, or by how much so, regular review is essential. Factors such as the severity of asthma, risk–benefit profile of treatment and patient preference should all be considered. Reduction of inhaled corticosteroids is best done slowly as patients can deteriorate at different rates and reductions in dose of between 25–50% every 3 months are suggested.

Assessment of acute asthma

Most acute episodes of asthma severe enough to require hospital admission actually develop relatively slowly over a period of hours or in some cases even days. It should therefore be possible to take action early in an attack and to reduce the potential number of attacks requiring admission. It is essential that any asthma patient experiencing worsening respiratory symptoms knows how and when to increase their medication and how and when to access medical advice and support.

All potential initial contact personnel need to be aware that anyone with asthma and worsening symptoms is potentially at risk and requires early assessment. The severity of the attack can be categorized as below:

Moderate asthma exacerbation
- Increased symptoms
- PEFR 50–75% best or predicted
- No features of acute severe asthma.

Acute severe asthma
Any one of:
- PEFR 33–50% best or predicted
- Too wheezy or breathless to complete a sentence in one breath
- In infants, too wheezy or breathless to feed
- Respiratory rate
  Adults >25 breaths/min
  Children (over 5yrs)>30 breaths/min
  Children (under 5 yrs)>50 breaths/min
- Pulse rate
  Adults >110 beats /min
  Children (over 5yrs)>120beats/min
  Children (under 5yrs) >130beats/min.

Life-threatening asthma
Any one of the following in a patient with severe asthma:
- PEFR<33% best or predicted
- SpO_2 <92%; PaO_2<8Kpa
- Normal $PaCo_2$ (4.6–6.0 Kpa)
- Silent chest
- Cyanosis
- Feeble respiratory effort
- Bradycardia
- Dysrhythmia
- Hypotension
- Exhaustion
- Confusion
- Coma.

Managing acute asthma—adults

The BTS/SIGN guidelines provide very clear information on how to deal with acute episodes. A summary is given below and algorithms provided at the end of the chapter.

Adults

Initial management

Moderate exacerbation (PEFR 50–75%)

- High-dose β_2 agonist via spacer (4–6 puffs inhaled separately repeated at 10–20 minute intervals) or nebulized (salbutamol 5mg or terbutaline 10mg) ideally oxygen driven
- Prednisolone 40–50mg daily for at least 5 days or until recovery complete.

Acute severe asthma (PEFR 33–50%)

- Oxygen 40–60% if available
- High dose β_2 agonist via spacer (4–6 puffs inhaled separately repeated at 10–20 minute intervals) or nebulized (salbutamol 5mg or terbutaline 10mg) ideally oxygen-driven
- Prednisolone 40–50mg daily and continue for at least 5 days or until recovery complete
- If good response and PEF improves to 50–75% repeat salbutamol via spacer or nebulizer.

Life-threatening asthma (PEFR<33%)

- Arrange immediate admission
- Oxygen 40–60%
- Prednisolone 40–50mg orally or IV hydrocortisone 100mg
- High dose β_2 agonist and ipratropium bromide via oxygen driven nebulizer (salbutamol 5mg or terbutaline 10mg and ipratropium 0.5mg).

Criteria for admission

- Any life-threatening features
- Previous near fatal asthma
- Little or no response to initial treatment
- Previous severe attacks
- Recent hospital admission for asthma
- Poor social circumstances
- Poor patient perception of severity
- Lower threshold for admission if afternoon or evening attack.

Hospital management

Life-threatening or severe acute asthma (PEFR<50%)

- Continue oxygen
- Continue nebulized β_2 agonist/ipratropium bromide 4–6 hrly
- Discuss with senior clinician and ICU team
- Arterial blood gasses
- Consider continuous salbutamol nebulisation 5–10mg per hour via suitable nebulizer system
- Consider single dose of magnesium sulphate if there has not been a good response to initial treatment.

- Consider IV β_2 agonist or IV aminophylline or progression to intermittent positive pressure ventilation (IPPV)
- Chest Xray if pneumothorax or consolidation suspected or if patient requires IPPV.

Monitor
- PEFR 15–30 minutes after starting treatment and then as dictated by response
- Continue to monitor PEFR during hospital stay and until controlled post discharge
- SPO_2 to keep at >92%
- Blood gasses 2 hours after starting treatment if:
  - Initial PaO_2 <8KPa unless SPo_2 >92%
  - Initial $PaCO_2$ is normal or raised
  - Patient's condition deteriorates
- Heart rate
- Serum potassium and blood glucose
- Serum theophylline if aminophylline is continued for more than 24 hours.

Criteria for referral to intensive care unit
- Deteriorating PEFR
- Persisting or worsening hypoxia
- Hypercapnia
- Blood gasses showing falling pH or rising H+ concentration
- Exhaustion, drowsiness, confusion
- Feeble respiratory effort
- Coma or respiratory arrest.

For further information, please see the following algorithms attached at the end of this chapter:
- BTS/SIGN algorithm for acute asthma in hospital (Adults)
- BTS/SIGN algorithm for acute asthma in general practice (Adults).

Managing acute asthma—children

Children over 2 years
Initial management
Moderate exacerbation
- β_2 agonist 2–4 puffs via spacer +/– facemask
- Titrate dose to response; increase β_2 agonist by 2 puffs every 2 mins up to 10 puffs
- Consider soluble prednisolone:
  - Age 2–5 years—20mg
  - Age 5–12 years—30–40mg

If good response:
- Continue prednisolone for up to 3 days
- Continue bronchodilator 4 hourly.

If poor response:
- Arrange admission.

Acute severe asthma
- Oxygen via facemask
- 4–6 puffs β_2 agonist via spacer (inhaled separately repeated at 10–20 minute intervals)or nebulized salbutamol:
  - Age 2–5 years—salbutamol 2.5mg or terbutaline 5mg
  - Age 5–10 years—salbutamol 2.5mg or terbutaline 5–10mg
- Soluble prednisolone:
  - Age 2–5 years—20mg
  - Age 5–12 years—30–40mg

If good response:
- Continue prednisolone for up to 3 days
- Continue bronchodilator 4 hourly.

If poor response:
- Repeat bronchodilator
- Arrange admission.

Life-threatening asthma (PEFR<33%)
- Arrange immediate admission
- Oxygen via facemask
- Soluble prednisolone:
  - Age 2–5 years-20mg
  - Age 5–12 years-30–40mg
- Or IV hydrocortisone 4mg/kg
- High dose β_2 agonist and ipratropium bromide via oxygen-driven nebulizer:
  - Age 2–5 years salbutamol 2.5mg or terbutaline 5mg and ipratropium 0.25mg
  - Age 5–12 years salbutamol 5mg or terbutaline 10mg and ipratropium 0.25mg.

Criteria for admission
- Any life-threatening features
- Little or no response to initial treatment
- Previous severe attacks

- Recent hospital admission for asthma
- Poor social circumstances
- Lower threshold for admission if afternoon or evening attack.

For further information, please see the following algorithm attached at the end of this chapter:

- BTS/SIGN algorithm for acute asthma in general practice (children).

Hospital management

- Continue β_2 agonists/ipratropium bromide every 20–30 mins
- Continue oxygen therapy to maintain SPO_2 >92%
- Discuss with senior clinician
- Monitor response to treatment using heart rate, respiratory rate and oxygen saturation.

Good response

- Continue bronchodilators 1–4 hrly prn
- Continue prednisolone for up to 3 days.

Poor response

- Arrange transfer to high dependency unit paediatric intensive care unit
- Repeat bronchodilators every 20–30 mins and consider:
  - Bolus IV salbutamol 15mcg/kg over 10 mins
  - Continous Iv salbutamol infusion 1–5 mcg/kg/min (200mcg/ml solution)
  - IV aminophylline 5mg/kg loading dose over 20 minutes (omit in those receiving oral theophyllines) followed by continuous infusion 1mg/kg/hr
  - Children >5 years bolus IV infusion of magnesium sulphate 40mg/kg (max 2g) over 20 minutes
  - Chest X-ray and blood gasses

For further information, please see the following algorithm attached at the end of this chapter:

- BTS/SIGN algorithm for acute asthma in hospital (children).

Discharge planning

It is important that discharge from hospital or an ED is planned and adequate follow up arranged. There are no definitive criteria for discharge and timing will depend on a combination of clinical improvement and adequate social support. It would be good practice to ensure that:

- PEFR >75% best or predicted
- Diurnal variability <25%
- Patient has been stable for 24 h on discharge medication with β_2 agonists no more than 4 hrly.

Prior to discharge it essential that patients have adequate supplies of all their medications and understand:

- When to use their inhaled and other medication
- How to monitor their condition
- How and when to seek medical help
- A written action plan to support verbal advice can help to reduce the need for further admission.

Follow-up with the patient's own GP or practice nurse should be arranged prior to discharge and ideally patients should be reviewed within two working days of discharge. Follow-up with a hospital respiratory specialist nurse or a respiratory physician is recommended within one month of discharge.

When a patient has been treated entirely within primary care without a hospital admission it is equally important to ensure that patients are able to manage their condition and that adequate follow up is provided. Even patients with less severe exacerbations need to understand how and when to take their medications, how to monitor their condition and when to call for extra help.

Follow-up after an acute episode

It is important that a thorough review is undertaken after any acute event so that where possible further occurrences can be prevented. Every opportunity should be taken to reinforce educational messages and promote improved asthma management. Issues to cover at review after an acute episode include:

- Events leading up to the attack
- Any triggers for attack
- Potential warning signs to enable patient to spot similar attacks in the future
- Actions to take in case of future attacks
- Review medication use
- Response to treatment given at attack
- Current symptoms
- Review need to step up regular medication
- Discuss and agree action plan.

Asthma in pregnancy

Asthma is one of the most common diseases to complicate pregnancy. Asthma affects around 7% of women during their childbearing years and is thought to complicate 1–4% of all pregnancies. Pregnancy can affect asthma but asthma may also affect pregnancy outcomes.

Effect of pregnancy on asthma

The course of asthma during pregnancy is unpredictable but in general more severe asthma is more likely to worsen than mild asthma. Some women, however, with severe asthma do experience a significant improvement in their symptoms during pregnancy whilst it is also possible for those with previously mild disease to experience significant deterioration. As a general rule in pregnant women with asthma:

- One third experience an improvement in their asthma
- One third experience a deterioration in their asthma
- One third have no change in their asthma.

The reasons why asthma severity may change during pregnancy are not absolutely clear but it is likely to be a combination of factors. Many of these factors are related to hormonal changes that occur but there are also significant cardiovascular and physiological changes in pregnancy that may potentially influence asthma control.

Factors that may worsen asthma in pregnancy

- Reduced response to corticosteroid treatments due to competitive binding to glucocorticosteroid receptors by progesterone, aldosterone or deoxycorticosterone
- Prostaglandin F2 mediated bronchoconstriction
- Decreased functional reserve capacity of the lung
- Increased placental major basic protein reaching the lung
- Increased sensitivity to viral or bacterial respiratory infections as triggers
- Increased gastro-oesophageal reflux
- Increased stress.

Factors that may improve asthma in pregnancy

- Progesterone-mediated bronchodilation
- Greater sensitivity to β_2 due to oestrogen or progesterone or increased free cortisol levels
- Decreased plasma histamine mediated bronchoconstriction
- Prostaglandin E-mediated bronchodilation
- Prostaglandin I2-mediated bronchial stabilization.

Hormonal changes

The interaction of the hormonal changes in pregnancy is complex and the impact on asthma not completely understood. The rising levels of free cortisol may improve asthma symptoms but this may be counterbalanced by increased levels of serum progesterone, aldosterone and deoxycorticosterone.

It is thought that in those with improvement of symptoms the balance lies with the free cortisol and in those with deteriorating symptoms it is being pushed the other way. This is in part supported by the fact that asthma tends to improve in the last 4 weeks of pregnancy and is rarely of any bother during labour, a time when circulating levels of free cortisol are at their highest.

Cardiovascular changes

Due to changes in the cardiopulmonary system most pregnant women will experience some shortness of breath regardless of whether they have asthma or not. Elevated progesterone levels are responsible for stimulating increased depth of respiration and relative hyperventilation. Oxygen consumption is increased by 20% during pregnancy and metabolic rate increases by 15% affecting the rate and depth of breathing.

Physiological changes

As pregnancy progresses there is an increase in abdominal pressure and the diaphragm is pushed upwards causing a restrictive effect on lung function. Breathlessness results from the physiological hyperventilation that occurs. It is most common in the third trimester and is thought to be experienced by up to 75% of women in pregnancy.

Effect of asthma on pregnancy

Providing asthma remains well controlled throughout the pregnancy there is little or no increased risk to mother or child. The risk of poorly controlled asthma carries more risk to the fetus than the effects of treatment. It is therefore important not to withhold appropriate treatment on the grounds of pregnancy. The greatest risk posed to the development of the fetus is likely to be as a result of fetal hypoxia as a consequence of an asthma exacerbation. Fetal hypoxia can result in:
• Poor intrauterine growth
• Preterm birth
• Increased risk of low birthweight
• Increased risk of Caesarian delivery.
Women with poorly controlled asthma have a 2–3 times greater risk for premature delivery than those without asthma. Maternal complications associated with poorly controlled asthma include:
• Hyperemesis
• High blood pressure
• Pre-eclampsia
• Vaginal haemorrhage.
Fetal complications associated with poorly controlled asthma include:
• Stillbirth
• Prematurity
• Neonatal hypoxaemia
• Low newborn assessment scores
• Increased perinatal mortality.

Asthma management in pregnancy

The main aims of asthma management in pregnancy should be to:
- Optimize asthma therapy
- Maximize lung function
- Reduce the risk of acute exacerbations
- Minimize the risks of fetal hypoxia.

Overall asthma in pregnancy should be managed and treated according to the usual management guidelines. It is important to emphasize the need for close monitoring and maintenance of good control in order to avoid acute exacerbations and potential fetal hypoxia. A lower threshold for referral or admission in cases of acute or difficult to manage asthma may also be required. Women with difficult to manage asthma should be co-managed by obstetric and respiratory specialists.

Asthma medications during pregnancy

Overall the medications used to treat asthma are safe in pregnancy and the potential risk of harm to the fetus from under treated asthma outweighs any small risk from medications used.

All medications should therefore be used in pregnancy as they are in the usual management of asthma. The only exception is that due to lack of information on their use it is not recommended to start leukotriene receptor antagonists during pregnancy (p.422). If started before pregnancy and required to maintain ongoing control they should be continued.

As with any asthma management, the principle should be to monitor asthma carefully and to titrate the medication to needs of the moment, aiming to achieve maximum control with the minimum of medication.

Management of acute exacerbation

- Give drug therapy as for the non-pregnant patient
- Give oxygen to maintain saturations above 95%
- Acute severe asthma in pregnancy is a medical emergency and requires continuous fetal monitoring and treatment in hospital.

Management during labour

Acute attacks of asthma are very rare during delivery due to the high levels of circulating endogenous corticosteroids. It is safe to continue all usual asthma medication throughout labour.

For women who have been taking oral corticosteroids at doses of more than prednisolone 7.5mg daily for more than two weeks prior to labour there is a theoretical risk of hypothalamic–pituitary–adrenal axis suppression. For these women it is recommended that intravenous hydrocortisone 100mg should be given 6–8 hrly during labour.

It is safe for women with asthma to use all usual forms of pain relief during asthma.

Management of premenstrual asthma

Women who have asthma triggered by the hormonal changes of their menstrual cycle should have their overall asthma management optimized. If symptoms still occur around the time of their period then there are some different strategies that can be tried although the evidence to support them is limited.

Some women report that it is helpful to increase the dose of their inhaled steroid for the week prior to their period but there is no robust evidence to support this. It may be possible that it is the improved compliance with medication which results in an improvement of symptoms.

Use of either the progesterone-only or the combined oral contraceptive pill has been found to be helpful in reducing symptoms for some women. The contraceptive pill reduces the fluctuations in hormonal levels which may be responsible for the reduction in symptoms. Studies are small and some have reported contradictory evidence where women on oral contraceptives reported greater problems with asthma control, but it still may be a worthwhile option to try if symptoms are significantly interfering with lifestyle.

Patient education

Most patients will receive asthma education as part of an individual consultation with a health professional. In some areas, however, there may also be access to more formal asthma education programmes which may involve group sessions. There is little evidence to suggest that one method is superior to another, the key is to ensure that every opportunity is taken to work with patients to develop appropriate knowledge and skills to promote good asthma control. It is also important to remember that in an attempt to understand more about their condition patients may also access information from other sources such as patient groups or charities, the internet, popular press, friends and family etc.

Improved asthma control will not result simply as a result of improved knowledge, and asthma education is not a single event to be ticked off on a checklist, but rather an ongoing process. Over time, review and reinforcement of key issues and concerns will enable people with asthma to develop the skills necessary to recognize changes in their condition and to be able to act appropriately on those changes. Every asthma consultation provides an opportunity to:
• Review asthma control
• Explore the patient's issues and concerns
• Reinforce important messages about asthma
• Review treatment strategies
• Negotiate appropriate actions to take in case of deteriorating asthma.
The type of information that could be covered through asthma education sessions includes:
• Disease process
• Types and actions of treatments
• How to use treatment
• Identification of patient concerns
• Identification of patient goals and desired outcomes for asthma management
• Development of self assessment skills
• Negotiation of asthma action plan in line with identified patient goals
• Recognition and treatment of acute episodes
• Appropriate allergen or trigger avoidance.
It is essential that the way in which this information is conveyed is tailored to the individual patient's circumstances. The purpose of education is to empower patients and/or carers to undertake self-management more effectively within their own capabilities and at a level with which they feel comfortable and confident. Attention needs to be paid to factors such as the patient's age, social circumstances, personal support networks, emotional status, intellectual capabilities, literacy, culture, language and disease state.

Asthma action plans

The aim of asthma education is to provide patients with the knowledge and skills to enable them to take control of their asthma. Written personalized asthma action plans (formerly known as self-management plans) have been shown to improve outcomes when used as part of an overall education package.

Current guidelines recommend that:

- Patients with asthma should be offered self-management education that should focus on individual needs and be reinforced by a written action plan
- Prior to discharge, inpatients should receive individualized asthma action plans given by a clinician with appropriate training in asthma management.

Patients need to be involved in drawing up their own action plan to ensure that it meets their personal circumstances. The level and complexity of the plan is likely to depend on:

- Willingness of the patient to take control of their asthma
- The level of control that they feel comfortable with
- Ability to follow the plan.

Although asthma action plans can help to give patients a feeling of control over their asthma it is important to ensure that patients are comfortable with the level of responsibility being given to them. Patients will vary in the level of their desire to be actively involved in decision-making about their treatment or management and this must be acknowledged when negotiating the action plan.

To be effective action plans must be regularly reviewed and amended in light of changing circumstances. Asthma is a dynamic and variable condition and an action plan needs to be updated to reflect this.

Asthma action plans should be reviewed at scheduled review appointments, but even more importantly they must be reviewed following an acute exacerbation. It is essential to consider what went wrong and how the action plan could be amended to avoid similar events in the future. It may require, for example, greater information on how to spot deterioration or a different threshold for commencing extra treatment or seeking medical advice; if the action plan is not reviewed and amended then the problem may continue to arise in the future.

An action plan needs to contain information on adjustments to therapy that a patient can make in response to specific action points such as changes in symptoms or PEFR measurement. There is insufficient evidence to recommend a preference for either symptom or PEFR monitoring and the precise method of monitoring will need to be agreed with the individual. It is important that the plan is clear and those that focus on two to four key action points only seem to be the most effective.

Symptom-based plans

For many people with asthma this will be the easiest method of monitoring control. The plan should outline the patient's usual medication and then provide clear instructions on what to do in the event of increasing symptoms. Indicators for action might include:

- Night-time waking with cough or wheeze
- Increased exercise symptoms
- Requiring to use bronchodilator more frequently
- Reduced effectiveness of bronchodilator.

For many patients with an increase in symptoms it will be sufficient to use their bronchodilator therapy regularly and to continue with their usual doses of inhaled steroid whilst monitoring carefully.

If asthma continues to deteriorate then they may have a supply of oral steroids that they can commence themselves or alternatively they may be instructed to seek urgent medical review at this point.

In the past many plans focused on 'doubling' the dose of inhaled steroids at the first signs of an exacerbation, however although anecdotally this may appear to work current guidelines state that there is insufficient evidence to make a robust recommendation for its use.

Often the level at which action needs to be taken and the exact changes in treatment will reflect the past history of the patient. It may be known that at a certain level of symptoms in previous exacerbations that a particular individual required emergency treatment with oral steroids and it would therefore be reasonable to incorporate this into future plans.

Peak flow-based plans

A PEFR-based plan may be more appropriate for those who:

- Have more severe asthma
- Require frequent doses of oral steroids
- Have required hospital admission for asthma.

Action points are calculated as a certain level of the patient's best peak flow reading. A general guide to these action points is given below, but as with symptoms the exact levels for action may be determined by the individual's past history and experiences in previous exacerbation.

- 75% and above—continue usual treatment
- 50–75% regular bronchodilators (possibly increase inhaled steroids but limited evidence)
- 33–50% commence oral steroids and seek medical advice
- 33% and below—urgent medical attention/admission.

Compliance, concordance and adherence

In asthma the term compliance usually refers to the extent to which a patient takes regular prophylactic therapy in line with advised doses. Failure to take adequate prophylactic therapy is likely to be a common cause of poor asthma control. For this reason it is important to ensure that before stepping up therapy the patient's compliance with the pre-scribed regime is always discussed. Compliance or adherence tends to suggest a regime imposed by another, and does not allow for negotiation and shared decision-making or responsibility. The concept of concordance is now more popular. The patient and the health professional have an equal role in agreeing an appropriate treatment or management plan.

The reasons why individuals do not take treatments as advised are complex but can be broadly split into three main categories.

Erratic non-compliance
This is possibly the most common reason why people do not exactly follow treatment regimes. Patients know what they should take and when they should take it but other lifestyle factors get in the way. Hectic lives with competing demands may mean that they simply forget! Even those who normally follow the prescribed routine can experience this if their usual routine is disturbed, for example during holidays or periods of social upheaval.

Unintentional non-compliance
In this case the patient may not understand how or why they are sup-posed to take medication. They may therefore believe that they are fol-lowing the advised regime and be unaware of any problem. For example, some patients will be using the bronchodilator inhaler regularly and only using an inhaled steroid as required for symptom relief believing this to be correct.

Intentional non-compliance
This is where patients make a conscious decision not to follow the advised treatment regime. They may stop prophylactic medications, reduce doses, alter times of administration or actually never start therapy at all. It is important to establish the reasons behind the individual's decisions before you can explore how to address this.

Assessing adherence to treatment
It is not easy to assess adherence to treatment regimes and there is no typical non-compliant patient. Counting prescriptions obtained may give some indication but still does not actually assess how many doses are actually taken. Open and honest communication with support rather than

blame for the patient who does not take medication as advised is likely to be the best method. It may be helpful to:

- Ask how often a patient forgets their medication
- Assess the level of symptoms and use of reliever therapy
- Ask if the patient feels that their treatment is of benefit
- Discuss the practicalities of being able to follow the advised treatment regime.

Improving adherence to treatment

Improving communications and adopting a more patient-centred approach to consultations where the patient's views and feelings are given equal weight to those of the health professional are crucial to increasing the use of prophylactic medication. Practical issues which may also help to improve the ability to follow agreed plans include:

- Ensuring that a suitable device is chosen that the patient is willing and able to use
- Simplifying the treatment regime where possible by reducing number of inhalers or doses to be taken
- Paying attention to the patient's lifestyle and working out how treatments can best be fitted in
- Linking inhaler use to other routine activities, e.g. teeth cleaning; watching favourite TV programmes; making tea etc
- Providing supporting information, written instructions or asthma action plans.

Health beliefs

Asthma education and action plans have been demonstrated to be of benefit in improving outcomes for asthma control, but it is clear that they do not always result in changes in behaviour. There are still many patients who despite having good asthma knowledge still manage their condition in a suboptimal manner.

The health belief model has been used to explain why patients may not take their treatment as advised or may act in ways considered by the health professional to be detrimental to their health. The underlying principle is that health behaviours are rationally determined by the individual's feelings about being at risk from or vulnerable to a health threat. Three main beliefs are included:

- General health motivation
- Perception of how 'risky' a particular disease is
- Perception of the effectiveness of a particular behaviour in reducing the 'risk'.

There are two main influences on how vulnerable (how at risk) an individual may feel:

- How likely are they to develop ill health (susceptibility to disease)
- How much will this disease impact on their lifestyle (severity).

Even when a person feels significant vulnerability they may still not take action. They will be influenced by the perceived benefits and barriers of taking action:

- Benefits—what will improve if I take action
- Barriers—what problems might this action bring about.

There are also other factors which will act as drivers for action which include:

- Age
- Ethnicity
- Sex
- Personality
- Socio-economic status.

Finally, it will sometimes be a specific incident or pressure that will act as a spur to action, such as:

- A particular symptom
- Peer pressure
- Concern of a family member
- Media coverage of the disease.

Beliefs about asthma will influence patients' behaviour not only in terms of medication adherence but also in relation to other issues such as attendance at appointments. If an individual does not perceive asthma as a significant health risk or does not believe that they have asthma then it is not surprising that they would not take medication or attend appointments.

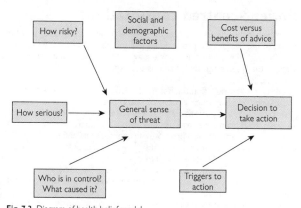

Fig. 7.3 Diagram of health belief model

Reproduced with permission from Education for Health http://www.educationforhealth.org.uk.

Patient-centred consultations

In order to achieve concordance there needs to be an acceptance that the views of the health care professional and the patient whilst different are equally valid. The health professional may be the expert in medical knowledge of the disease but the patient is the expert in their life, preferences and experiences.

In this type of consultation the health professional does not seek to direct the patient to a particular course of action but allows them to explore their own views and goals to arrive at a suitable course of action for them. In order to facilitate this type of interaction it is important to ensure a suitable environment which promotes an approachable and friendly feel:

- Arrange layout so patient and health professional appear as equals (e.g. health professional not behind large desk)
- Value the time by ensuring no interruptions (e.g. from telephone)
- Open friendly body language e.g. sit forward to convey listening, look at patient not at computer monitor.

In order to elicit and appreciate patient's views and to provide the patient with appropriate information so that shared decision making can take place requires certain key skills.

Asking

It is important to use open questions and to avoid a series of questions that require only brief answers. Use words or phrases such as, 'why,' 'how' or 'tell me more about' to enquire further into the patient's perspective. Consider the choice of words to ensure that meaning is understood by patients and avoid jargon. Tone of voice and pace of speech will also affect how the patient perceives the interaction overall.

Listening

It is important that the health professional is seen to be listening attentively and does not interrupt the patient early by assuming where the conversation is going. It is important that the health professional reflects back to the patient what they have heard in order to ensure that there is mutual understanding of the issue. Acknowledgement of any efforts the patient has demonstrated in dealing with the issue will promote the supportive climate of the consultation. Regular summarizing of the conversation also enables the patient to feel that their contribution is being valued.

Informing

Even in this type of patient focused consultation there is a role for the health professional in giving appropriate information in order that the patient may make decisions based on all relevant facts. The aim of giving information in this way is not to dictate a particular course of action but rather to provide sufficient information so that an informed discussion can take place.

Patients' views about asthma and its treatment may differ significantly from those of the health professional and so it is important to uncover the patient perspective. When exploring the patient perspective it is important that the balance of conversation lies with the patient. It should not be the health professional who does most of the talking. Their role is to facilitate the patient in telling their own story.

The type of issues which might be covered when exploring the patient perspective include:

- Beliefs and attitudes about asthma
- Knowledge about disease processes
- Fears or worries about consequences of having asthma
- Fears or worries about whether successful outcomes are achievable
- Understanding of need for treatment
- Fears or worries about treatment side effects
- Past experiences of health services
- Expectations of outcome of treatment
- Cultural perspectives
- Practical issues such as financial, employment, family commitments etc
- Ability to manage.

Understanding the patient perspective forms the basis on which to build further discussion and the context within which the health professional can provide further information. It is important to give information in a clear and easy to understand manner. All options for treatment including taking no action should be presented and consideration given to both positive and negative outcomes. Health professionals can still contribute their expertise and experiences to the discussion by providing information on what is in their clinical judgment the best option and provide a rationale for their recommendation. Although not all patients want to be involved to the same extent in decision making about treatment it is important to give them the opportunity to make decisions.

Sometimes patients will arrive at decisions that are in direct conflict with what the health professional may believe to be best practice or the most suitable treatment option. This is a difficult situation to manage and the health professional will need to address this conflict in a constructive way. Considerable negotiation may be required to try to find a way forward that is acceptable to all parties but ultimately the health professional must accept that the decision lies with the patient. Once the patient leaves the consulting room they will follow their own path and so enforced treatment regimes are unlikely to succeed. It is better to have an open understanding of what treatment is or is not being taken rather than a relationship in which one party or the other is constantly hiding issues from the other.

Once a decision has been made then it needs to be documented along with the basis for the decision. An action plan can then be drawn up which outlines the treatment regime that has been agreed and the arrangements for follow up that have been made.

Key steps in a patient centered consultation

- Establish rapport
- Elicit the patient's ideas, concerns and expectations
- Establish patients information needs
- Explore pros and cons of treatment options
- Facilitate patients assessment of options in light of their own personal circumstances
- Establish how far the patient wants to be involved in decision making
- Resolve any conflict and reach a decision
- Agree action plan and make follow up arrangements.

Inhaler devices and delivery systems

The majority of asthma medications are delivered by inhalation, so it is essential for successful asthma treatment that optimum delivery of the chosen drug to the lung is achieved (📖 p.391). If an inhaler is used incorrectly it can result in drug wastage and unnecessary cost, both in direct financial costs and indirectly in loss of quality of life and increased disability. Although poorly controlled asthma may indicate a need for an increase in therapy it is also important to remember that it can result from inadequate use of medication as a result of poor inhaler technique.

Nebulizers driven by either compressed air or oxygen can be used to deliver a high dose of medication without any inspiratory manoeuvre by the patient but are rarely necessary in routine asthma management. Most people with asthma can be taught to use some type of inhaler device adequately and before commencing regular nebulized therapy referral to a specialist for assessment is required.

Whilst nebulizers have traditionally been popular for the treatment of acute asthma attacks there is now good evidence to show that in all but life-threatening episodes a pressurised metered dose inhaler plus a spacer is at least as effective as a nebulizer.

There are a wide range of inhaler devices to choose from, varying from MDI, large- and small-volume spacers with or without the addition of a facemask, dry powder inhalers and breath-activated aerosol inhalers. This can be confusing and make it difficult for the health professional to become familiar with all the individual inhaler characteristics and available drug formulations.

The selection of an appropriate inhaler device for an individual patient requires collaborative working between the health professional and the patient and/or carer. If patients are unhappy with their device or embarrassed at using it then they may be more reluctant to continue with regular therapy.

When selecting devices the health professional should have an understanding of:
- The drug required
- The range of available therapies
- The range of available inhaler devices
- How various inhalers work
- Local drug formulary
- Cost-effectiveness.

When selecting an inhaler device consideration also needs to be given to a range of patient considerations. These include:
- Patient preference
- Past experiences of the patient with inhalers
- The patient's expectations of treatment and inhaler device
- Patient's ability to use different inhaler devices
- Any fears or misconceptions about diagnosis or treatments
- The influence of peer pressure
- Age
- Physical and intellectual capability
- Lifestyle characteristics.

The key point is that for inhaled therapy to be effective people with asthma must have a device that they can and will use.

Practical considerations when choosing an inhaler device

- Ease of use—consider manual dexterity and level of understanding
- Is it quick and easy to teach how to use?
- Situations for use—will the inhaler be used solely at home? Or is patient a regular traveller? Is it required to be used during activity or need to withstand the humidity of a sports changing room?
- Is the device going to be needed in an acute episode? If yes, will need to consider potential reduction in ability to inhale deeply and that complex instructions can be hard to follow during stressful situations
- Does the patient require assurance that dose has been successfully administered?
- How important is it that the patient or carer is able to know how many doses have been taken?
- Can the patient or carer easily tell if the device is running out or empty?
- How easy is it for the patient to distinguish one inhaler from another? Some devices have Braille indicators to assist those with poor vision.

Introduction to allergy

Allergy is a common and important cause of respiratory symptoms, particularly in children and young adults. Atopy, defined as one or more positive skin prick or specific IgE blood tests to common aeroallergens, is a risk factor for the development of both asthma and rhinitis. Food allergy, particularly egg allergy in infancy, is also a predictor of respiratory symptoms in later life.

In atopic individuals, allergic symptoms typically begin in childhood with eczema and progress with age, with rhinitis and asthma being the most common manifestations. It is important to remember that allergy is a systemic disease, and, as such, can manifest itself in several different organ systems, often at the same time. Conditions which have an important allergic component include:

• Asthma
• Rhinitis
• Acute (but not chronic, i.e. lasting longer than 6 weeks) urticaria and/or angioedema
• Conjunctivitis
• Anaphylaxis.

Diagnosis can often be made by taking a good allergy history as allergy symptoms are often related to exposure to an allergen. Although diagnostic testing can be crucial to securing a diagnosis of allergy, it must be undertaken in a considered manner as there are time and cost implications. There is good evidence that the majority of patients presenting in primary care with suspected allergic disorders can be managed without formal identification of the specific allergen trigger. This is a function of three factors:

• The pre-test likelihood of correctly diagnosing or excluding an allergic disorder is high if appropriate clinical questions are asked
• Existing treatment options for managing allergic problems are relatively safe
• There is insufficient evidence from randomized controlled trials to support current approaches which attempt to avoid aeroallergen exposure.

The position is more complex for the smaller numbers of patients who exhibit more serious potentially life-threatening systemic allergic reactions in response to food, drug and venom exposure.

Allergy and the allergic response

Allergy is a systemic disease resulting in symptoms in multiple organ systems in the same patients. Allergic reactions are classic examples of Type 1 hypersensitivity, characterized by the interaction between allergen (e.g. grass pollen, peanut) and mast cells (cells which are ubiquitous in the peripheral blood and tissues and which contain granules which in turn contain histamine, a potent chemical which causes itching due to irritation of nerve endings, redness due to vasodilatation of blood vessels, and swelling due to increased vascular permeability) via an antibody, subsequently named immunoglobulin E (IgE).

The inhalation (via the nose or mouth), ingestion or injection of allergen results in a classic sequence of events: allergen quickly forms a bridge between two allergen-specific IgE antibody molecules and mast cells, which then degranulate (break open) and release their contents. Histamine, amongst other chemicals such as leukotrienes, prostaglandins, heparin and platelet-activating factor (PAF), is released into the local and general circulation causing the characteristic symptoms of allergy in one or more organ systems. The classic signs of allergy are itching, redness and swelling: its classic time course (immediate symptoms, usually occurring within 15 mins of exposure) mark the cornerstone of allergy diagnosis, and, at a simplistic level, allow you to quickly differentiate between allergic and non-allergic symptoms.

Examples of conditions in which allergy plays a major part include:

- Asthma
- Rhinitis (runny, blocked, itchy nose)
- Conjunctivitis
- Acute (but not chronic [lasting for >6 weeks]) urticaria
- Anaphylaxis.

And to a lesser extent:

- Eczema.

It is important to remember, however, that all of the above conditions can also be driven by non-allergic mechanisms, and that differentiating between the two has implications in terms of avoidance and, less importantly, treatment.

Triggers of allergic (IgE-mediated) symptoms

- Pollens (grass, tree, weed)
- House dust mites
- Furry animals (cats, dogs, horses)
- Foods (nuts, peanuts, eggs, milk, shellfish, fruit and vegetables)
- Drugs (antibiotics, muscle relaxants)
- Insect venom (wasp, bee, hornet).

Non-allergic triggers
- Infection
- Cold air
- Pressure/trauma
- Drugs
- Hormones
- Emotion/stress.

Atopy

'Atopy' is described as an inherited predisposition to develop allergic symptoms and is defined clinically as a positive skin-prick test or specific IgE blood test to one or more common aeroallergens (in the UK this includes house dust mite, cat, dog or grass pollen). Atopy occurs as a result of sensitization and simply describes the potential for developing symptoms on exposure to the offending allergen. Identification (by skin-prick test or blood test) of allergen sensitization does not predict symptom on exposure and so it is important to remember that patients with a positive skin test/blood test to a particular allergen may not have symptoms on exposure to that allergen, and so a causal trigger cannot be demonstrated by the results of a skin-prick test/blood test alone.

Individuals with a family history of atopy have an increased risk of developing IgE sensitization, and the atopic constitution is also a major risk factor for the development of allergic diseases such allergic asthma, rhinitis or atopic dermatitis. The contribution of genetic factors to the development of IgE sensitization and to family history of an IgE-mediated disease is between 70–80%. The risk of developing allergic disease in a particular organ is related to family history of that organ-based disease.

Early signs of allergic disease, especially the atopic dermatitis in infancy, and the presence of IgE antibodies specific to inhalant allergens, are important risk factors for later respiratory allergy.

Diagnosis of allergy

Accurate allergy diagnosis depends on the concordance (or lack of it) between the history and the results of an objective measurement of allergen-specific IgE antibodies. Accurate history taking is of primary importance in establishing the role of allergy, and it is important to question patients closely. Particular questions to ask include:

Do the symptoms seem to fit the pattern of histamine release: i.e. do symptoms include redness, itching or swelling?

It is important to look out for the manifestation of histamine release in different organ systems; for example, histamine-induced nerve irritation manifests in the nose as sneezing, in the skin as itching and in the lungs as wheezing; increased vascular permeability manifests in the skin as a wheal similar in appearance to a nettle rash, in the nose as nasal blockage and systemically as hypotension (due to sudden and excessive leakage from major vessels).

What is the relationship between allergen exposure and symptoms?

As mentioned previously, typical IgE-mediated allergic symptoms occur within approximately 15 mins of allergen exposure. This is helpful to remember when trying to interpret a history of possible food-related symptoms: early signs of food-related anaphylaxis include a histamine-induced generalized itchy rash occurring immediately after the ingestion of a food; abdominal pain, flatulence and general malaise (with no sign of itching, redness or swelling) occurring 6–8 hours after a meal are more likely to be the result of a food intolerance.

Is there more than one organ system involved?

Because mast cells are present at many different sites throughout the body, IgE-mediated allergy tends to occur in more than one organ system. Thus a patient who wheezes when near a cat is also likely to develop a runny nose and sneezing, a rash attributed to penicillin is more likely to be IgE-mediated if it is accompanied by symptoms in other organ systems such as wheezing, vomiting or diarrhoea. Allergy is a systemic disease, and thus patients are likely to present with symptoms in more than one organ system during their lifetimes. Babies who have food-related eczema often have asthma as a child and then hay fever as an adolescent and it is important to be on the look out for new manifestations of allergic symptoms in subsequent consultations.

Is there an obvious allergic trigger?

In a situation where the history points to an obvious allergic trigger, an objective test of specific IgE may not be necessary. In patients where the relationship between exposure and symptoms is unclear, a skin-prick test or blood test may be helpful, although it is important to remember that evidence of specific IgE does not imply causality. Allergen avoidance underpins both the asthma and rhinitis management guidelines, advice which cannot be given with any confidence unless a causal relationship is established.

Is there a past history of allergic disease?

True (IgE-mediated) food or drug allergy is much more likely in patients who have seasonal or perennial hay fever (an exception to this is wasp or bee venom allergy which occurs similarly in atopic and non-atopic patients).

• Other questions should include family history (allergy is more common in children of (an) atopic parent(s)), environmental history (exposure to furry animals, house dust mite) and occupation/hobbies.

The need for an objective diagnostic test depends on whether the suspected allergen is likely to be avoidable, and whether there is an allergen-specific treatment available.

Diagnosis of allergic rhinitis and asthma

Rhinitis is one of the most common manifestations of allergic disease, and treatment is rarely allergen-specific, the most effective treatment being a combination of antihistamine and topical anti-inflammatory drugs. The probability of rhinitis symptoms being allergic in nature is significantly increased if symptoms are triggered by animals or pollen, or if the patient has a personal history or a family history of allergy. The need for a diagnostic test should therefore depend on whether or not the identification of an allergen trigger will influence the treatment decision. Given the challenges in avoiding exposure to these allergen triggers, there is in most individuals little merit in identifying the underlying allergenic trigger. Empirical treatment is therefore justified as an initial step for rhinitis patients with a convincing history of allergy.

In contrast, if allergen avoidance is both effective and possible (in the case of food or drug allergy) or an allergen-specific treatment such as immunotherapy is being considered, then identification of the specific allergen trigger is essential, although again, accurate history taking is of primary importance in establishing the role of allergy and interpreting test results.

Allergic rhinitis 1

Symptoms of allergic rhinitis:
- Itching
- Sneezing
- Watery rhinorrhoea (runny nose)
- Nasal blockage.

Rhinitis is extremely common, its prevalence ranging between 15–30% depending on age, and is a particular problem in young children and adolescents where symptoms may lead to sleep disturbance, practical problems, activity limitations and emotional problems. Trigger factors include grass pollens, tree pollens, house dust mites and moulds, most of which are ubiquitous in the UK and largely unavoidable. Accurate identification of the responsible trigger is possible by performing a skin-prick test/sIgE test, although this may not be necessary given that successful pharmacotherapy is not allergen-dependent. Management depends on avoidance (where possible) and the regular administration of appropriate pharmacotherapy.

Management of allergic rhinitis

Allergen avoidance

Avoidance of pollens is difficult although taking a holiday abroad or by the sea (where the pollen count is likely to be lower) during the peak pollen season (usually the last 2 weeks in June) may be helpful. Pollens differ by country and climate, and sufferers seeking low pollen exposure should aim for hotter drier climates such as those found in southern Europe. House dust mite avoidance is also difficult; strategies centre on the use of impregnable mattress covers, pillowcases and duvet covers, although conclusive evidence that such measures reduce asthma or rhinitis symptoms is lacking.

Management of allergic rhinitis is dependent upon diagnosis, education and pharmacological treatment using a stepwise approach. Nurses can play a crucial role in the provision of this treatment by providing the following:
- Diagnosis of allergic rhinitis (positive history and positive skin-prick tests/sIgE tests)
- Diagnosis of comorbidities such as asthma
- Allergen avoidance advice
- Availability of drug treatments and training in their use to ensure optimum response
- Follow-up in patients suffering from persistent rhinitis and severe intermittent rhinitis
- Referral to specialist centres for patients who are unresponsive to treatment.

Treatment choices and patient management should depend on efficacy of treatment, safety and compliance, which is then guided by patient preference.

The following recommendations are based on guidelines from the British Society for Allergy and Clinical Immunology and highlight the key issues that are of importance to the treatment of rhinitis.

Mild, intermittent symptoms

Drug treatment should include a non-sedating antihistamine taken as required to control symptoms. First generation antihistamines (e.g. chlorphenamine) cause sedation in approximately 50% of people, and should be avoided, particularly in children, in whom they have been shown to impair learning ability. If symptoms are confined to the eyes or nose, topical application of an antihistamine (e.g. azelastine) or sodium cromoglicate may be sufficient to control symptoms.

Persistent symptoms (moderate/severe)

For persistent, moderate or severe symptoms, the choice of drug treatment should be based on the primary symptom, although optimal symptom control is likely to be achieved with a combination of treatments.

Nasal blockage

Whilst a non-sedating antihistamine alone taken as required is often sufficient to control mild, intermittent symptoms, moderate or severe symptoms warrant a combined treatment approach (topical nasal steroid and non-sedating antihistamine) which should be started at least two weeks before the symptoms are expected to start for maximal effect. Patients should be educated about the need for regular steroid treatment and advised that the benefit may not be noticed immediately. They should also be shown how to use the appropriate nasal spray device. Important advice when prescribing aqueous sprays should include:

- Stand up, fixing the eyes on a point on the floor about 3 feet away
- Using the right hand for the left nostril and vice versa, insert the tip of the nasal spray as far as is comfortable
- Use the required number of sprays according to instructions
- Do not sniff! (sniffing may result in the drug going to the stomach instead of the nose; this may be the biggest reason for treatment failure).

Rhinorrhoea, itching, sneezing

These symptoms usually respond best to a combination of a daily topical nasal steroid and a non-sedating antihistamine. Again, if symptoms are unresponsive, try an alternative antihistamine, check compliance and nasal spray technique. Alternatively consider increasing the dose of nasal steroid, or try another nasal steroid. Another alternative is to add ipratropium bromide, which may be helpful in controlling symptoms of watery rhinorrhoea.

Allergic rhinitis 2

Uncontrolled symptoms

If symptoms remain uncontrolled, a short course of oral prednisolone (20mg/day for 5 days) may relieve acute symptoms, although there is limited evidence to support such an intervention. Depot triamcinolone is no longer recommended in the UK because of concerns regarding adverse events associated with its use. Grass pollen immunotherapy is effective at reducing symptoms and medication scores in those patients with seasonal allergic rhinitis symptoms that are unresponsive to treatment and is available from specialist centres (http://www.bsac.org).

Anaphylaxis

Anaphylaxis is an acute potentially life-threatening medical condition that is commonly due to a systemic allergic reaction to an allergen, e.g. a food, drug or insect sting. Its onset is immediate and rapid. Recent estimates suggest that anaphylaxis is responsible for between 20–30 deaths each year in the UK, many of which are potentially preventable. It is important to consider anaphylaxis not only as an acute episode but as a chronic condition requiring long-term follow-up and detailed health education.

Clinical features

Crucial to effective management is quick and accurate diagnosis and being able to identify those at greatest risk of adverse outcomes. Any of a number of organ systems may be affected, the most important of which are the respiratory and the cardiovascular systems. Early signs of anaphylaxis (which are often ignored or misinterpreted) include flushing and systemic urticaria. Death is due usually to either cardiovascular collapse or suffocation (especially in younger children). Treatment may be delayed due to non-recognition of early signs and delayed administration of adrenaline is associated with increased mortality.

Symptoms typically begin within minutes of exposure, and as a rule of thumb the quicker that symptoms begin, the more severe the clinical reaction is likely to be. Latex-induced anaphylaxis is however known to develop more slowly—normally over a period of about 30 mins or so. The main clinical features that characterise anaphylaxis are summarized in Table 7.1, differential diagnoses are shown in Table 7.2.

Diagnosis

Diagnosis of specific triggers may be possible using skin-prick tests (not recommended in primary care for reasons of safety) or measurement of specific IgE antibodies in the blood. Measurement of specific IgE in the blood can be arranged via a local laboratory; measurement of *total* IgE is not related to *specific* IgE and so is not helpful for diagnosis. In non-IgE-mediated reactions, however, there are no tests which are able to identify specific triggers and the diagnosis must be made from taking a detailed history of the reaction.

Raised serum tryptase levels can be observed in ~50% of patients presenting with acute allergic reactions, and may be helpful in providing evidence of histamine release if measured at the time of the reaction. Results should be interpreted with caution as raised tryptase levels have been identified in patients without respiratory, cardiovascular or abdominal signs.

Table 7.1 Clinical features of anaphylaxis

Organ	Symptoms and signs
Skin	Pruritis, flushing, urticaria, and angioedema
Respiratory system	Rhinitis, sneezing, stridor and hoarseness as features of upper airways inflammation and oedema Cough, wheezing, and dyspnoea due to lower airway obstruction. If untreated cyanosis and asphyxia may develop
Cardiovascular system	Vasodilatation, tachycardia, hypotension, circulatory collapse, leading to shock and infarction of tissues
Gastrointestinal	Tingling and swelling of the lips and tongue, palatal itch, nausea, vomiting, abdominal cramps and diarrhoea
Neurological	Anxiety, headache, convulsions and loss of consciousness

Table 7.2 Differential diagnosis of anaphylaxis

Condition	Comment
Vasovagal attack	Bradycardia not tachycardia No urticaria, pruritis, angiodema, upper respiratory obstruction. Pallor instead of flushing Nausea without abdominal pain
Serum sickness	Slower onset (over days instead of minutes) No upper respiratory obstruction, brochospasm or hypotension
Mastocytosis	No upper respiratory obstruction Slower onset Chronic low-level symptoms between attacks
Angiodema and C1-esterase inhibitor deficiency	No flushing, pruritis, urticaria, bronchospasm or hypotension History of C1-esterase inhibitor deficiency
Globus hystericus	No clinical evidence of upper respiratory obstruction No flushing, pruritis, urticaria, angiodema, bronchospasm, hypotension
Acute or chronic urticaria	Generalized rash without respiratory symptoms or hypotension

Acute and longer-term care of anaphylaxis

Treatment of anaphylaxis can be considered as a two-stage process: immediate treatment and longer-term care. In primary care, immediate treatment consists of:

- Basic and advanced life support (if required)
- Restoring blood pressure (by lying the patient flat, and raising the feet)
- Adrenaline given by intramuscular injection: the dose of adrenaline that should be given is 0.5 ml of 1:1000 in adults, but varies with age and body weight in children
- Administering high-flow oxygen (if available) (📖 p.359)
- Arranging emergency admission to hospital.

Doses of adrenaline may be repeated every 10 minutes, according to blood pressure and pulse, until improvement occurs. In those who are moribund and if there is doubt about the adequacy of the circulation, a dilute solution of adrenaline (1:10,000) may need to be given by the intravenous route. Intravenous administration should be given whilst undergoing cardiac monitoring because of the risk of cardiac arrhythmias. It is important to give adrenaline promptly as delayed administration is associated with an increased risk of mortality.

Additional treatment measures that should be considered in those failing to respond include chlorphenamine 10–20mg by slow intravenous injection and hydrocortisone 200mg by intravenous injection. Other treatments that may be of value in resistant cases include intravenous fluids, nebulized adrenaline and/or salbutamol and vasopressors.

Longer-term care should involve identification of the trigger, advice on avoidance and instructions on the immediate management of further episodes. For those individuals where the likelihood of an anaphylactic reaction is recognized the patient and carers should be taught to use an adrenaline auto-injector such as an EpiPen® or Anapen® for prompt treatment of symptoms and referred to a specialist centre. Identification of the triggers most likely to be responsible for provoking anaphylaxis in different age groups may prevent future reactions by making allergen avoidance possible. An anaphylaxis management plan has been shown to improve reduce the number and severity of reactions in children with peanut or nut allergy and such plans should be developed and tailored to individual patient use.

Triggers of anaphylaxis

Foods

Commonly implicated foods are:
- Dairy products (egg, milk and cheese)
- Nuts (ground and tree nuts)
- Pulses
- Fruits (strawberries and kiwi fruit, for example)
- Seafood.

Drugs

- Antibiotics (penicillin and cephalosporins). (NB It is important to formally identify true, IgE-mediated allergy to antibiotics as life-long avoidance is often necessary. The majority of rashes which occur during antibiotic therapy are not mediated by IgE and do not recur on subsequent exposure.)
- Anaesthetic agents (particularly muscle relaxants)
- Peptide hormones (e.g. insulin and antidiuretic hormone)
- Enzymes (e.g. streptokinase)
- Aspirin and other NSAIDs
- Opioid analgesics
- Immunizations.

Insect venoms

- Bee and wasp venoms
- Latex.

Other triggers

Blood, plasma, immunoglobulins, and in very rare cases seminal fluid exposure (during coitus), have been identified as triggers of anaphylaxis reactions. Less common causes include physical stimuli such as exercise and exposure to cold weather. Idiopathic anaphylaxis also occurs, although mastocytosis and the carcinoid syndrome should be excluded as occult causes.

Immunotherapy

Immunotherapy targets the causes of allergic responses by desensitizing the patient to the allergen, usually through a course of injections in an attempt to change the immune response. Sublingual immunotherapy may be effective in many patients although the effect is recognized as less effective than by injecton.

As well as reducing symptoms in allergic disease, desensitization may protect against the onset of asthma in patients treated for rhinitis and may reduce new sensitizations to other allergens. Subcutaneous immunotherapy is only available in specialist allergy centres (see http://www.bsaci.org) because of the risk of anaphylaxis, although sublingual immunotherapy can be used in primary care.

Monoclonal antibodies

Anti-IgE in the form of omalizamub is a humanized anti-IgE antibody which in selected patients appears to reduce asthma symptoms and exacerbations and reduce inhaled steroid load. It is given subcutaneously in individually prescribed doses. The National Institute for Health and Clinical Excellence (NICE) recommend the use of omalizumab in adolescents (12 years of age and over) and adults with severe, persistent allergic asthma. It should only be initiated if the patient fulfils the criteria of severe unstable allergic asthma:

- Clinical confirmation of allergic (IgE-mediated) asthma
- Either two or more severe exacerbations of asthma requiring hospital admission within the previous year, or three or more severe exacerbations of asthma within the previous year, at least one of which required admission to hospital, and a further two which required treatment or monitoring in excess of the patient's usual regimen, in an accident and emergency unit.

A full trial and documented compliance with inhaled high-dose corticosteroids and long acting β_2 agonists in addition to leukotriene receptor antagonists, theophyllines, oral corticosteroids and β_2 agonist tablets and smoking cessation where applicable.

Recommended reading

Asthma UK *Living on a knife edge*. Asthma UK (2004) London.

Asthma UK *Where do we stand?* Asthma in the UK today. Asthma UK (2004) London.

British Thoracic Society, Scottish Intercollegiate Guidelines Network British Guideline on the Management of Asthma. Revised edition. Edinburgh: SIGN (SIGN publication no. 63) 2008. Available from http://www.sign.ac.uk/guidelines/fulltext/63/Index.html

British Thoracic Society *The Burden of Lung Disease*, 2nd Edition. British Thoracic Society (2006) London.

Gibson et al. *Self-management education and regular practitioner review for adults with asthma* (Cochrane review). In The Cochrane library Issue 3, (2001) Chichester, UK. Wiley and Sons Ltd.

Algorithms

1. Summary of Stepwise management in adults
2. Summary of Stepwise management in children aged 5–12 years
3. Summary of Stepwise management in children less than 5 years
4. Summary of British Thoracic Society/Scottish Intercollegiate Guideline Network (BTS/SIGN) Guidelines for Management of Asthma 2008.
5. Management of acute severe asthma in adults in hospital
6. Management of acute asthma in children in general practice
7. Management of acute asthma in children in hospital

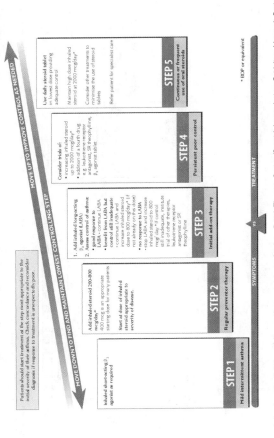

Reproduced with permission from the British guideline on the management of asthma, British Thoracic Society/Scottish Intercolegiate Guidelines Network. Revised May 2008. (Sign publications no. 101.) Available from http://www.sign.ac.uk

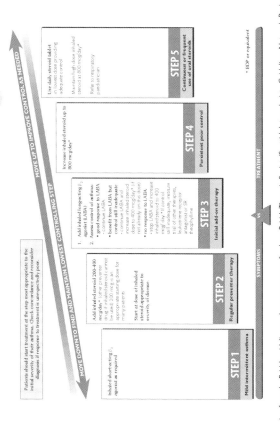

MOVE UP TO IMPROVE CONTROL AS NEEDED

MOVE DOWN TO FIND AND MAINTAIN LOWEST CONTROLLING STEP

Patients should start treatment at the step most appropriate to the initial severity of their asthma. Check concordance and reconsider diagnosis if response to treatment is unexpectedly poor.

STEP 1
Mild intermittent asthma

Inhaled short-acting β₂ agonist as required

STEP 2
Regular preventer therapy

Add inhaled steroid 200–400 mcg/day* (other preventer drug if inhaled steroid cannot be used) 200 mcg is an appropriate starting dose for many patients.

Start at dose of inhaled steroid appropriate to severity of disease.

STEP 3
Initial add-on therapy

1. Add inhaled long-acting β₂ agonist (LABA)
2. Assess control of asthma:
 • good response to LABA – continue LABA
 • benefit from LABA but control still inadequate – continue LABA and increase inhaled steroid dose to 400 mcg/day* (if not already on this dose)
 • no response to LABA – stop LABA and increase inhaled steroid to 400 mcg/day.* If control still inadequate, institute trial of other therapies, leukotriene receptor antagonist or SR theophylline

STEP 4
Persistent poor control

Increase inhaled steroid up to 800 mcg/day*

STEP 5
Continuous or frequent use of oral steroids

Use daily steroid tablet in lowest dose providing adequate control

Maintain high dose inhaled steroid at 800 mcg/day*

Refer to respiratory paediatrician

SYMPTOMS vs TREATMENT

* BDP or equivalent

Reproduced with permission from the British guideline on the management of asthma, British Thoracic Society/Scottish Intercollegiate Guidelines Network. Revised May 2008. (Sign publications no. 101.) Available from http://www.sign.ac.uk

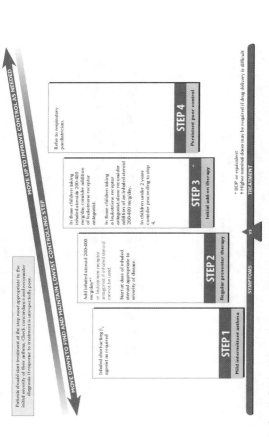

Patients should start treatment at the step most appropriate to the initial severity of their asthma. Check concordance and reconsider diagnosis if response to treatment is unexpectedly poor.

MOVE UP TO IMPROVE CONTROL AS NEEDED

MOVE DOWN TO FIND AND MAINTAIN LOWEST CONTROLLING STEP

STEP 1
Mild intermittent asthma

Inhaled short-acting β₂ agonist as required

STEP 2
Regular preventer therapy

Add inhaled steroid 200–400 mcg/day**

or leukotriene receptor antagonist if inhaled steroid cannot be used.

Start at dose of inhaled steroid appropriate to severity of disease.

STEP 3
Initial add-on therapy

In those children taking inhaled steroids 200–400 mcg/day consider addition of leukotriene receptor antagonist.

In those children taking a leukotriene receptor antagonist alone reconsider addition of an inhaled steroid 200–400 mcg/day.

In children under 2 years consider proceeding to step 4.

STEP 4
Persistent poor control

Refer to respiratory paediatrician.

SYMPTOMS   vs   TREATMENT

* BDP or equivalent
† Higher nominal doses may be required if drug delivery is difficult

Annex 2

Management of acute severe asthma in adults in general practice

Many deaths from asthma are preventable. Delay can be fatal. Factors leading to poor outcome include:

- Clinical staff failing to assess severity by objective measurement
- Patients or relatives failing to appreciate severity
- Underuse of corticosteroids

Regard each emergency asthma consultation as for acute severe asthma until shown otherwise.

Assess and record:

- Peak expiratory flow (PEF)
- Symptoms and response to self treatment
- Heart and respiratory rates
- Oxygen saturation (by pulse oximetry, if available)

Caution: Patients with severe or life threatening attacks may not be distressed and may not have all the abnormalities listed below. The presence of any should alert the doctor

Moderate asthma	Acute severe asthma	Life threatening asthma
	INITIAL ASSESSMENT	
PEF >50% best or predicted	PEF 33–50% best or predicted	PEF <33% best or predicted
	FURTHER ASSESSMENT	
■ Speech normal	■ Can't complete sentences	■ SpO2 <92%
■ Respiration <25 breaths/min	■ Respiration ≥25 breaths/min	■ Silent chest, cyanosis or feeble respiratory effort
■ Pulse <110 beats/min	■ Pulse ≥110 beats/min	■ Bradycardia, dysrhythmia or hypotension
		■ Exhaustion, confusion or coma

Reproduced with permission from the British guideline on the management of asthma, British Thoracic Society/Scottish Intercollegiate Guidelines Network. Revised May 2008. (Sign publications no. 101.) Available from http://www.sign.ac.uk

(continued)

MANAGEMENT		
Treat at home or in surgery and ASSESS RESPONSE TO TREATMENT	**Consider admission**	**Arrange immediate ADMISSION**

TREATMENT

Treat at home or in surgery and ASSESS RESPONSE TO TREATMENT

- High-dose β_2 bronchodilator:
  - Via oxygen-driven nebuliser (salbutamol 5 mg or terbutaline 10 mg)
  - Or via a spacer (4-10 puffs [given one at a time single puffs, tidal breathing and inhaled separately] repeated at intervals of 10-20 minutes) or air-driven nebuliser

If PEF >50-75% predicted/best:
- Give prednisolone 40-50 mg
- Continue or step up usual treatment

If good response to first nebulised treatment (symptoms improved, respiration and pulse settling and PEF >50%) continue or step up usual treatment and continue prednisolone

Admit to hospital if any:
- life threatening features
- features of acute severe asthma present after initial treatment
- previous near-fatal asthma

Lower threshold for admission if afternoon or evening symptoms or hospital admission, previous severe attacks, patient unable to assess own conditions, or concern over social circumstances.

Consider admission

- Oxygen 40-60% if available
- High-dose β_2 bronchodilator:
  - Via oxygen-driven nebuliser (salbutamol 5 mg or terbutaline 10 mg)
  - Or via a spacer (4-10 puffs [given one at a time single puffs, tidal breathing and inhaled separately] repeated at intervals of 10-20 minutes)
- Prednisolone 40-50 mg or IV hydrocortisone 100 mg
- **If no response in acute severe asthma: ADMIT**

If admitting the patient to hospital:
- Stay with patient until ambulance arrives
- Send written assessment and referral details to hospital
- Give high-dose β_2 bronchodilator via an oxygen-driven nebuliser in ambulance

Arrange immediate ADMISSION

- Oxygen 40-60%
- Prednisolone 40-50 mg or IV hydrocortisone 100 mg immediately
- High-dose β_2 bronchodilator and ipratropium:
  - Via oxygen-driven nebuliser (salbutamol 5 mg or terbutaline 10 mg) and ipratropium 0.5mg)
  - Or via a spacer (4-10 puffs [given one at a time single puffs, tidal breathing and inhaled separately] repeated at intervals of 10-20 minutes)

Follow up after treatment or discharge from hospital:
- GP review within 48 hours
- Monitor symptoms and PEF
- Check inhaler technique
- Written asthma action plan
- Modify treatment according to guidelines for chronic persistent asthma
- Address potentially preventable contributors to admission

Annex 4

Management of acute severe asthma in adults in hospital

IMMEDIATE TREATMENT

Features of acute severe asthma

- Peak expiratory flow (PEF) 33–50% of best (use % predicted if recent best unknown)
- Can't complete sentences in one breath
- Respirations ≥ 25 breaths/min
- Pulse ≥ 110 beats/min

Life threatening features

- PEF < 33% of best or predicted
- SpO₂ < 92%
- Silent chest, cyanosis, or feeble respiratory effort
- Bradycardia, dysrhythmia, or hypotension
- Exhaustion, confusion or coma

If a patient has any life threatening feature, measure arterial blood gases. No other investigations are needed for immediate management

Blood gas markers of a life threatening attack:

- Normal (4.6–6 kPa, 35–45 mmHg) PaCO₂
- Severe hypoxia PaO₂ < 8 kPa (60mmHg) irrespective of treatment with oxygen
- A low pH (or high H⁺)

Caution: Patients with severe or life threatening attacks may not be distressed and may not have all these abnormalities. The presence of any should alert the doctor.

- Oxygen 40–60% (CO₂ retention is not usually aggravated by oxygen therapy in asthma)
- Salbutamol 5 mg or terbutaline 10 mg via an oxygen-driven nebuliser
- Ipratropium bromide 0.5 mg via an oxygen-driven nebuliser
- Prednisolone tablets 40–50 mg or IV hydrocortisone 100 mg or both if very ill
- No sedatives of any kind
- Chest X ray if pneumothorax or consolidation are suspected or patient requires mechanical ventilation

IF LIFE THREATENING FEATURES ARE PRESENT:

- Discuss with senior clinician and ICU team.
- Add IV magnesium sulphate 1.2–2 g infusion over 20 minutes (unless already given)
- Give nebulised β₂ agonist more frequently e.g. salbutamol 5 mg up to every 15–30 minutes or 10 mg continuously hourly.

→

SUBSEQUENT MANAGEMENT

IF PATIENT IS IMPROVING, continue:

- 40–60% oxygen
- Prednisolone 40–50mg daily or IV hydrocortisone 100 mg 6 hourly
- Nebulised β₂ agonist and ipratropium 4–6 hourly

IF PATIENT NOT IMPROVING AFTER 15–30 MINUTES:

- Continue oxygen and steroids
- Give nebulised β₂ agonist more frequently e.g. salbutamol 5 mg up to every 15–30 minute or 10 mg continuously hourly
- Continue ipratropium 0.5 mg 4–6 hourly until patient is improving

IF PATIENT IS STILL NOT IMPROVING:

- Discuss patient with senior clinician and ICU team.
- IV magnesium sulphate 1.2–2 g over 20 minutes (unless already given)
- Senior clinician may consider use of IV β₂ agonist or IV aminophylline or progression to mechanical ventilation

Reproduced with permission from the British guideline on the management of asthma, British Thoracic Society/Scottish Intercollegiate Guidelines Network. Revised May 2008. (Sign publications no. 101.) Available from http://www.sign.ac.uk

(continued)

- Near fatal asthma
- Raised $PaCO_2$
- Requiring mechanical ventilation with raised inflation pressures

Peak expiratory flow in normal adults

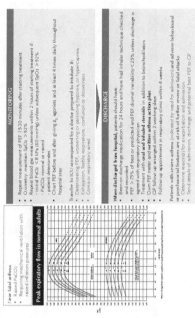

Mean ± standard error; number, age in years; and the predicted values are shown

MONITORING

- Repeat measurement of PEF 15-30 minutes after starting treatment
- Oximetry: maintain $SpO_2 > 92\%$
- Repeat blood gas measurements within 2 hours of starting treatment if:
  - initial $PaO_2 < 8$ kPa (60 mmHg) unless subsequent $SpO_2 > 92\%$
  - $PaCO_2$ normal or raised
  - patient deteriorates
- Chart PEF before and after giving β_2 agonists and at least 4 times daily throughout hospital stay

Transfer to ICU accompanied by a doctor prepared to intubate if:

- Deteriorating PEF, worsening or persisting hypoxia, or hypercapnoea
- Exhaustion, feeble respiration, confusion or drowsiness
- Coma or respiratory arrest

DISCHARGE

When discharged from hospital, patients should have:

- Been on discharge medication for 24 hours and have had inhaler technique checked and recorded
- PEF > 75% of best or predicted and PEF diurnal variability < 25% unless discharge is agreed with respiratory physician
- Treatment with **oral and inhaled steroids** in addition to bronchodilators
- Own PEF meter and **written asthma action plan**
- GP follow up arranged within 2 working days
- Follow up appointment in respiratory clinic within 4 weeks

Patients with severe asthma (indicated by need for admission) and severe behavioural or psychosocial features are at risk of further severe or fatal attacks

- Determine reason(s) for exacerbation and admission
- Send details of admission, discharge and potential best PEF to GP

Annex 5

Management of acute asthma in children in general practice

Age 2–5 years

ASSESS ASTHMA SEVERITY

Moderate exacerbation	Severe exacerbation	Life threatening asthma
■ SpO_2 ≥92%	■ SpO_2 <92%	■ SpO_2 <92%, plus any of:
■ Able to talk	■ Too breathless to talk	■ Silent chest
■ Heart rate ≤130/min	■ Heart rate >130/min	■ Poor respiratory effort
■ Respiratory rate ≤50/min	■ Respiratory rate >50/min	■ Agitation
	■ Use of accessory neck muscles	■ Altered consciousness
		■ Cyanosis
■ β_2 agonist 4–6 puffs via spacer ± facemask	■ Oxygen via face mask	■ Oxygen via face mask
■ Consider soluble prednisolone 20 mg	■ 4–6 puffs of β_2 agonist given one at a time single puffs; trial breathing and inhaled separately) at intervals of 10/20 minutes or nebulised salbutamol 2.5 mg or terbutaline 5 mg	■ Nebulise: • salbutamol 2.5 mg • or terbutaline 5 mg + ipratropium 0.25 mg
	■ Soluble prednisolone 20 mg	■ Soluble prednisolone 20 mg or IV hydrocortisone 50 mg
Increase β_2 agonist dose by 2 puffs every 2 minutes up to 10 puffs according to response	**Assess response to treatment 15 mins after β_2 agonist**	

Age >5 years

ASSESS ASTHMA SEVERITY

Moderate exacerbation	Severe exacerbation	Life threatening asthma
■ SpO_2 ≥92%	■ SpO_2 ≥92%	■ SpO_2 <92%, plus any of:
■ PEF ≥50% best or predicted	■ PEF ≥50% best or predicted	■ PEF <33% best or predicted
■ Able to talk	■ Too breathless to talk	■ Silent chest
■ Heart rate ≤120/min	■ Heart rate >120/min	■ Poor respiratory effort
■ Respiratory rate ≤30/min	■ Respiratory rate >30/min	■ Agitation
	■ Use of accessory neck muscles	■ Altered consciousness
		■ Cyanosis
■ β_2 agonist 4–6 puffs via spacer	■ Oxygen via face mask	■ Oxygen via face mask
■ Consider soluble prednisolone 30–40 mg	■ 4–6 puffs of β_2 agonist given one at a time single puffs; trial breathing and inhaled separately) at intervals of 10/20 minutes or nebulised salbutamol 2.5–5 mg or terbutaline 5–10 mg	■ Nebulise: • salbutamol 5 mg • or terbutaline 10 mg + ipratropium 0.25 mg
	■ Soluble prednisolone 30–40 mg	■ Soluble prednisolone 30–40 mg or IV hydrocortisone 100 mg
Increase β_2 agonist dose by 2 puffs every 2 minutes up to 10 puffs according to response	**Assess response to treatment 15 mins after β_2 agonist**	

(continued)

IF POOR RESPONSE ARRANGE ADMISSION	IF POOR RESPONSE REPEAT β_2 AGONIST AND ARRANGE ADMISSION	REPEAT β_2 AGONIST VIA OXYGEN-DRIVEN NEBULISER WHILST ARRANGING IMMEDIATE HOSPITAL ADMISSION

GOOD RESPONSE
- Continue β_2 agonist via spacer or nebuliser, as needed but not exceeding 4-hourly
- **If symptoms are not controlled repeat β_2 agonist and refer to hospital**
- Continue prednisolone for up to 3 days
- Arrange follow-up clinic visit

POOR RESPONSE
- Stay with patient until ambulance arrives
- Send written assessment and referral details
- Repeat β_2 agonist via oxygen-driven nebuliser in ambulance

LOWER THRESHOLD FOR ADMISSION IF:
- Attack in late afternoon or at night
- Recent hospital admission or previous severe attack
- Concern over social circumstances or ability to cope at home

NB: If a patient has signs and symptoms across categories, always treat according to their most severe features

---

IF POOR RESPONSE ARRANGE ADMISSION	IF POOR RESPONSE REPEAT β_2 AGONIST AND ARRANGE ADMISSION	REPEAT β_2 AGONIST VIA OXYGEN-DRIVEN NEBULISER WHILST ARRANGING IMMEDIATE HOSPITAL ADMISSION

GOOD RESPONSE
- Continue β_2 agonist via spacer or nebuliser, as needed but not exceeding 4-hourly
- **If symptoms are not controlled repeat β_2 agonist and refer to hospital**
- Continue prednisolone for up to 3 days
- Arrange follow-up clinic visit

POOR RESPONSE
- Stay with patient until ambulance arrives
- Send written assessment and referral details
- Repeat β_2 agonist via oxygen-driven nebuliser in ambulance

LOWER THRESHOLD FOR ADMISSION IF:
- Attack in late afternoon or at night
- Recent hospital admission or previous severe attack
- Concern over social circumstances or ability to cope at home

NB: If a patient has signs and symptoms across categories, always treat according to their most severe features

Annex 7

Management of acute asthma in children in hospital

Age 2–5 years	Age > 5 years
ASSESS ASTHMA SEVERITY	**ASSESS ASTHMA SEVERITY**

Age 2–5 years — ASSESS ASTHMA SEVERITY

Moderate exacerbation
- SpO₂ ≥ 92%
- No clinical features of severe asthma

NB: If a patient has signs and symptoms across categories, always treat according to their most severe features

Severe exacerbation
- SpO₂ < 92%
- Too breathless to talk or eat
- Heart rate > 130/min
- Respiratory rate > 50/min
- Use of accessory neck muscles

Life threatening asthma
- SpO₂ < 92% plus any of:
- Silent chest
- Poor respiratory effort
- Agitation
- Altered consciousness
- Cyanosis

Oxygen via face mask/nasal prongs to achieve normal saturations

- β₂ agonist 4–6 puffs via spacer + facemask (given one at a time single puffs, tidal breathing and inhaled separately)
- Increase β₂ agonist dose by 2 puffs every 2 minutes up to 10 puffs according to response
- Consider soluble oral prednisolone 20 mg

Reassess within 1 hour

- Nebulised β₂ agonist: salbutamol 2.5 mg or terbutaline 5 mg plus nebulised salbutamol 2.5 mg or terbutaline 5 mg
- Soluble prednisolone 20 mg or IV hydrocortisone 4 mg/kg
- Repeat β₂ agonist up to every 20–30 minutes according to response
- If poor response add 0.25 mg nebulised ipratropium bromide

Discuss with senior clinician, PICU team or paediatrician

Age > 5 years — ASSESS ASTHMA SEVERITY

Moderate exacerbation
- SpO₂ ≥ 92%
- PEF ≥ 50% best or predicted
- No clinical features of severe asthma

NB: If a patient has signs and symptoms across categories, always treat according to their most severe features

Severe exacerbation
- SpO₂ < 92%
- PEF < 50% best or predicted
- Heart rate > 120/min
- Respiratory rate > 30/min
- Use of accessory neck muscles

Life threatening asthma
- SpO₂ < 92% plus any of:
- PEF < 33% best or predicted
- Silent chest
- Poor respiratory effort
- Altered consciousness
- Cyanosis

Oxygen via face mask/nasal prongs to achieve normal saturations

- β₂ agonist 4–10 puffs via spacer or nebulised salbutamol 2.5–5 mg or terbutaline 5–10 mg
- Oral prednisolone 30–40 mg or IV hydrocortisone 4 mg/kg if vomiting

- If poor response nebulised β₂ agonist plus ipratropium bromide 0.25 mg
- Repeat β₂ agonist and ipratropium up to every 20–30 minutes according to response

Reassess within 1 hour

Life threatening asthma
- Nebulised β₂ agonist: salbutamol 5 mg plus ipratropium bromide 0.25 mg nebulised
- IV hydrocortisone 4 mg/kg

Discuss with senior clinician, PICU team or paediatrician
- Repeat bronchodilators every 20–30 minutes

Reproduced with permission from the British guideline on the management of asthma, British Thoracic Network. Revised May 2008. (Sign publications no. 101.) Available from http://www.sign.ac.uk

(continued)

ASSESS RESPONSE TO TREATMENT
Record respiratory rate, heart rate and oxygen saturation every 1-4 hours

RESPONDING
- Continue bronchodilation 1-4 hours prn
- Discharge when stable on 4 hourly treatment
- Continue oral prednisolone for up to 3 days

At discharge
- Ensure stable on 4 hourly inhaled treatment
- Review the need for regular treatment and the use of inhaled steroids
- Review inhaler technique
- Provide a written asthma action plan for treating future attacks
- Arrange follow-up according to local policy

NOT RESPONDING
- Arrange HDU/PICU transfer

Consider:
- Chest X-ray and blood gases
- IV salbutamol 15 mcg/kg bolus over 10 minutes followed by continuous infusion 1-5 mcg/kg/min (titrate to 200 mcg/ml)
- IV aminophylline 5 mg/kg loading dose over 20 minutes (omit in those receiving oral theophylline) followed by continuous infusion 1 mg/kg/hour

ASSESS RESPONSE TO TREATMENT
Record respiratory rate, heart rate, oxygen saturation and PEF/FEV every 1-4 hours

RESPONDING
- Continue bronchodilation 1-4 hours prn
- Discharge when stable on 4 hourly treatment
- Continue oral prednisolone 30-40 mg for up to 3 days

At discharge
- Ensure stable on 4 hourly inhaled treatment
- Review the need for regular treatment and the use of inhaled steroids
- Review inhaler technique
- Provide a written asthma action plan for treating future attacks
- Arrange follow-up according to local policy

NOT RESPONDING
- Continue 20-30 minute nebulisers and arrange HDU/PICU transfer
- Consider: Chest X-ray and blood gases
- Consider risks and benefits of:
- Bolus IV salbutamol 15 mcg/kg if not already given
- Continuous IV salbutamol infusion 1-5 mcg/kg/hour (200 mcg/ml solution)
- IV aminophylline 5 mg/kg loading dose over 20 minutes (omit in those receiving oral theophyllines) followed by continuous infusion 1 mg/kg/hour
- Bolus IV infusion of magnesium sulphate 40 mg/kg (max 2 g) over 20 minutes

Bronchiectasis

Introduction

Bronchiectasis is defined as irreversible bronchial wall dilatation and thickening. It may present clinically with recurrent chest infections, cough, chronic sputum production, shortness of breath, pleuritic chest pain, fatigue and malaise. It occurs as a result of a primary infection or toxic insult occurring at anytime from childhood to late adulthood, but in approximately 50% of cases no underlying cause is found.

There is no recent data outlining the incidence of this lung disease within the general population within the UK. Data from before the 1950s estimated the prevalence of bronchiectasis within the UK from 0.77–1.3 per 1000 population.

Causes of bronchiectasis

There are a number of different causes and underlying conditions associated with bronchiectasis. A primary insult causes bronchial wall inflammation and destruction, leading to ciliary dysfunction and impaired clearance of mucus; this may result in infection becoming chronic or reoccurring which in turn leads to further bronchial wall inflammation and destruction. Thus a vicious circle of damage and infection is established.

Table 8.1 Causes of bronchiectasis

Types of cause	Example
Developmental defects	Structural—tracheobronchomegaly
	Biochemical—α1 antitrypsin deficiency
Mucociliary clearance defects	Primary ciliary dyskinesia
	Young's syndrome
	Cystic fibrosis
Immune deficiency	Primary
	Hypogammaglobuliaemia
	Specific antibody deficiency
	Secondary
	Malignancy—chronic lymphocytic leukaemia
	HIV infection
Excessive immune response	Allergic bronchopulmonary aspergillus
	Post lung transplantation
Toxic insult	Gastro-oesophageal reflux/aspiration
	Inhalation of toxic gases or chemicals
Mechanical obstruction	Intrinsic—tumour or foreign body
	Extrinsic—tuberculous lymph node
Post infective	Bordella pertussis (whooping cough)
	Measles
	Tuberculosis
	Atypical mycobacteria
Associated conditions	Chronic rhinosinusitis
	Rheumatoid arthritis
	Ulcerative colitis
	Connective tissue disorders and vasculitis
Idiopathic	

Reproduced from Bilton D, Warrell DA, Cox JD, Firth JD, Benz EJ, *Oxford Textbook of Medicine*, 2003, Chapter 17.9 Bronchiectasis, 1421. Volume 2; 4th Edition, with permission from Oxford University Press.

Clinical features 1

History

Each patient's history will differ, depending on the underlying cause and disease severity, with presentation occurring at any time throughout life. Usually there is a history of cough productive of purulent sputum and/or a history of recurrent chest infections which may be slow to respond to conventional courses of antibiotics. Chronic malaise is often a prominent feature, particularly in severe disease.

A detailed history of child and adult health is essential to gain a clinical insight into this multifaceted disease. Some patients may give a history of childhood pneumonia or whooping cough with subsequent recurrent infections. Severe pneumonia in adulthood may lead to bronchiectasis in the affected lobar distribution. A history of treatment for tuberculosis should always be sought. A history of recurrent chest infections with no obvious initiating event may reflect an underlying cause such as an immunodeficiency. Underlying inflammatory conditions such as connective tissue diseases or inflammatory bowel disease should be considered in those with a known diagnosis or suggestive symptoms.

Symptoms of bronchiectasis include:
- Cough
- Sputum production—usually daily, can be purulent
- Pleuritic chest pain—usually associated with an infection
- Intermittent haemoptysis
- Shortness of breath
- Lethargy and malaise
- Recurrent chest infections
- Upper respiratory symptoms.

Cough with sputum production is a common feature of bronchiectasis. At an early stage of the disease the patients may produce sputum only during an exacerbation. However, as the disease progresses the patient often becomes productive on a daily basis with mucoid sputum becoming purulent during exacerbations. An exacerbation of this disease may follow a viral upper respiratory tract infection, and often presents with increased sputum volume and purulence, fever, increased malaise, pleuritic chest pain, increasing breathlessness with or without wheezing, and occasionally with haemoptysis. In the later stages of the disease, patients may expectorate large volumes of purulent sputum on a daily basis (📖 p.31).

In addition to symptoms referable to the chest, approximately 30% of cases have a history of chronic sinusitis or rhinosinusitis, and post-nasal drip is a commonly associated symptom.

Examination

In patients presenting in the early stages of the disease, clinical examination may be entirely normal. Coarse crackles may be audible over bronchiectatic areas of lung. Patients with extensive disease may have widespread coarse crackles and finger clubbing (📖 p.31). Some patients may have expiratory wheeze indicating hyperreactivity and/or inflammation related to infection within the airways. Signs of an underlying disease may be present, for example joint disease in rheumatoid arthritis.

Signs:
- Coarse inspiratory crackles +/– expiratory crackles on auscultation
- Finger clubbing depending on the severity of the disease
- Airflow obstruction and +/– wheeze.

Investigations

The aims of investigations are:
- To establish the diagnosis of bronchiectasis
- To document the distribution and severity of the disease
- To establish the underlying cause if possible
- To monitor the patient for disease progression and the development of complications.

If bronchiectasis is suspected on clinical grounds, radiological imaging is appropriate. The sensitivity of plain chest X-ray is limited, and this investigation is frequently normal or non-diagnostic; in more severe cases cystic cavities may be apparent, with enlarged and non-tapered airways giving the appearance of tram lines (Figure 8.1) (📖 p.75).

In most cases, the diagnosis of bronchiectasis made by high-resolution computerized tomography (HRCT) (📖 p.75) which demonstrates bronchial dilation. The bronchial wall may become thickened and mucus impaction may be seen. HRCT documents the extent and severity of bronchiectasis, and may give important clues to suggest an underlying cause; for example, a dilated oesophagus associated with bibasal bronchiectasis may suggest aspiration as a possible aetiology.

Clinical Features 2

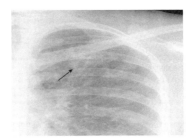

Fig. 8.1 Chest X-ray. Arrow indicating tram line

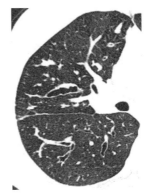

Fig. 8.2 Cystic lesions on CT scan

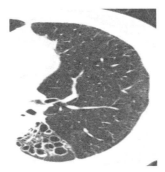

Fig. 8.3 Severe cystic bronchiectasis in the left lower lobe

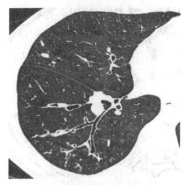

Fig. 8.4 Mild cylindrical bronchiectasis in the right lower lobe with loss of tapering and mild dilatation

Table 8.2 Investigation of underlying cause of bronchiectasis

Potential cause	Investigation
Idiopathic (40–50%)	Diagnosis of exclusion
Aspiration: reflux, or chronic aspiration which may be silent	• HRCT appearance (lower lobe distribution of bronchiectasis, dilated oesophagus) • Oesophageal manometry • Gastroscopy
Mechanical obstruction	HRCT +/– bronchoscopy to exclude foreign body/mechanical obstruction
Allergic broncho pulmonary Aspergillosis	Aspergillus RAST, total Ig E, Aspergillus skin prick test, eosinophil count, sputum culture for fungi
Immunodeficiency Common variable immunodeficiency Specific antibody deficiency Other immunodeficiency	• IGG, IgA, and IgM levels • Antibody response to vaccines (e.g pneumo-coccal vaccine, tetanus toxoid and haemophilus influenza B • Neutrophil and lymphocyte function studies
α1 anti-trypsin deficiency	α1 anti-trypsin levels
Connective tissue disease, vasculitis	Antinuclear antibody (ANA), antinuclear cytoplasmic antibody (ANCA), atrial natriuretic factor (ANF) and rheumatoid factor
Post-tuberculous	Radiological appearance. Sputum culture for acid fast bacilli
Primary ciliary dyskinesia	Nasal brushings/biopsy and electron microscopy. Nasal nitric oxide
Cystic fibrosis (CF)	Sweat test, genetic testing, faecal elastase, sperm count

Adapted from Bilton D, Warrell DA, Cox JD, Firth JD, Benz EJ, Oxford Textbook of Medicine, 2003, Chapter 17.9, Bronchiectasis 1424, Volume 2: 4th edition with permission from Oxford University Press.

Management of bronchiectasis

General management principles

- Management of underlying or predisposing condition e.g. rheumatoid arthritis, immunodeficiency, gastro-oesophageal reflux
- Physiotherapy and exercise
- Upper respiratory tract management
- Optimize nutrition
- Education of patient—self-management plan
- Ascertain appropriate antibiotic treatment with sputum cultures (📖 p.75)
- Early treatment of chest exacerbations, prevention of frequent or severe exacerbation
- Treatment of airways obstruction and regular monitoring of lung function
- Ongoing monitoring of clinical state, sputum cultures, inflammatory indices and radiological parameters to identify patients in whom the disease is progressing despite the measures above. Such patients may require re-evaluation and/or more aggressive therapy.

Physiotherapy, airway clearance and exercise

Chest physiotherapy aims to improve the clearance of secretions, allowing the patient to breathe more freely during everyday activities. Clearing secretions reduces the patient's need to cough in public (often a problem at the workplace or in social situations) and prevent sleep disturbance.

There are a number of techniques:

- Active cycle of breathing techniques and autogenic drainage
- Mechanical aids: Positive end expiratory pressure (PEEP), flutter, acapella, and the cornet
- Postural drainage: in conjunction with breathing techniques or mechanical aids. Manual techniques may be added.

The use of pharmacological agents (such as inhaled mannitol or hypertonic saline, plus oral carbocysteine) to promote clearance of secretions is currently under evaluation in bronchiectasis. Results from trials in cystic fibrosis cannot automatically be extrapolated to non-CF bronchiectasis (for example, nebulized DNAase was found to be counter-productive in non-CF bronchiectasis).

Exercise

- Assists clearance of secretions, especially if used before chest physiotherapy
- Should not replace chest-clearing techniques
- Increases muscle strength, flexibility and circulation
- Improves well-being and self-confidence
- May reduce the feeling and fear of breathlessness.

Some patients with severely impaired exercise tolerance may benefit from formal pulmonary rehabilitation (📖 p.531).

Education

Patients should have a clear understanding of their disease and the underlying cause if known. They should be involved in formulating a management plan. In particular, all patients should have clear guidelines on what constitutes an infective exacerbation (see below), and what action they should take when they experience an exacerbation.

To aid compliance with treatment the patient needs to understand the multiple factors that will help the patient manage their disease. For example:

- Understanding of the disease, potential cause and its long-term influence on the patient's health
- Potential benefit of physical exercise and chest physiotherapy in terms of the active cycle of breathing and/or postural drainage
- Susceptibility of the patient to an exacerbation of the disease and the influence of common colds/viral illnesses
- How to access medical care in the event of an exacerbation
- Understanding of the symptoms of an exacerbation in terms of increasing sputum colour, volume and associated by increasing wheeze and breathlessness and/or systemic upset
- The usefulness of sending a sputum sample for culture and sensitivity to aid appropriate management with antibiotics
- The use of reserve antibiotics (and in some cases inhalers and even corticosteroids) in the treatment of an exacerbation understanding when to access further advice if the patient is not responding to the treatment
- Education and help from support groups
- Regular review and monitoring of the disease
- Vaccination with influenza vaccine, and in some cases pneumococcal vaccine
- Travel abroad – fitness to fly, provision of regular and reserve medication, adequate insurance (📖 p.613).

Antibiotic management of bronchiectasis 1

General principles

Whilst working on establishing the underlying cause it is important to establish the organism(s) present in patients' sputum and ascertain their daily sputum amount. The aim is to maximize clinical well-being and reduce sputum to a minimal volume and mucoid state. Patients may often have accepted purulent sputum and malaise as usual, but after appropriate high-dose targeted antibiotic therapy (oral therapy for 2 weeks or longer, with recourse to intravenous therapy if oral treatment is not successful) they may achieve mucoid sputum and a marked reduction in malaise. Having achieved this state the aim is to establish the individual patient's requirements for antibiotics to maintain this stable state. An algorithm for the antibiotic management of patients with bronchiectasis is shown below Figure 8.5.

A relapse or exacerbation may be defined as increased sputum volume, purulence or viscosity PLUS 2 of the following:

• Increase in cough
• Increase in shortness of breath (SOB)
• Fever
• New chest pain
• Increased malaise
• New crackles on examination.

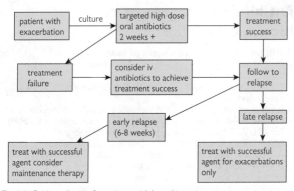

Fig. 8.5 Guide to therapy for patients with bronchiectasis

Adapted from Bilton D, Warrell DA, Cox JD, Firth JD, Benz EJ, *Oxford Textbook of Medicine*, Chapter 17.9 Bronchietasis, 1426, Volume 2, 4th Edition with permission from Oxford University Press.

Antibiotic management of bronchiectasis 2

Antibiotics for initial treatment of exacerbations

- Positive sputum cultures alone do not justify treatment—treat the patient, not the culture
- Ensure adequate physiotherapy and treatment of reversible airways obstruction
- Establish causative organism and antibiotic sensitivities if possible
- Institute antibiotic therapy appropriate to the clinical isolate (if available) for AT LEAST 2 weeks (some patients may require longer)
- Check history for antibiotic allergy or side-effects
- Avoid broad spectrum antibiotics where possible. Ciprofloxacin is the only effective oral antibiotic for treatment of exacerbations with *Pseudomonas aeruginosa* and thus should be used for other infections only if there is a failure or intolerance of first-line agents
- Consider drug interactions (e.g. with anticoagulants, oral theophyllines and cytotoxic agents) and warn patients of possible side effects (e.g. tendonitis with quinolones, photosensitivity with tetracyclines)
- If the patient improves ie: mucoid sputum, reduced malaise, then follow until the next relapse
- If no relapse for >3 months or suffers less than 4–6 exacerbations per year, then the patient requires exacerbation-only treatment
- If the patient is severely unwell (e.g. profound shortness of breath, hypoxia, haemoptysis) hospital admission for intravenous antibiotics, physiotherapy, bronchodilator therapy etc may be required
- Antibiotics should be chosen empirically and then adjusted based on sputum culture if the patient fails to respond. In the absence of previous *Pseudomonas* colonization, amoxicillin 500–1g three times a day is a common first-line treatment. In cases of penicillin sensitivity clarithromycin 500mg twice a day or trimethoprim 200mg twice a day is an alternative antibiotic
- Antibiotic guidelines depend on local bacterial sensitivity patterns and local antimicrobial.

Maintenance antibiotic therapy in bronchiectasis
Consider antibiotic prophylaxis if:
- Frequent oral antibiotic courses are greater than four exacerbations per year
- Rapid relapse (<8 weeks) after a course of antibiotics
- > 2 admissions to hospital for IV antibiotics per year

In general, prophylaxis should only be instituted following successful treatment of exacerbation. Treatment should be in accordance with local antibiotic sensitivity patterns and antibiotic policies; national guidelines are currently in preparation.

Table 8.3 Potential therapies for maintenance prophylaxis

Sputum culture	Medicine
Haemophilus Influenzae	Doxycycline 100mg daily (od), amoxicillin 500mg twice a day (bd) nebulized amoxicillin 500mg bd
Streptococcus pneumoniae	Penicillin V 500mg bd, trimethoprim 200mg bd
Staphylococcus Aureus	Flucloxacillin 500mg bd or 1g bd
Moraxella catarrhalis	Unusual for it to be colonizing the respiratory tract—usually an exacerbating organism
Pseudomonas aeruginosa	After effective intravenous antibiotics—nebulized colomycin 2 mega units bd

Other infections in bronchiectasis

Viral infections

Viral upper respiratory tract infections may increase susceptibility to bacterial exacerbations, but in general specific treatment is not available or indicated. Patients with bronchiectasis should be vaccinated against influenza. Infection with human immunodeficiency virus (HIV) has been identified as a potential cause of bronchiectasis, but in the UK it is infrequently found in the bronchiectatic population.

Atypical mycobacterial infections

Atypical mycobacteria are related to the organism that causes tuberculosis, but are found in the general environment. *Mycobacterium avium intracellulare* (MAI) has been identified as a cause of bronchiectasis, most frequently affecting slim, middle-aged women and causing middle lobe and lingular bronchiectasis with a characteristic appearance on HRCT (nodular bronchiectasis with florid 'tree-in-bud' inflammation). MAI and other atypical mycobacteria may also transiently colonize patients with bronchiectasis, and in some cases cause chronic infection. These organisms are difficult to treat, requiring lengthy courses of several, sometimes toxic drugs. The decision whether or not to treat a patient is influenced by whether the same organism is repeatedly isolated, whether the patient is clinically unwell, and whether there are signs (on HRCT) of ongoing lung damage. These infections should be treated by lung specialists.

Monitoring

Patients with bronchiectasis require follow-up to ensure their infections are adequately controlled, and that their disease is not progressing. Clinical appraisal is the most important form of monitoring. Lung function, blood testing and radiological investigations are also relevant.

Clinical review

- Review regularly—frequency depending on the severity of the disease
- Monitor rate of exacerbations and number of antibiotic courses; assess the effectiveness of antibiotic courses
- Question patients about their day to day symptoms, general well-being/ quality of life. A decline should prompt further assessment to establish cause and plan intervention
- Record sputum volume and bacteriology
- Check physiotherapy regimen, re-evaluation by a physiotherapist if concordance is poor
- Regular education of patient about their medicines and self-management plan
- Encourage patient to send sputum sample for culture and analysis, with each exacerbation to aid appropriate antibiotic treatment of an exacerbation
- Offer access to advice (telephone support line if available) and review
- Assess concordance with the prescribed treatment
- Be aware that each patient's symptoms are different for each patient
- Address patient's or carers' specific concerns.

Lung function

Spirometry is a valuable clinical indicator for monitoring this chronic disease but should be evaluated alongside other markers such as exacerbation frequency, sputum volume, bacteriology and general well-being (📖 p.75).

The forced expired volume in one second (FEV_1) correlates with the extent of disease severity on HRCT, sputum production and the patient's quality of life. Obstructive ventilatory defects are common, with some patients having evidence of small airways disease apparent on a flow volume loop and expiratory images on HRCT (📖 p.75). Depending on the degree of airflow obstruction and clinical symptoms, bronchodilators plus a trial of inhaled or oral steroids may improve the degree of airflow obstruction.

Acute decline in lung function may reflect an intercurrent exacerbation, and should recover with treatment of the exacerbation. A chronic and persistent decline may reflect disease progression. In mild to moderate disease the decline in lung function should be slow. More rapid decline may indicate the need for more aggressive investigation and management.

Blood testing

In general, blood testing does not play a major role in the monitoring of bronchiectatic patients. Inflammatory markers such as C-reactive protein may rise during exacerbations and return to baseline with treatment; ongoing elevations may suggest chronic sepsis or inflammation. In some cases, monitoring of underlying disease states may be appropriate; for example, a patient with a subtle immune defect such as specific antibody deficiency may develop common variable immunodeficiency and require immunoglobulin replacement. Patients on long-term medication may require monitoring through blood tests, and patients who take courses of antibiotics which react with regular medications such as anticoagulants may require additional measurements of their clotting.

Radiology

Baseline plain chest X-rays are useful as they may be compared with films taken during exacerbations, which may reveal new shadowing suggestive of acute consolidation or lobar collapse. Accurate assessment of disease progression requires HRCT, but these investigations expose the patient to a significant radiation doses and are expensive; hence in clinically stable patients they are performed infrequently (every 3–5 years); deterioration in clinical state may prompt earlier investigation.

Chronic obstructive pulmonary disease

Introduction

Chronic obstructive pulmonary disease (COPD) is a common respiratory disorder that causes considerable morbidity and mortality throughout the world. COPD is predominantly caused by smoking.

COPD is characterized by fixed airflow obstruction. Significant airflow obstruction may be present before the individual is aware of it. Airflow obstruction is slowly progressive, with minimal or no reversibility to bronchodilators.

COPD is an 'umbrella' term comprising chronic bronchitis, emphysema and long-standing, irreversible asthma. These conditions are an enormous burden to society, both in terms of the direct cost to healthcare services, and the indirect costs through loss of productivity.

The prevalence of COPD is difficult to determine because of problems with definition and coding. Sometimes it is difficult to differentiate between COPD and chronic severe asthma; and patients with mild to moderate disease may not be identified as suffering from COPD.

Causes and risk factors for COPD

Smoking

Tobacco smoking is the most important risk factor; it is responsible for 90% of COPD. More than 20 pack years (p.31) are usually required to develop COPD. However, not all people who smoke develop COPD; and not all patients with COPD are smokers or have smoked in the past. Approximately 25% of smokers are susceptible to COPD, indicating a possible genetic susceptibility. These smokers experience an accelerated decline in lung function as a result of smoking. In susceptible smokers, the more tobacco they smoke, the more rapid the decline in lung function. Susceptible people have an accelerated rate of decline of lung function (50–90ml of FEV_1/yr compared with 20–30ml of FEV_1/yr after the age of 25 in non-smokers)[1]. People with COPD, who stop smoking, slow down the progression of disease and may return to normal levels of FEV_1 decline. By the time they are symptomatic with breathlessness, they will already have impaired lung function, and stopping smoking at this stage may extend their life expectancy but may not improve their symptoms. Passive smoking is weakly associated with COPD.

Stopping smoking will reduce the rate of decline in lung function to that of a non-smoker or a non-susceptible smoker, but lung function already lost cannot be regained by stopping smoking. The earlier a susceptible smoker stops, the better the prognosis. By the time patients develop breathlessness, they will already have severe impairment of lung function. Stopping smoking at this stage may extend their life expectancy, but may not improve their symptoms.

Tobacco smoke acts as a bronchial irritant; and the body responds by producing additional mucus. This results in the characteristic 'smoker's cough' which can evolve into chronic bronchitis. The presence of smoke particles in the alveoli attracts white blood cells, as part of the body's natural defences. Enzymes called proteases are released to try to dissolve the invading particles. The long-term result is destruction of the alveolar wall, resulting in emphysema.

Occupational factors

Occupational exposure to dust and fumes (such as coal or silica) and solvents has been associated with COPD. Exposure to cadmium is associated with emphysema.

Coal mining is the most well-recognized occupational risk factor, and is the only occupational cause of COPD for which compensation may be paid. Welding fumes, especially welding in enclosed areas, are a suspected risk factor. The impact of occupational dust depends on intensity and/or prolonged exposure in order to be a risk factor independent of tobacco smoking.

1 Fletcher, C., Peto, R. The natural history of chronic airflow obstruction. *BMJ* 1977; i:1643–8.

It may be difficult to assess the exact contribution of occupation to the disease in people that also smoke.

Environment

Air pollution, particularly sulphur dioxide, carbon and other particulates which are produced by burning coal and petroleum fossil fuels are associated with COPD, but the role of air pollution is probably small. There may be interactions between smoking and air pollution.

The most common pollution is from vehicle exhaust emissions and photochemical pollutants such as ozone, produced by the action of sunlight on exhaust fumes (📖 p.541).

The incidence of COPD is higher in industrialized, polluted environments than in rural environments. Increased mortality from COPD is seen when particulate carbon and sulphuric acid levels are high, suggesting a direct toxic effect of environmental pollutants.

Socio-economic status

The prevalence of COPD is higher in lower socio-economic groups. Smoking rates are higher in these groups, but this may not be the sole causative factor. Maternal smoking has been linked with low birthweight and recurrent lower respiratory tract infection (LRTI), both of which are associated with COPD in later life. LRTIs are also associated with poor housing and social deprivation.

Poor diet is associated with socio-economic deprivation. Antioxidants in the diet protect against the harmful effects of smoking. A diet low in antioxidant vitamins such as vitamin C is associated with decreased lung function and increased risk of COPD.

α1- antitrypsin deficiency

This is a rare, inherited condition affecting about one person in 4000. Both parents will be carriers and there is usually a strong family history of COPD.

Family members should be tested for α1-antitryspin deficiency. This deficiency results in complete absence of one of the key antiprotease protection systems in the lung. The consequence is the early development of emphysema between the ages of 20 and 40 years, especially in smokers. Family members should be strongly encouraged not to start smoking or encouraged to stop.

Pathophysiology

COPD is an inflammatory condition, and all airway generations may be affected.

Chronic bronchitis

Chronic bronchitis is defined as the presence of a productive cough that occurs on most days, for at least 3 months in at least 2 consecutive years.

It is characterized by an increase in the size (hypertrophy) and number (hyperplasia) of mucus glands and leads to increased mucus production. Hypersecretion causes goblet cells in the airway to multiply and secrete excessive amounts of mucus, causing a chronic cough and sputum production. Loss of cilial function impairs the normal functioning of the mucociliary escalator.

The combination of excessive mucus production and reduced ciliary action leads to mucus plugging of the smaller airways. These become swollen (oedematous) and are infiltrated with inflammatory cells such as lymphocytes, neutrophils, and macrophages. The airways eventually lose their structural integrity as the supporting structures (cartilage) are damaged and close prematurely during expiration.

Inflammation of the small airways results in airway narrowing, increased airway resistance and hyperinflation. This in turn leads to reduced airflow, the hallmark feature of COPD. In severe cases there may be sustained hypoxia, which stimulates the kidneys to produce erythropoietin. Erythropoietin release stimulates red blood cell production, which eventually leads to an increase in the number of circulating red blood cells. These red blood cells attempt to increase oxygen delivery to the tissues to offset hypoxaemia imposed by underlying pulmonary disease. The extra red blood cells increase blood viscosity and can interfere with circulation.

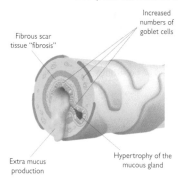

Increased numbers of goblet cells

Fibrous scar tissue "fibrosis"

Extra mucus production

Hypertrophy of the mucous gland

Fig. 9.1 Airway in chronic bronchitis
Reproduced with permission from Boehringer Ingelheim

Emphysema

Emphysema is defined as abnormal permanent enlargement of the air spaces distal to the terminal bronchiole (alveoli) accompanied by destruction of their walls.

The damaged alveoli merge into larger sacs called bullae. The bullae are relatively inefficient for gas exchange. As emphysema progresses, loss of the fine structure of the lungs causes collapse of small bronchioles, making air entry more difficult.

Emphysematous damage to the lung is not always evenly distributed. Two patterns have been described: centrilobular and panlobular.

- Centrilobular emphysema tends to be focused on the air spaces around the more proximal bronchioles, leaving the distal alveoli relatively undamaged
- Panlobular emphysema is a diffusely scattered disease, with no obvious preference for proximal or distal lung tissue.

Loss of the alveolar area leads to impaired gas exchange, and reduces the radial traction applied to the small airways. Loss of radial traction means that the airways are not supported and they tend to close. Closure of the small airways leads to impaired gas exchange because areas that are being perfused are not being ventilated.

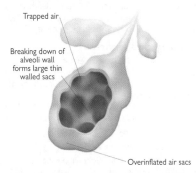

Trapped air

Breaking down of alveoli wall forms large thin walled sacs

Overinflated air sacs

Fig. 9.2 Changes in emphysema
Reproduced with permission from Boehringer Ingelheim

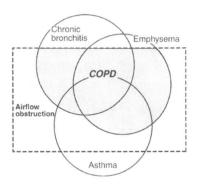

Chronic bronchitis

Emphysema

COPD

Airflow obstruction

Asthma

Fig. 9.3 Interrelationships of chronic bronchitis, emphysema, and asthma

Epidemiology

Prevalence

About 900,000 people in the UK have been diagnosed with COPD; 1.5% of the population. Some 32,000 people die from COPD each year in the UK. Physician-diagnosed COPD rates are seen as an underestimate of the true prevalence of the disease. Studies have indicated that as few as one person in four with COPD has been formally diagnosed.

COPD is currently more common in men and its prevalence increases with age: 2% of men aged 45–65 and 7% of men over the age of 75 have COPD in the UK, and the global mortality rate is higher in men. It has been proposed that men are heavier smokers and inhale more deeply than women, leading to more severe disease. Both the prevalence and the mortality rate for COPD are rising in women and the mortality rate for men is falling.

Worldwide, the prevalence of COPD is estimated to be 600 million; it is currently the fifth most common cause of death globally. COPD is predicted to be the third commonest health problem by 2020, with developing countries, especially in the Far East, being most affected.

Impact on primary care services

Only 10% of people with COPD are referred to hospital, the remainder are managed by their general practice. This results in a considerable workload for the General Practitioner (GP) and Practice Nurse (PN).

In an average health district serving 250,000 people there will be 14,500 GP consultations per year for COPD—approximately 2.4 consultations per patient per year. Consultation rates for COPD are four times more common than those for angina.

Impact on secondary care services

As many as one in eight hospital admissions may be due to COPD. This is approximately 220,000 hospital admissions per year. In an average health district, the annual inpatient bed days amount to 9,600 compared with 1,800 for asthma. The average length of stay is 7.5 days.

Impact on the patient

COPD results in progressive, disabling breathlessness. Breathlessness causes physical problems for patients, such as shopping, housework, walking up inclines and stairs. It also causes psychological problems such as loss of confidence, anxiety, and depression.

Financial hardship is suffered by many because of early retirement or need for help around the home.

Economic impact

COPD costs the health service approximately £100 million per annum in the UK. Secondary care management accounts for half this total. The average cost per patient per annum is £810.42. This is at least three times the cost of a person with asthma. The cost increases with disease severity from £150 per year for mild disease, £308 for moderate disease, to £1,307 for severe disease.

COPD causes considerable time lost from work, with 22,000 million working days lost each year.

Differential diagnosis

Often the diagnosis of COPD is suggested by the patient's history. The characteristic features of COPD are breathlessness, wheeze, persistent cough, and sputum production (📖 p.31). A diagnosis of COPD needs to be considered in any patient, especially smokers over the age of 35, if they have any of these symptoms. However, many other diseases can cause all or some of these symptoms. The most difficult condition to distinguish from COPD is chronic asthma.

Breathlessness

Breathlessness is defined as a sensation of difficult or uncomfortable breathing. It may be physically induced in response to exertion, or psychologically, as a response to stress. It is important to consider whether the breathlessness is a feature of:
• Lung disease
• Heart disease
• Pulmonary vascular disease such as pulmonary hypertension
• Systemic disorder such as anaemia, hyperthyroidism
• Obesity
• Respiratory muscle weakness diseases such as muscular dystrophy.

Wheeze

Wheeze is a musical note produced by airflow vibrating in narrowed or compressed airways. It is a feature of:
• Airway disorders such as COPD and asthma
• Congestive cardiac failure.

Cough

Cough is one of the most frequent symptoms seen in patients with cardio-pulmonary disease. It occurs when the cough receptors are stimulated. It can be a feature of many conditions such as:
• Airway disorders such as COPD, asthma, lung cancer, cystic fibrosis or bronchiectasis
• Parenchymal lung diseases such as fibrosing alveolitis, asbestosis
• Pneumonia
• Upper airway disorders such as post nasal drip, rhinitis
• Gastro-oesophageal reflux
• Heart failure
• Drugs such as angiotensin-converting enzyme inhibitors.

Sputum

Sputum refers to excessive production of secretions from the lung. Mucus is normally produced in small amounts in the airways as part of the lung's defence against invasion by irritants. It is moved to the larynx by the cilia and is not normally noticed by healthy people. Increased mucus production is a feature of:
• Airway disorders such as COPD and asthma
• Pneumonia
• Bronchiectasis
• Cystic fibrosis.

A good patient history along with other investigations is required to diagnose the cause of a patient's respiratory symptoms. Lung-function testing, assessing a response to therapeutic trials (📖 p.75), and a clinical and social history are central to the confirmation of COPD from asthma.

Clinical features differentiating asthma from COPD

Asthma and COPD are common diseases and may coexist in the same patient. However, both diseases manifest in different ways, and in most cases it is possible to differentiate asthma from COPD.

- Nearly all patients with COPD are or were smokers, whereas many patients with asthma have never smoked
- It is uncommon to have symptoms under the age of 35 in COPD, but asthma symptoms can start at any age
- Patients with COPD often have a productive cough, whereas asthmatics generally have an unproductive cough
- Patients with COPD tend not to have night-time symptoms of breathlessness, cough and wheeze, whereas these symptoms are common in those with asthma
- Patients with COPD tend to have little variation on a day to day basis in their symptoms, whereas asthmatics may have a lot of variation.

Investigations

Lung function testing

Objective testing of lung function is required to diagnose COPD and differentiate between COPD, asthma and other diseases causing similar symptomatology. Two basic measures of lung function are used in patients with COPD. These are the peak expiratory flow rate (PEFR), measured using a peak flow meter, and the forced expiratory volume in one second (FEV_1)/forced vital capacity (FVC) ratio and FEV_1 measured using a spirometer (📖 p.75).

Peak flow v. spirometry

The peak flow meter acts as a guide to the degree of obstruction occurring in large airways. This makes it more applicable to patients with asthma, where the prime focus of inflammation lies in the larger airways.

Whilst there may be a reduction in PEFR readings in COPD, peak flow is a poor guide to disease severity, and may seriously underestimate the degree of obstruction in more severe disease. Therefore measurement of airflow (FEV_1/FVC ratio and FEV_1) and lung volumes (FVC) using spirometry is the preferred lung function test in COPD.

The British, American, European, and international COPD guidelines all use FEV_1 percentage of predicted value as a basis for estimating the severity of the disease. The BTS/NICE COPD (2004) guidelines use the following scale:

• FEV_1% predicted 50–80%—mild disease
• FEV_1% predicted 30–49%—moderate disease
• FEV_1% predicted below 30%—severe disease.

Further investigations should be done if the diagnosis remains in doubt or symptoms are disproportionate to the spirometry readings.

Chest X-ray

This is taken
• To exclude lung cancer
• To detect enlargement of the heart and pulmonary oedema
• To detect bullae
• To detect hyperinflation, often seen in COPD but also seen in chronic, severe asthma.

Additional investigations may be undertaken as in Table 9.1.

Additional investigations

Further investigations may be carried out to ensure that the diagnosis is accurate, especially if the patient has symptoms that are disproportionate to their spirometry results. These tests would include:

- Full pulmonary function tests, including gas transfer (📖 p.75)
- High-resolution CT scan of the thorax
- Blood tests to identify α1-antitryspin enzyme deficiency, polycythaemia, anaemia, thyroid problems
- ECG and echocardiogram
- Sputum culture
- Pulse oximetry
- Body mass index.

Assessment of the COPD patient

The most common symptoms of COPD are breathlessness on exertion and cough, both productive and unproductive (📖 p.31). Some patients with COPD also experience wheezing, especially on exertion.

Breathlessness

This is COPD's most common feature and the main cause of disability. It is caused by hyperinflation of the lungs, with air trapping in the alveoli, leading to increased residual volumes and resulting in breathlessness.

Dynamic airway collapse due to destruction of the alveolar attachments ('guy ropes') in emphysema causes further air trapping, adding to the residual volumes of air trapped in the lungs. When hyperinflation is present, the diaphragm may become flattened. This results in the accessory muscles of respiration being utilized to assist with breathing.

Activities that use the accessory muscles other than for breathing, such as carrying shopping, stretching or bending over will make breathlessness worse. Patients often modify their activities to avoid becoming breathless. A person's subjective perception of breathlessness does not always correlate with the actual degree of airflow obstruction.

Breathlessness does not vary markedly from day to day although it may vary according to the weather, getting worse in very hot/cold/damp weather. It usually develops insidiously, and the patient may regard it as part of the ageing process.

Questions to ask the patient:
- When did you first notice you were getting breathless?
- How often do you get breathless?
- Is it getting worse?
- How far can you walk before you get breathless?
- What else makes you breathless?

Cough

Cough is the first symptom that is reported in 75% of patients with COPD. It may be intermittent at first, but it tends to become more severe as the disease progresses. Sputum is common, but not all patients produce it. The sputum tends to be clear, white or grey in colour, but may become green or yellow with exacerbations. It tends to be worse in the morning.

Questions to ask the patient:
- How often and when do you cough?
- How long have you been coughing?
- Is it getting worse?
- Do you cough up sputum?
- What colour is it?
- Is it easy to expectorate?
- Have you ever coughed up blood?

Wheeze

COPD patients often have wheeze that is associated with temperature change, especially in cold air. Patients are not usually wheezy at rest, and are rarely woken at night with wheeze, unlike asthma. The wheeze is more often heard on expiration. It may be audible or heard on auscultation.

It is often 'polyphonic'—a whistling sound of varying pitch caused by narrowing of the airways

Smoking history

Ask about the patient's use of tobacco—establishing how long the patient has smoked for, and how much tobacco a day is smoked. Also ask about any passive smoking history. If they are an ex-smoker, find out how long ago they stopped smoking. If they are still smoking, assess their motivation to quit. Have they used nicotine replacement therapy in the past?

The patient should be asked about:

- Exposure to airborne irritants, such as dust or chemicals
- Occupational exposure
- Childhood respiratory illnesses
- Family history of respiratory disease
- Other medical conditions, and what treatment the patient is on.

Assessing disability

It is important to measure the impact of the disease on the patient's life. An assessment of the level of disability and handicap experienced by the patient should include the following factors:

- Breathlessness, using the MRC dyspnoea scale, 'oxygen cost' diagram, or the BORG scale (p.75)
- Walking distance, using 6-minute walk test and/or shuttle walk test
- Health status, using questionnaires such as St George's Respiratory Questionnaire, or the Chronic Respiratory Questionnaire
- The impact of the disease on the person's daily activities
- The impact of the disease on the person's psychosocial functioning, for example, anxiety, depression, loss of independence, low self-esteem, and self-destructive behaviour such as continuing to smoke, not adhering to prescribed medications, sexual problems (p.571).

Clinical signs

In mild and moderate COPD, clinical signs may be absent. It is important to detect early COPD objectively, using spirometry to measure lung function. Nursing assessment of the COPD patient should include observing the following:

- Signs of hyperinflation; the typical barrel-shaped chest of patients with severe disease
- The use of the accessory respiratory muscles in the neck and abdomen
- Signs of hypercapnia (flapping tremor of the hands when the arms are outstretched, bounding pulse, drowsiness)
- A raised respiratory rate on effort, such as walking into the consulting room
- 'Pursed lip' breathing
- Ability to talk in complete sentences
- Prolonged expiration
- Low body weight
- Cyanosis
- Ankle oedema.

All of the above are poor prognostic features, and must be taken seriously.

COPD management strategies

The first UK guidelines for COPD were published in 1997. In 2004 new evidence-based guidelines were compiled and published by the National Institute for Health and Clinical Excellence (NICE). Other global guidelines have also been compiled and updated (Global Initiative for Obstructive Lung Disease). These guidelines offer the most up to date knowledge and recommend best practice.

Managing stable COPD

The management of COPD includes drug therapy, exercise, and psycho-social support. It is important not to treat the patient in isolation, but to address the needs of the family and carer as well. The NICE COPD guidelines recommended the following seven priorities:

- Diagnosis
- Smoking cessation
- Inhaled therapy
- Pulmonary rehabilitation
- Non-invasive ventilation
- Exacerbations
- Multidisciplinary working.

Diagnosis

A diagnosis of COPD is to be considered in smokers and ex-smokers over the age of 35, who have one or more of:

- Breathlessness on exertion
- Chronic cough
- Regular sputum production
- Frequent winter 'bronchitis'
- Wheeze.

Spirometry should be offered to all this group of patients to confirm the diagnosis.

Smoking cessation (☐ p.541)

Smoking cessation is one of the most significant interventions in slowing the more rapid decline in FEV_1 in patients with COPD. Advice and support should be offered at every opportunity. People that have smoked for many years may think that the damage has already been done and it is too late to stop smoking. It is important to stress that it is never too late to stop. Combining pharmacological therapies such as nicotine replacement therapy, bupropion, or varenicline (☐ p.391) with appropriate support leads to more success in stopping smoking.

Pharmacotherapy 1

No drug therapy to date has been shown to alter the underlying disease progression in COPD. However, patients can experience symptomatic relief from the appropriate use of inhaled, nebulized and oral therapies (📖 p.391).

Bronchodilators

Bronchodilators are the cornerstone of pharmacotherapy for COPD. They offer symptom control and treat any reversible component of airflow obstruction. However, no significant improvements in FEV_1 will be observed when bronchodilators are used.

The choice of therapy depends on the individual patient's response. Bronchodilators can help patients by:
• Reducing perception of breathlessness
• Improving exercise capacity
• Increasing perception of well-being.

In COPD, bronchodilators work by:
• Relaxing bronchial smooth muscle, reducing airway resistance
• Reducing hyperinflation, thus reducing breathlessness and the effort of breathing, so enabling patients to walk further
• Changing mucociliary clearance.

Inhaled bronchodilators

There are two classes of inhaled bronchodilators: β_2 agonists and antimuscarinics, both short- and long-acting.

For mild COPD (FEV_1 between 50–80% of predicted) short-acting inhaled bronchodilators—such as salbutamol, terbutaline, ipratropium bromide—should be used for symptom relief.

Long-acting bronchodilators (tiotropium, salmeterol, formoterol) should be tried in patients with moderate and/or severe disease and those in whom short-acting drugs do not give adequate symptom relief.

Oral bronchodilators

Oral preparations such as theophyllines produce only small amounts of bronchodilation in COPD. However, it has been shown to improve symptoms, such as breathlessness in COPD.

The value of theophyllines for COPD patients is limited because:
• They have a narrow therapeutic range, and to be effective need to be given in the higher part of the range. The toxic dose is only a little higher than the effective one
• They have many drug interactions and an unpredictable metabolism in the elderly
• Blood levels are influenced by smoking, viral infections, and the influenza vaccination. All these are commonly experienced by COPD patients
• At toxic levels, it can cause life-threatening arrhythmias.

The benefits of improvement in symptoms compared to the risk of side-effects must be considered by independent non-medical prescribers before prescribing, and they should only be considered in patients who cannot use inhaled therapies, or who remain symptomatic despite maximal inhaled therapy.

Inhaled steroids

The use of inhaled steroids in COPD remains controversial. Four large clinical trials conducted in the 1990s failed to demonstrate a decline in lung function over time. These studies concluded that for patients with mild COPD, these drugs were of no benefit. However, some benefits were found. Patients on inhaled steroids were found to have less frequent exacerbations.

The current guidance from NICE is that a select group of COPD patients should be given inhaled steroids. These guidelines state that:
• Oral corticosteroid reversibility tests do not predict response to inhaled steroids
• Those patients with moderate to severe COPD (FEV$_1$ <50% of predicted) who have frequent exacerbations (two or more per year) should be prescribed inhaled steroids
• The aim of the treatment is to reduce exacerbations, thus slowing the rate of decline in health status.

The optimal dose of inhaled steroids remains unclear. Trials suggest that high doses (800–1200 micrograms of budesonide, 1000 micrograms of fluticasone, and 2000 micrograms of beclometasone daily) are required. The following factors also need to be considered:
• Although these drugs are commonly prescribed for patients with COPD, they are not currently licensed in the UK, unless combined with a long-acting bronchodilator in a single inhaler
• Patients on high doses should be told of the potential risk of developing osteoporosis, and other side-effects associated with high-dose inhaled steroids
• Does the benefit of reduced exacerbations and symptom control outweigh the cost and possible side-effects of long-term high-dose inhaled steroids?

Pharmacotherapy 2

Oral corticosteroids

The use of oral corticosteroids as maintenance therapy is not recommended by the NICE nor the GOLD guidelines. This is because:
- There is a dose-dependent and duration-dependent risk of side-effects (☐ p.266)
- They produce a sustained reduction in symptoms in a very small proportion of patients
- Patients often deteriorate rapidly when oral steroids are gradually stopped, with worsening breathlessness, wheeze or cough.

If oral steroids cannot be withdrawn, the dose should be kept as low as possible; patients should be monitored for osteoporosis, and prophylaxis prescribed.

In acute exacerbations of COPD, oral steroids are recommended; there is clear evidence that oral steroids improve the rate of recovery. How they work in acute exacerbations, when they cannot control stable COPD, is unexplained. It is possible that there is a different pattern of inflammation in exacerbations, which is steroid-sensitive. An eosinophil increase has been reported in exacerbations, and these cells are potentially suppressed by steroids.

The NICE/GOLD COPD guidelines recommend 30 mg of prednisolone for 7–14 days for an acute exacerbation. Any patient considered for long-term maintenance oral steroids should be referred to a respiratory physician for further assessment.

Combination therapies

Short-acting bronchodilators

If neither antimuscarinics nor β-agonists can control the patient's symptoms, a combination of the two may be more effective than either drug individually. The reasons for this are:
- The combined effect of both drugs produces a greater degree of relaxation than can be achieved by either on its own
- It may be that the two drugs, by acting on the different receptors attain a greater degree of bronchodilation throughout the conducting airways, resulting in improvements in exercise tolerance.

Other advantages of combination therapy are greater convenience of use, and possible enhanced compliance. The guidelines state that combination therapy should be tried if patients remain symptomatic on monotherapy.

Long-acting bronchodilators and inhaled steroids

There are two currently licensed for COPD combinations on the market: fluticasone and salmeterol (Seretide®) and budesonide and formoterol (Symbicort®). Studies using these combinations in COPD patients showed:
- Benefits of the combination over each constituent part
- Improvement in health status
- Reduction in exacerbations
- Improvements in lung function.

Combination inhalers may be more convenient for COPD patients. As with all inhaled steroids, they should be considered for patients with an FEV_1 <50% of predicted who are experiencing two or more exacerbations a year; as well as in those patients who have demonstrated either a subjective or objective improvements to a long-acting β-agonist.

Mucolytics

Mucus hypersecretion is a prominent feature of COPD. Mucolytics are thought to make expectorating mucus easier. There is also evidence to suggest that they reduce exacerbation rates.

Both NICE and GOLD recommend the use of mucolytic drugs such as carbocisteine and mecysteine in patients with COPD who have a chronic productive cough. Therapy should only be continued if there is a symptomatic improvement.

Drug delivery systems in COPD

Inhaled therapy is the preferred method of drug delivery in COPD. The NICE guidelines state:

- Most patients, whatever their age, can learn how to use an inhaler unless they have significant cognitive impairment
- Hand-held devices are usually best, with a spacer if appropriate
- If a patient cannot use a particular device, try another
- Teach technique before prescribing an inhaler and check regularly
- Titrate the dose of drug against response for each patient.

When considering delivery devices, factors to consider are:

- Coexisting diseases such as arthritis, and subsequent poor hand grip strength; this may cause the patient difficulties using the inhaler device
- Inspiratory flow rate of the patient; some devices require higher inspiratory flow rates than others
- Cost of the inhaler; metered dose inhalers are generally cheap but unless they are used with a spacer device they give poor pulmonary deposition. Up to 75% of COPD patients cannot use them correctly
- Dry powder devices can be used by up to 90% of COPD patients but are generally more expensive.

For some patients who cannot manage inhaled therapies, or who are on very high doses of bronchodilators, nebulized therapies can be considered. There is little evidence to support nebulized bronchodilators over inhaled therapies. The NICE guidelines recommend:

- Considering a nebulizer for patients with distressing or disabling breathlessness despite maximal therapy with inhalers
- Assessing the patient and/or carer's ability to use the nebulizer before prescribing, and arranging access to equipment, servicing, advice, and support
- Allowing the patient to choose whether to use a facemask or mouthpiece, unless inhaling a drug (such as an antimuscarinic) where a mouthpiece is required
- Continuing nebulized therapy only if there is a reduction in symptoms, or an improvement in activities of daily living, exercise capacity or lung function
- Referring to a respiratory specialist doctor or nurse if long-term nebulized therapy is being considered.

Other therapies 1

Guidelines from NICE and GOLD recommend an annual influenza vaccine and a pneumococcal vaccine for all patients with COPD.

Oxygen

COPD is usually accompanied by some degree of ventilation–perfusion (V/Q) mismatch (📖 p.13). This results in arterial hypoxia when the patient is breathing room air. This makes the patient feel breathless, and it can also bring about changes in the pulmonary circulation leading to the development of pulmonary hypertension and right-sided heart failure (cor pulmonale). However, only a small number of patients with COPD need oxygen to manage their chronic condition.

Patients with chronic hypoxia need long-term supplementary oxygen therapy (📖 p.359). The NICE/GOLD COPD guidelines have strict criteria for which patients should be prescribed this therapy.

Pulmonary rehabilitation (📖 p.471)

Breathlessness on exertion often means that COPD patients avoid physical activity. This can lead to deconditioning of the skeletal muscles, and increased disability. COPD patients often say that leg tiredness rather than breathlessness limits their activity, as well as fear of breathlessness. This can lead to lack of confidence, social isolation and the phenomenon known as the 'emotional straitjacket' of COPD.

Pulmonary rehabilitation is very effective in patients with COPD, and the benefits can last at least two years. Patients with moderate to severe disease and who are motivated to attend should be considered for a pulmonary rehabilitation programme, which includes exercise and educational advice.

Nutrition (📖 p.541)

COPD has a significant effect on nutritional status. Patients with COPD have three common nutritional problems:
- Malnutrition
- Obesity
- Diabetes.

Diabetes commonly coexists in patients with COPD, as both are age-related and are linked with obesity and oral steroid use.

Malnutrition

Weight loss and nutritional depletion is associated with a greater mortality and morbidity, resulting in:
- More frequent exacerbations and hospitalizations
- Poorer exercise capacity
- Poorer quality of life.

Factors that contribute to weight loss in COPD are:
- Energy cost of recurrent infections
- Increased energy expenditure due to increased work of breathing
- Reduced oral intake related to breathlessness and/or depression
- Hypoxia related to deranged gas exchange

- Metabolic effect of pharmacotherapy (β-agonists, theophyllines causing an increase in energy expenditure, steroid effect causing a reduction in muscle mass).

Other factors that should be considered by health professionals are:
- Access to fresh food may be limited because of social circumstances
- Economic factors; patients with COPD are more likely to come from lower socio-economic groups and may have limited finances
- COPD patients may have problems preparing food due to breathlessness. Bending or stretching to reach cupboards induces breathlessness in many patients with severe disease
- Some COPD patients have a reduced appetite due to physical inactivity.

All patients with COPD should have their BMI (📖 p.75) calculated. Patients with a BMI <21 are either at risk or are malnourished, and should be referred for dietetic advice. Nutritional supplements are recommended in the NICE guidelines if the BMI is low, but this should be combined with advice on energy conservation and an exercise programme.

Obesity

Obesity occurs because of inactivity, and may be a result of the increased appetite from oral steroid use. What may be only a minor degree of obesity in a non-COPD patient may result in an increase in the respiratory work of a COPD patient causing:
- An increase in breathlessness on exertion
- Reduced exercise capacity and activity levels
- An increase in symptoms.

Achieving significant weight reduction is often difficult, and this subject should be handled sensitively. Patients need to agree a common goal for weight reduction and be motivated to change their eating habits. Encouraging them to participate in an exercise programme such as pulmonary rehabilitation may help. Patients with a BMI >30 should be referred to a dietician for specialist advice.

Patients with a normal or high BMI, who are losing weight unintentionally, should also be referred to a dietician as they may be losing fat-free mass (which is mostly composed of skeletal muscle). This is important as it correlates well with peripheral and respiratory muscle performance and exercise intolerance. These patients should also be considered for a chest X-ray to exclude malignancy, as a common feature of lung cancer is weight loss, and both COPD and lung cancer are common in smokers and ex-smokers.

Other therapies 2

Anxiety and depression

Many patients with COPD have anxiety and/or depression. This is possibly because of the limitations imposed on them by their disease. It is more prevalent in patients who:

- Have severe disease
- Are hypoxic
- Have severe breathlessness
- Are hospitalized frequently.

Patients with moderate or severe COPD should be screened for anxiety and depression. Many patients may find it difficult to approach their doctor or nurse about feeling depressed or anxious. The medical practitioner should ensure that they ask their patient how they are coping with their disease.

The NICE COPD guidelines advise that anxiety and depression should be treated with medication, with time being taken to explain to the patient why this is needed.

Travel and leisure

Patients with COPD should be encouraged to maintain as independent a life as possible. Social isolation is common in people with moderate or severe COPD, and many need help to remain mobile. The health practitioner should inform patients of what help is available from social services and voluntary agencies. These may include:

- A 'blue badge' for their own car, or to be used by someone driving the patient (who must be unable to walk more than 100 m)
- Attendance allowance/disability living allowance
- Dial-a-ride
- Local initiatives for disabled people.

The local Citizen's Advice Bureau can help patients complete the claim forms for allowances. Some advisers will visit patients at home.

Patients who want to travel in the UK can often get help from local travel agents who will advise on suitable accommodation with disabled access and facilities. Some larger train stations will provide a porter to assist with luggage, and many now have a lift to make access to platforms easier.

Oxygen-dependent patients now have access to oxygen equipment free of charge for the duration of their holiday in the UK (📖 p.386).

Travel abroad may be more problematic, but with forward planning it is achievable for most patients. Patients should be advised that:

- 'Blue Badges' are recognized and are valid throughout Europe
- Oxygen-dependent patients can hire equipment such as cylinders and concentrators in many parts of the world
- Portable oxygen concentrators and nebulizers are available to buy which run on rechargeable batteries and via a car cigarette lighter
- Wheelchairs and/or buggies can be pre-booked at many airports to transport patients and their luggage to their aircraft.

Some areas are more difficult to manage:
- Insurance cover for a COPD patient tends to be very high, and the patient may need to shop around for an affordable policy
- A reciprocal agreement in the European Union (European Health Insurance Card) will provide basic health cover if the patient becomes unwell, but it will not cover anything additional or repatriation costs
- Patients who are hypoxic may need additional oxygen on a flight, which requires pre-booking and frequently incurs additional costs (📖 p.613).

Acute exacerbations of COPD

An exacerbation is:

> A sustained worsening of the patient's symptoms from his or her usual stable state that is beyond normal day-to-day variations, and is acute in onset. (NICE COPD guidelines 2004).

Commonly reported symptoms are:

- Worsening breathlessness
- Cough
- Increased sputum production
- Change in sputum production.

The change in these symptoms often necessitates a change in medication.

Prevention and management of exacerbations is important because:

- Frequent exacerbations increase the rate of decline in lung function and increase mortality
- Frequent exacerbations result in a decline in health-related quality of life
- Exacerbations may cause an increase in disability and often take many weeks to resolve
- Many patients will be admitted to hospital for management of their exacerbation
- The average length of stay is 7.6 days and up to 34% of patients will be readmitted within 3 months
- This is a heavy burden on the NHS, and accounts for a significant proportion of the costs of caring for COPD patients.

The causes of exacerbations:

- Viral infections:
  - Rhinovirus
  - Influenza
  - Parainfluenza
  - Adenovirus
  - Respiratory syncitial virus (RSV)
  - Coronavirus
- Bacterial Infections:
  - *Haemophilus influenza*
  - *Streptococcus pneumonia*
  - *Moraxella catarrhalis*
- Increase in air pollution and environmental irritants
- 30% of exacerbations have an unidentifiable cause.

Exacerbations are more common in patients:

- With severe disease
- Who continue to smoke
- With worse health status scores
- With a low BMI (<18.5)
- Who are depressed.

Management of exacerbations

The severity and range of symptoms is variable. The following symptoms are common in many patients; indicating an exacerbation that may be managed in the community:
• Increasing breathlessness
• Increasing cough associated with sputum production and or purulence
• Increased wheeze
• Reduced exercise tolerance
• Fatigue
• Fluid retention.

Symptoms of a severe exacerbation that may need hospital management include:
• Increased respiratory rate
• Severe breathlessness, especially if breathless at rest
• Use of accessory muscles when resting
• New onset of ankle oedema
• New onset of cyanosis
• Significant reduction in ability to self-care and/or self-medicate
• Acute confusion and/or drowsiness.

The decision to admit a patient to hospital depends not only on their physical symptoms but also on social factors. Other factors to consider when a decision to admit a patient to hospital include:
• Whether the patient and family can cope at home and what their social circumstances are
• What the patient's general condition and level of activity is like
• Whether the patient has any other comorbidity such as diabetes or heart disease
• If the patient's saturated oxygen levels are falling despite already receiving long-term oxygen therapy
• If arterial blood gases indicate respiratory failure
• If a chest X-ray is abnormal.

The more factors for hospital admission that apply to an individual the more likely they should be managed in hospital. Many areas throughout the UK are running 'hospital at home' services (📖 p.330). This service provides a safe alternative to hospital admission for certain patients and is one that is preferred by many patients and their carers.

Treatment of exacerbations of COPD

Treatment of acute exacerbations primarily consists of bronchodilators, antibiotics, corticosteroids, diuretics, and oxygen therapy. Patients with severe exacerbations who have developed respiratory failure may need non-invasive or invasive ventilation (📖 p.494).

Bronchodilators

Primary care

- Patients should be started on a β_2 agonist and/or antimuscarinic if not already taking one regularly
- During an acute exacerbation, the dose and frequency of the drug may need to be increased if already on regular bronchodilators
- Patients should have their inhaler technique checked. Technique may be compromised in an acutely ill patient and a change in delivery system may be required
- Some patients may require nebulized therapy, but this is rare as high doses of bronchodilator can be delivered via a spacer device (📖 p.266).

Secondary care

- Short-acting bronchodilators are given 2–4 hourly
- Patients are routinely given both β_2 agonists and antimuscarinics in combination
- Drug delivery tends to be via a nebulizer rather than a hand-held device, as severely breathless patients may need large doses of drugs, resulting in unacceptably large number of inhalations from an inhaler
- Oxygen should not be used to drive the nebulizer in patients with hypercapnia or respiratory acidosis (📖 p.494), as this may result in worsening CO_2 retention
- Intravenous aminophylline may be given in patients who have not responded to maximal nebulized bronchodilator therapy
- In addition to their bronchodilator effect, aminophylline increases respiratory drive and may avoid the need for ventilatory support
- Patients receiving intravenous aminophylline need careful monitoring because of the wide range of side-effects, drug interactions, and drug toxicity that can occur (📖 p.266).

In both primary and secondary care, patients should have their bronchodilator therapy gradually stepped down to their normal maintenance dose once their clinical condition has improved.

Antibiotics

Most exacerbations are viral in nature, but a significant number are caused by bacteria. This makes the use of routine antibiotic prescribing in exacerbations of COPD controversial. Antibiotics have been shown to be effective only in patients with at least two of the following features:

- Increased breathlessness
- Increased sputum production
- Increased sputum purulence
- Features of infection (raised white cell count, C-reactive protein).

For those patients who do need antibiotics, the specific antibiotic prescribed will depend on sensitivities. Generally, broad spectrum antibiotics such as amoxicillin or erythromycin should be prescribed first-line. If there is a lack of clinical response, or a sputum sample sent for culture and sensitivity testing has shown bacteriological evidence of resistance, then second-line antibiotics such as co-amoxiclav or ciprofloxacin should be considered (📖 p.75).

Mucolytics

Erdosteine is a mucolytic which has a licence for use to treat the symptoms of acute (bronchitic) exacerbations of COPD (📖 p.391). It is given at a dose of 300mg twice daily for 10 days.

Corticosteroids

The NICE COPD Guidelines (2004) recommend a course of oral corticosteroids unless they are contraindicated in the individual patient. It is believed that this results in a faster improvement in lung function back to baseline, and for those patients admitted to hospital a shorter length of stay. A dose of 30 mg of prednisolone daily for 7–14 days should be given. The oral route is as good as the parental route in those that are able to take tablets, and nebulized steroids are not recommended. Other points to consider are:

- It is important that the steroids are discontinued after the initial course has been completed. There is little evidence to support the use of maintenance oral steroids
- If the steroids are given for 7–14 days only the dose does not need to be tapered off and can be stopped (📖 p.266).

Diuretics

Diuretics are not routinely indicated in the management of an acute exacerbation. They may be of use to patients who have associated heart failure causing peripheral oedema. Removing the oedema will make the patient feel more comfortable and reduce the load on the failing heart. If too much diuretic is given the patient may become dehydrated and may develop renal failure. This is more common in elderly patients.

Oxygen

The aim of oxygen therapy is to prevent life-threatening hypoxia by keeping oxygen saturations over 90% ($\square$ p.359).

Primary care

Patients who require oxygen to manage an acute exacerbation should be referred to hospital for assessment. If a 'hospital at home' scheme is in operation, a fully trained respiratory nursing team may organize controlled oxygen for the patient to use at home during the exacerbation.

Patients who are already receiving longterm oxygen therapy (LTOT) may need admission to hospital. The dose of oxygen should not be adjusted whilst awaiting transfer to hospital.

During ambulance transfer, saturated oxygen levels should be maintained around between 88 and 92%. Special care needs to be taken in patients with known type II respiratory failure.

Secondary care

On arrival at hospital, it may be helpful to give a breathless patient up to 28% oxygen, initially via a venturi mask. Higher concentrations should not be given until arterial bloods have been taken. This is because patients may be in 'Type II' respiratory failure ($\square$ p.494). Most patients will need between 24–35% oxygen.

Other points to remember are:

- The flow rate of oxygen should be prescribed on the inpatient drug chart to maintain saturated oxygen levels between 82–92%
- Venturi masks should always be used
- Too little oxygen (SaO_2 <80%) causes anaerobic metabolism—the creation of energy through the combustion of carbohydrates in the absence of oxygen. This occurs when the lungs cannot put enough oxygen into the bloodstream to keep up with the demands from the muscles' energy—and metabolic acidosis
- Too much oxygen (SaO_2 >90%) can cause CO_2 retention and respiratory acidosis
- A falling level of consciousness is the best clinical marker of significant CO_2 retention and respiratory acidosis
- Patients may need consideration for non-invasive ventilation if respiratory acidosis is not responding ($\square$ p.494)
- Oxygen therapy should be continued during other forms of therapy such as nebulized drugs. Patients can use nasal cannulae for their oxygen, whilst a mask or mouthpiece can be used for the nebulizer
- Nasal cannulae are better tolerated by patients than Venturi masks, and can be used once the patient is stabilized
- Oxygen should be discontinued once the SaO_2 is stable at <90% breathing room air
- Patients should not be routinely discharged with oxygen to have at home until a formal oxygen assessment has been undertaken ($\square$ p.359).

Assisted ventilation

The majority of patients with an acute exacerbation of COPD respond to maximal pharmacological therapy and will not need assisted ventilation. Some patients will develop severe respiratory failure that requires ventilatory support. Non-invasive ventilation (📖 p.494) (NIV) is indicated in patients who:

• Are not responding to maximal medical therapy
• Are conscious and cooperative
• Can clear secretions.

The advantages of NIV are:

• It improves quality of life, arterial blood gas tensions, and sleep quality in hypercapnic patients
• As it does not require intubation, it avoids swallowing impairment
• It reduces mortality rates
• It can be performed on a general ward by trained nurses or physiotherapists.

The disadvantages are:

• The mask has to be fitted tightly to the face and patients may find it uncomfortable to wear
• The patient has to be conscious and cooperative
• Patients have difficulty talking whilst on the machine and will need a lot of reassurance to maintain the treatment
• Some patients feel claustrophobic whilst on the machine.

Before NIV is started, it is important that a decision has been made, and documented in the patient's notes, regarding what will happen if NIV is ineffective or if it is not tolerated by the patient. Some patients will require invasive ventilation, but before this is considered, the patient's own wishes, if known, should be taken into account. Many patients now have a 'living will' where they have documented what they wish to happen in the event of a severe deterioration in their COPD. Any decision regarding resuscitation should also be documented in the patient's notes.

Factors that would encourage the use of invasive ventilation are:

• A demonstrable treatable reason for current decline for example, radiographic evidence of pneumonia
• The first episode of respiratory failure
• An acceptable quality of life.

Factors that are likely to discourage the use of invasive ventilation are:

• Previously documented severe COPD that has been fully assessed and found to be unresponsive to therapy
• Severe comorbidities such as pulmonary oedema or cancer
• A poor quality of life, for example, being housebound, in spite of maximal therapy.

Invasive therapy is seen as a final resort in worsening respiratory failure; but in-hospital mortality in ventilated COPD patients is no higher than those patients ventilated for other conditions, and the five-year survival rates are better than many people believe.

Nursing care

When patients are admitted to hospital with an exacerbation they are often frightened, anxious, and tired. Nursing involves caring and supporting patients through the exacerbation, and allowing trust to develop between the patient and nurse. The patient and their carer/family will need reassurance that they are going to be made to feel more comfortable.

The role of the ward respiratory nurse

The care of the COPD patient includes:

- *Positioning of the patient.* A patient, who is sitting upright, with shoulders hunched, is working hard to breathe. The nurse's aim is to position the patient in such a way to maximize respiratory function while reducing physical effort
- The patient should be comfortable and well supported, with pillows supporting the small of the back. Too many pillows can restrict chest movement. Some patients are more comfortable sitting on the edge of the bed or in an armchair, leaning forward with their arms resting on a bed table or pillows.
- *Assessment of breathing including*:
  - Respiratory rate: between 12 and 18 breaths per minute (BPM) is regarded as normal. This should be recorded 4-hourly initially, more frequently if the patients' condition deteriorates
  - Rhythm and depth: alterations may indicate hyperventilation, caused by fear, anxiety or alterations in blood gas concentrations
  - Effort to breathe: known as the work of breathing is dependent on rate, depth and airway resistance. COPD patients may use the accessory muscles to assist with breathing—lifting the shoulders and using the intercostal muscles during inspiration. The patient's breathing may also be shallow and rapid due to increased airway resistance caused by bronchospasm. Healthy, spontaneous breathing is quiet with minimal effort
  - Ability to speak without breathlessness
- *Skin colour and perfusion.* Cyanosis is most noticeable around the lips, earlobes, mouth and fingers. Measurement of SaO_2 should be recorded and documented 4-hourly, more frequently if the patient appears to be deteriorating. Medical assistance should be called for if levels are falling, despite controlled oxygen being given
- Pressure areas. Hypoxia is a risk factor associated with skin breakdown
- Communication. Patients who are very breathless may only be able to speak a few words at a time. Closed questions will help them to answer, using a shake or nod of the head if necessary. It is important that the nurse does not make assumptions on behalf of the patient. Oxygen or NIV masks also hinder communication
- Hygiene. Patients may become more breathless when washing. Adequate time or assistance should be offered. Some patients may need oxygen during washing and bathing
  - An increased breathing rate may result in a drying effect on the mucous membrane. Fluids should be encouraged, along with regular mouth care

- Oral candidiasis is a common side-effect from inhaled corticosteroids and rinsing the mouth after using a steroid inhaler should be encouraged
- Patients may need help with denture care
- Eating and drinking. Patients who are acutely breathless may have difficulty in eating and drinking. This can result in dehydration, malnourishment and weight loss
  - Unless contraindicated, patients should be encouraged to drink plenty of water to minimize the risk of a dry mouth (common when antimuscarinic drugs are given) constipation and sputum retention
  - Patients should be offered small meals and frequent snacks as they often complain of feeling more breathless following a large meal. Oxygen should be delivered via nasal cannulae during meal times
- Medication. Patients may need additional help with their routine medication when unwell; this particularly applies to inhaled therapies. Bronchodilators should be given regularly, as prescribed. Patients often find it beneficial to receive their bronchodilators prior to any exertion, such as washing or eating. Patients receiving intravenous aminophylline should receive cardiac monitoring and those on diuretic therapy may need assistance with toileting requirements
- Psychological care. Patients may appear very anxious about their condition and anxiety can increase breathlessness. Allowing time, talking calmly, and reassuring them can be very effective. Stroking the patient's back or hand can sometimes help to relax them. Some people will not like this, so always ask permission. A well-ventilated room, with a fan blowing cool air onto the patient's face can also provide relief from anxiety. Providing distractions, such as television, radio or someone to talk to can also provide relief
- Discharge planning. Patients should be referred to the respiratory nurse specialist for review prior to discharge. Patients and carers should be given appropriate information so that they understand the correct use of their medication before discharge. Arrangements for follow-up and home care such as visiting nurse, referral to social service and voluntary agencies should be made. Patients who are oxygen-dependent may need ambulance transport to get home.

Respiratory nurse specialists

A respiratory nurse specialist should form part of the multidisciplinary approach to COPD management. Their role includes:
- Offering specialist nursing advice and support to ward-based and community nurses
- COPD assessments/reviews to patients admitted acutely, including spirometry and arterial or ear lobe capillary blood gases
- Initiating NIV if appropriate
- Giving advice on inhaler technique/nebulizer and oxygen use
- Offering smoking cessation support
- Advising patients on self-management strategies
- Identifying and monitoring patients at high risk of exacerbations and helping avoid further admission to hospital
- Offering follow-up to patients in nurse-led respiratory clinics to review how the patient is managing their disease
- Assessing patients who may benefit from LTOT and/or ambulatory oxygen and arranging for this service in the community
- Identifying patients who may benefit from an exercise programme.

Community respiratory nurse

Community nurses have a key role in the prevention and treatment of COPD in primary care. Many community nursing schemes have now been set up to support the COPD patient and help prevent hospital admissions. (📖 p.588). Their role includes:
- Home care provision including 'hospital at home' schemes
- Assessing and monitoring stable COPD over time
- Providing effective education and support to patients and their carers, enabling patients to adjust to their condition and be proactive in their management
- Encouraging the patient to maintain an active lifestyle
- Psychological and emotional support for patients and carers
- Monitoring patients on oxygen and/or home ventilation
- Education and training in primary care.

Follow-up post-exacerbation

Community treated exacerbations normally respond well to conventional therapy. Patients should be offered a routine appointment to ensure that they are recovering. Patients who have been admitted to hospital should be seen by either their GP or the hospital respiratory team. Patients who fail to respond need further examination and specialist review, especially if the diagnosis is in doubt.

A follow-up appointment should be offered to:

- Assess the patient's clinical state and perform baseline spirometry; an exacerbation may take many weeks to recover from
- Assess the patient's treatment and re-check their inhaler technique: optimize treatment if indicated
- Assess their social circumstances: care that may have been ordered in hospital, such as personal care, may need increasing
- Reinforce lifestyle messages such as smoking cessation, diet, and exercise
- Consider referral for oxygen assessments or pulmonary rehabilitation
- Educate the patient on self-management of future exacerbations
- Patients who have regular exacerbations can be given a course of antibiotics and corticosteroids to keep 'on standby'
- Encourage patients to seek medical help early in the course of any future exacerbations
- Ask patients who have received ventilation about their experience of this treatment. Document their views on the future use of ventilation.

Routine follow-up of COPD patients in primary care

Patients with mild or moderate COPD should be reviewed at least annually, and patients with severe disease should be reviewed at least twice a year, either at the surgery, or if the patient is unable to get to the surgery a home visit should be offered. Every review should consist of a clinical assessment including:

- Smoking status and determination of desire to quit
- Symptom control including breathlessness management, exercise tolerance levels, and frequency of exacerbations
- Medicines management including concordance, inhaler technique, and patient's understanding of their medicines
- Assessment of patient's ability to cope physically, psychologically, and socially with their disease
- Assessment of complications such as cor pulmonale, hypoxia, anxiety, and/or depression
- Referral to specialist services for oxygen/nebulizer assessment, for pulmonary rehabilitation, or for dietetic advice.

Each review should also include measurements of:

- FEV_1 and FVC and FEV_1/ FVC ratio
- Inhaler technique
- BMI
- MRC dyspnoea score
- SaO_2.

Patients should be considered for referral to a specialist respiratory service if:

- The diagnosis is in doubt
- The patient is suspected of having very severe disease
- The patient is suspected of having complications such as cor pulmonale or bullae
- The patient reports haemoptysis
- The patient is experiencing frequent exacerbations
- An assessment for pulmonary rehabilitation, oxygen or nebulized therapy is indicated
- The patient may be a candidate for surgery such as lung-volume reduction or lung transplantation
- There is a family history of α-1 antitrypsin deficiency or the patient is under 40 years of age
- The patient's symptoms are disproportionate to their lung function deficit or if the patient is demonstrating dysfunctional breathing.

Other treatment modalities

Surgery

Surgical treatment is infrequently used in COPD management. There are three surgical procedures that are currently offered in the aim of improving respiratory function:

• Bullectomy
• Lung-volume reduction
• Lung transplantation.

Bullectomy

This procedure is indicated in patients with advanced emphysema. Damaged alveoli may form large air spaces called bullae. Large bullae can be problematic because:

• They may rupture causing a pneumothorax
• They cause hyperinflation of the chest resulting in worsening breathlessness
• They occupy space that could be taken up by healthy lung
• The elastic recoil of the lung may be impaired.

Surgical removal of a bullae is indicated where a significant proportion of the lung is taken up by bullae.

Lung-volume reduction surgery

Most patients with emphysema have diffuse disease, and there are no obvious bullae. Lung-volume reduction surgery (LVRS) aims to remove the least functional part of the lungs in order to improve airflow, diaphragm and chest wall mechanics, and alveolar gas exchange in the remaining portion of the lung. Surgery aims to reduce the volume of each lung by between 20–30%. This leads to symptomatic improvement in breathlessness and objective improvement in lung function.

Lung transplantation

This rare operation is more commonly offered to young patients with α1-antitrypsin deficiency. Single-lung transplantation is offered and the results are generally good. Shortage of donor organs makes it unlikely that transplantation will make any impact on the management of COPD.

Complications of COPD

Cor pulmonale

Cor pulmonale, also known as right-sided heart failure, is an increase in bulk of the right ventricle of the heart, generally caused by chronic diseases or malfunction of the lungs. Cor pulmonale occurs in 25% of patients with COPD. High blood pressure in the blood vessels (pulmonary hypertension) causes the enlargement of the right ventricle.

Signs and symptoms
• Shortness of breath
• Oedema of the feet or ankles
• Exercise intolerance
• Cyanosis
• Distension of the neck veins indicating high right-heart pressures
• Abnormal heart sounds.

Investigations (📖 p.75)
• Echocardiogram
• Chest X-ray
• CT scan of the chest
• Pulmonary function tests
• V/Q scan
• Measurement of blood oxygen by arterial blood gas (ABG).

Treatment
• Supplemental oxygen
• Diuretics
• Anticoagulants are sometimes prescribed.

Polycythaemia

Chronically low levels of oxygen in the circulation may result in an increase in the number of red blood cells (polycythaemia). The reduction in the oxygen content of the blood will lead to increased levels of the red cell growth factor erythropoietin which stimulates the marrow to produce more red cells. Whilst the increase in red blood cells increases the oxygen-carrying capacity of the blood, it also increases its viscosity and increases the risks of pulmonary embolism.

Signs and symptoms
• Headaches and blurred vision
• Skin may appear much redder in colour than normal (plethora).

Investigations and treatment
• A full blood count including haematocrit and packed cell volume (PCV)
• Patients with a haematocrit >47% in women or >52 in men should be investigated for hypoxaemia
• Venesection should be considered if the PVC is >60% in men or >55% in women.

Pneumothorax

In COPD pneumothorax may occur spontaneously, as a specific result of emphysematous bullae (📖 p.465).

Pulmonary emboli

If polycythaemia is not corrected, pulmonary emboli (PE) may result. (📖 p.475). The causes of PE in COPD patients include immobility due to breathlessness and increased viscosity of the blood, resulting in deep-vein thrombosis (DVT). DVT are highly unstable and prone to breaking up. The resulting emboli pass back to the heart and are pumped into the pulmonary circulation. These clots then cut off the blood supply to part of the lung. In the long term the cutting-off of multiple small pulmonary arteries increases the workload of the heart, resulting in worsening cor pulmonale, which may ultimately prove fatal.

Pulmonary hypertension

When areas of the lungs are poorly ventilated—V/Q mismatch—the alveolar capillary bed becomes constricted, causing increased pressure in the pulmonary vasculature. This is known as pulmonary hypertension (📖 p.481). The right ventricle has to work harder to pump an increased circulating volume of blood. Initially it will enlarge to compensate for the extra workload, but will eventually fail, increasing the peripheral oedema.

The development of pulmonary hypertension, secondary to COPD, is associated with an increased morbidity and mortality. Treatment is rarely directed specifically at pulmonary hypertension, but at the underlying COPD.

Palliative care

The management of severe COPD has a large palliative element and focuses on symptom control and optimizing quality of life (📖 p.336, 521). Patients with COPD should therefore be considered as having a terminal illness; the disease is progressive with no cure, so any treatment offered is essentially palliative.

The interval from diagnosis to death can be many years; so choosing the right moment to discuss the prognosis of the disease and the patient's views on issues such as ventilatory support or advance directives can be difficult. Predicting when death may occur is very difficult.

Predictors of poor prognosis are:
- Patients with an FEV_1 <40% of predicted
- Patients with cor pulmonale
- Patients with a low or falling BMI
- Patients who have frequent exacerbations.

The concerns and issues faced by a patient with COPD are very similar to patients who have other terminal diseases such as cancer or heart failure; and patients should be encouraged to address and discuss their feelings and needs.

Multidisciplinary team 1

Caring for patients with COPD requires a multidisciplinary approach to ensure that optimal care is delivered. The MDT will encompass professionals working in both primary and secondary care (📖 p.330).

The multidisciplinary team should consist of:

- Patient and their family
- Respiratory physician
- GP
- Respiratory nurse
- Practice nurse
- Community nurse/matron
- Physiotherapist
- Occupational therapist
- Dietician
- Community psychiatric nurse/psychologist
- Pharmacist
- Social worker.

Access to professional support varies according to what facilities are available locally to the patient. However, if optimal care and maximal therapeutic gain is to be achieved, all these practitioners should be included in the respiratory care team.

Multidisciplinary team 2

Table 9.1 Roles of members in the multidisciplinary team

Team member	Role
Respiratory physician and GP	• Assess patients and diagnose COPD • Manage acute exacerbations • Order further investigations such as lung function tests, radiology • Prescribe appropriate medication • Educate patients and other health professionals

Respiratory nurses including community matrons	• Assess patients including:
	  • Perform spirometry
	  • Assess the need for oxygen
	  • Assess inhaler technique
	  • Prescribe medication (qualified non-medical prescribers only)
	• Manage patients including:
	  • Non-invasive ventilation
	  • Hospital at home/early discharge schemes
	  • Palliative care
	• Identify and manage anxiety and depression
	• Advise patients on self-management strategies
	• Identify patients at risk of further exacerbations
	• Undertake activities aimed at preventing hospital admissions
	• Educate patients and other health professionals
	• Offer palliative care

Physiotherapist	• Teach the patient management techniques including sputum clearance and breathing control • Reduce patients' and carers' fears of exercise and breathlessness • Exercise training such as pulmonary rehabilitation to increase functional independence • Patient education—improving their knowledge and understanding of COPD and non-pharmacological symptom management and control
Occupational therapist	• Assess patients' lifestyle and their needs • Assist patients to achieve maximum independence in their day-to-day activities • Contribute to patient education
Dietician	• Provide effective, evidence based nutritional assessment, dietary support, and advice to patients • Contribute to patient education

Table 9.1 Roles of members in the multidisciplinary team (*Continued*)

Team member	Role

Community psychiatric nurse or psychotherapist	• Support patients in dealing with the feelings and emotions surrounding their chronic condition
	• Identify issues of poor self-esteem and motivation and offer approaches to therapy such as:
	  • Behavioural
	  • Cognitive
	  • Counselling
	• Detect, and encourage patients to obtain treatment for the depression and anxiety often associated with COPD
	• Provide advice on the use of relaxation and counselling for stress management
	• Provide education to encourage independence and compliance with therapy
	• Counsel patients who have problems with sexual relationships

Pharmacist	• Often the first port of call for those wishing to stop smoking; has a key role in providing advice as well as providing replacement therapy • Identify problems that patients are having in taking their medicines • Ensure that patients are receiving the appropriate level of pharmacological intervention for their disease severity and guarantee the patient's medication is reviewed frequently
Medical social worker	• Assess patients' housing for accessibility and the need for aids or adaptation • Assess patient suitability for a nursing home, residential care or a package of care within their own home • Provide patients with advice on claiming benefits • Provide patients with advice on support services available through social services and community nursing services

Self-management

Education

Patients should understand their disease and its treatment. Patients who understand what their management consists of are more likely to comply with their therapy. The areas that should be covered in a patient education programme are:

- Disease process including:
  - Clinical features
  - Lung function
- Treatment of COPD including:
  - Smoking cessation
  - Pharmacological therapy
- Supportive therapy
- Oxygen therapy including:
  - When it is used
  - Short and long-term therapy
  - Methods of supply and delivery
- Rehabilitation therapy including:
  - Physiotherapy
  - Breathing techniques
  - Exercise conditioning
  - Psychosocial support.

Self-management strategies

COPD is a progressive lifelong disease, and patients need to be able to function as best they can within the constraints of the disease. As the COPD progresses, patients become increasingly symptomatic. This often leads to an increase in dependence on others and may also lead to a loss in confidence unless they learn to adapt to their situation.

Any form of self-management must be individualized for the particular patient, addressing their fears and concerns. Individual goals need to be identified and the management plan written in concordance with the patient. The plan should focus on lifestyle changes and treatment changes.

Patients and their carers should be advised about any local self-help clubs such as 'Breathe Easy' clubs, run by the British Lung Foundation. These clubs are run by patients for patients. Breathe Easy is free to join and provides access to information leaflets and booklets. The network has 22,000 supporters and over 130 patient support groups.

Lifestyle changes

Lifestyle changes aim to avoid further damage to the airways and enhance the patient's ability to cope with disability. Lifestyle changes should be based on the individual goals of each patient and could include advice on:

- Smoking cessation and avoiding smoky environments
- Using nicotine replacement therapies as recommended
- Eating a balanced diet, including plenty of fruit and vegetables
- Having an annual influenza vaccine and a pneumococcal vaccination
- Performing a task using the least possible energy
- Working through a task slowly and steadily
- Sitting down as much as possible when carrying out a task
- Breathing out when performing the most strenuous part of the task
- Resting during and between tasks
- Alternating easy and strenuous tasks
- Breaking activities down into easily achievable parts
- Avoiding lifting
- Using controlled breathing throughout an activity.

A wide range of equipment is available to help patients with everyday tasks such as stair lifts, grab rails over the bath, and raised toilet seats.

Treatment changes

There is overwhelming evidence to support the use of self-management plans in asthma, but very little evidence to support the use of them in COPD. This may be because no large randomized trials have been undertaken. The NICE guidelines suggest that patients should be given advice on how to respond promptly to the symptoms of an exacerbation.

Patients are advised, in the event of an exacerbation, to:

- Start oral steroids if breathlessness increases and interferes with activities of daily living
- Start antibiotics if sputum becomes purulent
- Adjust bronchodilator therapy to control symptoms.

Patients who feel confident to manage their COPD should be prescribed a supply of prednisolone and antibiotics to keep at home for use as part of a self-management strategy. They should also be advised to increase their bronchodilators to help relieve their breathlessness. Patients should be advised to call for medical assistance if these measures are ineffective or they fail to improve. They should be provided with a written plan to remind them what to do in the event of an exacerbation, specifying how much medication to take and when, and emergency telephone contact numbers.

Further information
NICE COPD Guidelines (2004) http://www.nice.org.uk
GOLD COPD Guidelines (2003) http://www.goldcopd.com
Breathe Easy Clubs, run by the British Lung Foundation, http://www.lunguk.org
Quit (Smoking quitlines) http://www.quit.org.uk
British Thoracic Society http://www.brit-thoracic.org.uk
General Practice Airways Group (GPIAG) http://www.gpiag.org

Cystic fibrosis

Cystic fibrosis: an overview

The facts

Cystic fibrosis is the most common, life-threatening, and recessively inherited disease in the Western world. It results from a gene mutation on the long arm of chromosome 7 of which there are over a 1,000 identified mutations. It is estimated that cystic fibrosis affects 1:2500 Caucasians.

Aetiology

- The CF gene causes an abnormality in the production and function of a protein called the cystic fibrosis transmembrane conductance regulator (CFTR)
- Abnormal CFTR function leads to abnormal ion composition and relative dehydration of the surface liquid covering the epithelial cells
- The two major organs affected are the lungs and the gastrointestinal tract
- The clinical severity of CF varies between patients even with the same mutations in CFTR.

Pathology

Thick secretions produced by the epithelial cells cause:

- Obstruction in the small airways, which leads to recurrent chest infections and bronchiectasis
- Obstruction of the pancreatic duct, which causes destruction of the pancreas leading to pancreatic insufficiency
- Sinus disease
- Failure of embryological development of the vas deferens leading to infertility in male patients
- Bowel obstruction—meconium ileus and distal intestinal obstruction syndrome (DIOS).

Genetics

- CF is an inherited disease
- The abnormal gene is autosomal recessive
- Both parents must be carriers of the defective CF gene. See Box 10.1.

Screening

Anyone recognized as having high risk of having a baby with CF and in whom pregnancy is contemplated, or who has a newborn with CF, should be offered screening and early genetic advice. (See Box 10.2.)

Box 10.1 Genetic risk associated with CF

If both parents are carriers, their child has:

- A one in four chance of being born with CF.
- A two in four chance of being a carrier but not having CF.
- A one in four chance of not having CF or being a carrier of the defective gene.

Box 10.2 Screening tests to diagnose CF

- Carrier testing—This can be carried out either by a blood sample or mouth brushing.
- Antenatal testing—Via chorionic villus sampling (CVS) or amniocenteses—determines early in the pregnancy if the fetus has CF, usually offered to mothers recognized as being of high risk of having a child with CF (i.e. where both parents are carriers or there is a family history of CF)
- Neonatal testing—This is done on the heel-prick test (Guthrie) however not all regions are undertaking this at present.

Source: http://www.cftrust.org.uk

Clinical presentations and diagnosis of cystic fibrosis

Clinical presentation

Presentation with CF depends on the age of presentation and also on the phenotype of the disease.

- Typically CF presents in infancy with a combination of failure to thrive, steatorrhoea and respiratory symptoms
- 10–20% of patients present at birth with meconium ileus
- However, CF can present and be diagnosed at any age, adult males have been diagnosed at infertility clinics due to the absence of the vas deferens.

Confirmation of diagnosis

Diagnosis is made on clinical presentation together with a positive sweat test. See Box 10.3.

- All patients should be screened for known common CF gene mutations. This is known as genotyping
- Identification of two CF gene mutations is absolute confirmation of the diagnosis
- Neonatal screening for common CF mutations can be performed on the Guthrie test, which all new borns will have performed soon after birth. This is a simple heel-prick test
- Positive results can be further evaluated by examining the same blood spot for the presence of the common CF mutations.

Box 10.3 Sweat test

The sweat test is the standard method of diagnosis. First described by Gibson and Cooke (1959), this comprises three components:

- Sweat induction
- Sweat collection
- Sweat analysis

Sweat chloride interpretation (mmol/l)

<40	Normal–low probability of cystic fibrosis
40–60	Intermediate—suggestive but not diagnostic of cystic fibrosis
> 60	Elevated – supports the diagnosis of cystic fibrosis
Source:	Hill (1998)

Complications of cystic fibrosis 1

CF is a multisystemic disease with many complications.

Respiratory

- The respiratory tract can be colonized with one or more bacteria (see Box 10.4)
- These are treated with individual or combinations of antibiotics depending on the bacteria grown and antibiotic sensitivities. Aggressive treatment with intravenous antibiotics to treat a respiratory exacerbation is advised
- Antibiotics can be given as a prophylactic measure in an attempt to prevent rather than treat inevitable respiratory infections
- In the lungs, poor clearance of thick secretions leads to recurrent infection, bronchial damage, bronchiectasis and eventual death from respiratory failure. Box 10.5 illustrates disease progression.

Box 10.4 Pathogens affecting the respiratory tract in CF

Bacteria	*Staphylococcus aureus*
	Haemophilus influenzae
	Streptococcus pneumonia
	Pseudomonas aeruginosa
	Burkhoderia cepacia
	Mycobacterium tuberculosis
	Klebsiella pneumoniae
	Atypical mycobacterium
	Stenotrophomonas maltophilia
Fungi	*Aspergillus*

Gastrointestinal

- Gastro-oesophageal reflux and oesophagitis are common in CF
- This may be due to lung disease, oesophageal dysmotility and delayed gastric emptying
- Patients may be asymptomatic or present with anorexia, heartburn or reflux
- Patients may be prescribed proton pump inhibitors (PPI's) or H_2 receptor antagonists (H_2A) to alleviate symptoms.

Pancreatic complications

- Approximately 90% of patients will have pancreatic insufficiency (PI)
- PI leads to malabsorption and maldigestion
- Without efficient pancreatic enzyme replacement, malabsorption leads to steatorrhoea, malnutrition, and stunted growth, fat-soluble vitamin deficiency and delayed puberty
- Patients are therefore routinely given enzyme replacement and vitamins A, D, and E.

Bowel obstruction syndrome

- As a result of poor water flow, hyperconcentration of protein can occur and can lead to obstruction leading to DIOS
- Thick mucofaeculent material forms and obstructs the distal ileum, caecum and proximal colon
- It is reported to occur in 9–40% of patients[1]. The incidence appears to increase with age and is more common in adolescent and adult patients
- Treatment, if the patients is tolerating oral intake, is a balanced intestinal lavage solution. In some cases surgical intervention is necessary.

Hepatic complications

- Cirrhosis can occur arising from plugging of the small bile duct
- Patients with liver disease are often asymptomatic
- Splenomegaly, prominent abdominal veins, and a history of haematemesis suggests portal hypertension
- There is no proven therapy for liver disease, medications such as ursodeoxycholic acid can improve biochemical dysfunction but does not slow down progression
- The incidence of gallstones and other gallbladder disease is increased in CF. Some patients may require surgery to correct biliary problems.

1. Corway SP *et al.* (2003). Cystic Fibrosis in Children and Adults. The Leads Method of Management. Revised edition No. 6, Forest Laboratories UK Ltd.

Complications of cystic fibrosis 2

Reproductive complications

- Almost all males with cystic fibrosis are infertile as a result of absence of the vas deferens, preventing transport of sperm from the epididymis to the prostate
- Sexual performance remains unaffected
- The exact fertility status of women with cystic fibrosis is unclear. There is an increased chance of infertility due to increased thickness of cervical mucous, they are considered fertile and therefore require contraception; it is recommended that the contraceptive depot injection or a high oestrogen oral contraceptive pill be prescribed.

Cystic fibrosis-related diabetes (CFRD)

Due to increasing survival in CF, pancreatic destruction resulting in insulin deficiency and diabetes mellitus is increasingly recognized.

- Prevalence of CFRD increases with age and occurs in up to 30% by age 25 with the average age of onset being 18–25[2]. It is slightly more common in females
- CFRD is distinct from types I and II diabetes but has features of each.
- It is associated with insulinopenia and insulin resistance
- Ketoacidosis is unusual but can occur
- CFRD should be considered in patients with clinical decline and weight loss, and if undiagnosed can lead to decline in lung function.
- Some patients can have raised blood sugars only when unwell or when on corticosteroid therapy
- Conflicts between dietary therapy of CF (📖 p.306) and diabetes mellitus should be resolved in favour of the CF diet, i.e. they should not decrease their carbohydrate or fat intake
- All patients with CFRD need to be reviewed by a CF specialist dietitian on a regular basis. It is also advisable that patients are reviewed by a diabetologist at least annually
- CFRD is usually treated with insulin. Insulin therapy should be tailored to individual needs rather than diet tailored to insulin.

It is recommended that patients over the age of 10 years should be screened for CFRD via an oral glucose tolerance test. This is the most accurate way of diagnosing diabetes.

2. Cystic Fibrosis Trust (2004). Management of Cystic Fibrosis Related Diabetes Mellitus, http://www.cftrusts.org.uk/

Care and management of cystic fibrosis

Nutrition in CF

- Adequate nutrition is vital both for quality of life and long-term survival
- Patients require a high-energy diet, they should try to eat between 20–50% more kilocalories than the national recommendations for their age and sex
- Protein requirements are double the recommended adult intake with many patients
- As lung function deteriorates nutritional support needs to become more aggressive, this may include overnight nasogastric or gastrostomy tube feeding
- Enzyme replacement needs to be optimal at all times and it is extremely important that the CF specialist dietitian reviews patients regularly.

Care and management

Physiotherapy

- Thick sputum causes recurrent infections and progressive lung damage
- Physiotherapy aims to clear the sputum and minimise infection. See Box 10.5
- Reduced ability to exercise and breathlessness are features of progressive lung disease which physiotherapy can target
- CF patients can also suffer with joint pains especially back problems
- Females can suffer with stress incontinence due to weak pelvic floor muscles, probably caused by excessive coughing
- Physiotherapy techniques should be tailored to each patient's individual need
- There are several techniques used to assist in chest clearance. See Box 10.6)
- Timing of medication with chest physiotherapy is another important aspect, for example taking nebulized DNAse and bronchodilators before physiotherapy and nebulised antibiotics after chest physiotherapy
- Maintenance of cardiovascular fitness is important to keep limitation by breathlessness to a minimum
- Maintaining muscle strength and function oxygen to be used more effectively. It is important that a specialist CF physiotherapist sees all patients and assesses them regularly[3].

3. Cystic Fibrosis Trust (2002). Clinical Guidelines for the Physiotherapy Management of Cystic Fibrosis. http://www.cftrust.org.uk/.

Infection control

Owing to concerns about cross-infection between patients, the recommendations for patients with CF now include segregation according to microbiological status, not only in the clinic environment but also on the CF ward.

Antibiotics

Antibiotic courses in patients with CF are at higher doses and for longer than would be used for non-CF patients. The choice of antibiotic is normally on clinical response rather than *in vitro* resistance although sputum cultures may guide therapy. As a general guide:

- If patients are unwell or commencing a new antibiotic they should be admitted to hospital
- Many patients will be able to self-administer their antibiotics at home after training and supervision
- Antibiotics are usually given for 2 weeks but progress should be checked after the first week and the antibiotic altered if there is little evidence of a response.

Transition to adult care

- Teenagers are usually transferred from paediatric to adult care between the ages of 16–18
- Transition itself should be gradual, well planned and coordinated, with full involvement of the patient and family
- Interaction of parents and children with the adult team before transfer allows successful transition from paediatric to adult care.

Box 10.5 The aims of physiotherapy in CF

- To enable the patient to clear their chest as easily and effectively as possible with minimal coughing
- To improve or maintain their exercise levels
- To manage breathlessness
- To minimize joint pains
- To reduce or eliminate urinary incontinence.

Box 10.6 Physiotherapy techniques

- Active cycle of breathing—a combination of gentle deep breathing exercise and huffing (forced expiration) to break up and move sputum
- Autogenic drainage—a complicated technique involving breathing at different lung volumes to clear sputum from all parts of the lungs
- Flutter—a pipe-shaped device that causes vibrating airflow when deep breathing through it, breaking up the sputum
- PEP—device that produces a positive pressure when breathed through. This allows air to get behind sputum and move it
- Acapella—causes an oscillating, vibrating airflow, like the flutter, vibrations generated using a magnetic mechanism
- Postural drainage and percussion—especially with young children. Postural drainage involves lying in various positions using gravity to drain sputum. Percussion involves clapping the chest wall with a cupped hand. This dislodges sputum from the airway walls (usually combined with postural drainage).

Organization of care

Unfortunately specialist centres do not yet exist everywhere. The bulk of CF care should be undertaken by a specialist CF centre. If this is difficult due to lack of a local specialist multidisciplinary team, or the reluctance of the patient to travel long distances, patients are looked after via a shared care arrangement between a local hospital and major centre. However patients should always be reviewed at least annually at a specialist CF centre. Box 10.7 highlights the optimum CF multidisciplinary team.

Transplant

- Transplant should be considered when end-stage lung disease develops
- Around 90% of patients die from respiratory failure and home oxygen may be required
- Nocturnal non-invasive ventilation may be necessary as a bridge to transplant
- To be considered for transplant patients must meet a certain criteria (see Box 10.8)
- Transplantation in itself is regarded as a palliative procedure not a cure
- Mean waiting time from acceptance onto a transplant programme to transplant itself is 12–24 months and 50% of patients will die whilst waiting for organs.

Box 10.8 Transplant criteria in CF

- $FEV_1 \leq 30\%$ predicted (📖 p.75)
- Other important factors:
- Rate of decline in respiratory function
- Quality of life
- Increased need for intravenous therapy
- Poor weight profile.
Source: Egan et al. 2002[4]

End of life care (📖 p.290, 336, 521)

Even with optimal medical care, cystic fibrosis remains a life-limiting condition. The terminal stage can occur at any time from infancy to late adulthood. It is usually recognized by increased severity and frequency of respiratory exacerbations, which can lead to oxygen dependence and declining lung function. Emphasis on care changes from aggressive treatment regimes to those focusing on symptom control. Patients deserve a pain-free and dignified death. Whilst lung transplantation is an option in a few cases this will not be a reality for the majority of patients. However, the prospect of lung transplantation should never prevent good end of life care.

4. Egar TM *et al.* (2002). Long term results of lung transplantation for cystic fibrosis European J of Cardiothoracic Surgery, **22**, 602–9

The future
With the isolation of the faulty gene, research in the past decade has centred on gene therapy to replace the defect, research is still currently underway and the results awaited.

Acknowledgements
Cystic Fibrosis Multidisciplinary Team, Glenfield Hospital
Leicester

Useful addresses
Cystic Fibrosis Trust
11 London Road
Bromley
Kent
BR1 1BY
E-mail: enquiries @cftrust.org.uk
http://www.cftrust.org.uk
http://www.cysticfibrosismedicine.com

Box 10.7 The core CF team (📖 p.330)

Essential	Desired
Consultant physician	Specialist social worker
Clinical nurse specialist	Psychologist
Specialist physiotherapist	Pharmacist
Specialist dietitian	
Source: CF Trust Guidelines[5]	

---

5. Cystic Fibrosis Trust (2001). National Consensus Standards for the Nursing Management of Cystic Fibrosis. http://www.cftrust.org.uk/.

Diffuse parenchymal lung disease (interstitial lung disease)

Overview

The term diffuse parenchymal lung disease (DPLD) refers to an extensive range of lung diseases, sometimes also referred to as interstitial lung diseases, rather than referring to a single disease entity. Diffuse basically describes any widespread pulmonary disease process. These diseases are often grouped together because they have similarities in clinical presentation, radiographic changes, physiological features, and symptoms. Many of them are caused by injury to the lung resulting in chronic inflammation and ultimately to progressive scarring known as fibrosis. However, although these diseases have similarities they also have a variety of aetiologies, treatments and varying prognoses.

Presentation

The patient with DPLD often presents with chronic progressive dyspnoea on exertion and a cough which is often non-productive. The patient should be closely examined for symptoms of underlying connective tissue disease such as joint pains, erythema and swelling of the joints of the hands, which is indicative of rheumatoid arthritis and which may or may not have been previously diagnosed. Rate of onset of symptoms is very variable. Some patients present with long-standing radiological symptoms often found opportunistically, whilst other patients present with acute onset of symptoms with rapidly developing respiratory failure and death.

Clinical findings

On examination bilateral inspiratory crackles may be heard at the bases of the lungs. Wheeze is not often a presenting symptom unless there is also underlying airways disease. In sarcoidosis wheeze may be symptomatic of airways involvement.

Clubbing of the digits is common in the latter stages of the disease.

Diagnosis

Diagnosis is made from a combination of clinical findings, high-resolution cat scan (HRCT) and histology.

Common causes

There are many various causes of DPLD and some of the better known are listed below. Whilst a good history taking may reveal a possible cause, in many cases a definitive causative agent often cannot be found.

Occupational related
- Asbestosis
- Silicosis
- Pneumoconiosis
- Hard metal fibrosis
- Berylliosis
- Talc pneumoconiosis.

Hypersensitivity
- Wet hay (Farmer's lung)
- Birds (pigeon fanciers, bird fanciers)
- Fungi (mushroom picker's lung)
- Allergic reactions.

Connective tissue disease
- Rheumatoid arthritis
- Scleroderma
- Systemic lupus erythematosus
- Ankylosing spondylitis
- Mixed connective tissue disease
- Sjogren's syndrome.

Idiopathic
- Idiopathic pulmonary fibrosis/cryptogenic fibrosing alveolitis
- Sarcoidosis
- Bronchioitis obliterans-organizing pneumonia (BOOP)
- Adult respiratory distress syndrome (ARDS)
- Inflammatory bowel disease
- Hepatic cirrhosis
- Neurofibromatosis
- Lymhangioleiemyomatosis (LAM)
- Respiratory bronchiolitis.

Drug-induced
- Antibiotics (nitrofurantoin, sulfasalazine)
- Anti-inflammatory agents (gold, aspirin, penicillamine, methotrexate)
- Cardiovascular (amiodarone, tocainide)
- Chemotherapeutic (bleomycin, mitomycin-c, busulfan, cyclophosphamide, azathioprine, methotrexate, etoposide, vinblastine)
- Illicit drugs (heroin, methadone)
- Other agents (isoniazid, oxygen, radiation, talc).

Investigations

Spirometry

The DPLDs are by nature restrictive, so the pattern seen on spirometry ($\square$ p.75) is of a reduced FEV_1 and FVC but with a preserved FEV_1/FVC ratio; the result of smaller stiffer lungs. There may be an obstructive pattern if the patient is also a smoker. The alveolar–capillary interface is abnormal resulting in a decreased diffusing capacity for carbon dioxide. Stiff, poorly compliant lungs often means the patient desaturates on exercise and eventually will have hypoxaemia, type 1 respiratory failure, as the disease develops.

Blood tests

Blood tests may show both raised ESR and CRP, positive rheumatoid factor and/or ANA may show at low levels even in the absence of associated connective tissue disease. Some patients may also have a mild anaemia.

Chest X-ray

Although chest X-ray appearance can vary between the various diseases there is often bilateral reticular or reticulonodular opacities and generalized smaller lung volumes. Evidence of disease involvement and volume loss is often more prevalent in the bases of the lungs and this may make the hilar regions appear closer to the diaphragm than on a normal X-ray. If there is calcification along the pleura this may be suggestive of asbestos exposure. In the latter stages of the disease process multiple small cysts may be apparent reflecting end-stage fibrosis and often referred to as 'honeycombing'. Chest X-ray may appear normal in the early stages of the disease

High-resolution CT scan

CT scans will often demonstrate the peripheral nature of the disease and can help confirm clinical findings. Usual interstitial pneumonia (UIP) may show a patchy, heterogeneous distribution. A ground glass appearance is more indicative of non-specific interstitial pneumonia (NSIP) which has a better prognosis than UIP. Honeycombing is indicative of end-stage fibrosis.

Histology

Histology will confirm the diagnosis and the particular disease process, although diagnosis can be made in most cases on clinical and HRCT findings. Lung biopsy is not advocated in UIP. Histology may be important for treatment and more particularly for prognosis.

Some common DPLDs

Asbestosis

This is the result of exposure to asbestos which often has been many years prior to the patient presenting with symptoms. This exposure results in scarring of the lung parenchyma. Often the presentation is with dyspnoea on exertion and crackles may be heard especially in the lung bases on examination. The chest X-ray will show bilateral lower zone reticulonodular infiltrates and there may be pleural plaques

Chronic hypersensitivity pneumonitis

Chronic hypersensitivity pneumonitis (CHP) is commonly cause by exposure to organic antigens such as mouldy hay (farmer's lung), animal proteins common in pigeon fanciers'/bird fanciers' lung, fungi (mushroom pickers' lung), and bacteria and chemicals such as isocynates. Patients often develop progressive shortness of breath and presentation is more common in non-smokers than smokers. A typical chest X-ray shows bilateral reticulonodular infiltrates which may be in the upper lobes. The patients' environmental history is important to ascertain exposure and CHP often responds well to systemic corticosteroids and removal from the causative agent.

Drug-induced

If the interstitial disease is drug-induced it may resolve on cessation of the offending agent, but occasionally systemic corticosteroids are needed.

Non-specific interstitial pneumonia

NSIP describes a histological pattern rather than a specific disease entity. It is poorly understood, although it has a tendency to occur in a younger age group than UIP and has a better response to corticosteroids and therefore a better prognosis.

Pneumoconiosis

Pneumoconioses develop as a consequence of the chronic inhalation of mineral dusts such as coal dust or organic dusts over the years. There may be multiple small opacities on the chest X-ray but the patient is often asymptomatic unless they develop progressive fibrosis.

Sarcoidosis

This is an idiopathic multisystemic inflammatory disorder which commonly involves the lung, although not all patients have lung involvement. Sarcoidosis has a characteristic inflammatory process where the inflammatory cells collect in microscopic nodules known as granulomas. It is more common in young adults and can spontaneously resolve or follow a benign course. Although patients may often be asymptomatic abnormalities may be incidental and found on chest X-ray, showing bilateral hilar lymphadenopathy without parenchymal opacities. Systemic corticosteroids are use in symptomatic patents commonly for cough, chest pain, wheezing, and dyspnoea.

Silicosis

Silicosis requires exposure to silica over many years and the disease can present in an acute and accelerated form when the exposure is more intense. The occupations in which silica is a likely causative agent are mining, tunnelling, foundry work and sandblasting. A chest X-ray often shows upper zone small nodular opacities which may merge together. There may also be enlargement and calcification of the hilar lymph nodes. Some patients have very few symptoms and may only have minor impairment on lung function testing.

Usual interstitial pneumonia

Also known as idiopathic pulmonary fibrosis (IPF) or cryptogenic fibrosing alveolitis. This is perhaps one of the commonest diseases in this category of diseases. It is most common in patients in their 50s to 70s and there may in some cases be a family history, although often there is no familial link. It is also a lung disease that does not have a causal link with tobacco smoking. Patients with IPF develop progressive dyspnoea on exertion and a non-productive cough. There may be evidence of slowly progressive disease before a diagnosis is possible. There are relatively few treatments with around 50% of patients responding either physiologically or subjectively to prednisolone, azathioprine, cyclophosphamide or colchicines. However, this often merely slows disease progression and the median survival is around 3–5 years from diagnosis.

Treatments

Pharmacological

Corticosteroids

These are often the treatment of choice for many types of DPLD. As the diseases demonstrate an uncontrolled inflammatory process an anti-iinflammatory may appear to be the logical choice, but not all patients respond to this treatment and the side-effects can be as problematic to the patient as the effects of treatment. There is little evidence for length of treatment and this will vary from a few weeks or months or a few years depending on response to treatment. As individual responses vary patients require monitoring for responses to treatment and side-effects.

Cytotoxic agents

A variety of cytotoxic medications have been tried in the management of DPLD. These include azathioprine, ciclosporin and cyclophosphamide, all of which have anti-inflammatory properties and are considered more potent than steroids. Side-effects include depression of the immune system, so patients require close monitoring.

Colchicine

This is an antifibrotic medicine that has been used previously to treat gout and may be a useful treatment for DPLDs.

N-acetylcysteine (NAC)

There is some evidence for trying NAC as an antioxidant to treat free radical, oxidant damage.

Oxygen therapy

The result of many DPLDs is hypoxaemia. Oxygen therapy is widely used in the treatment although there is little evidence of its benefits. It is recommended that oxygen is given for generalized hypoxaemia, hypoxia on exercise and during sleep if clinically indicated. Maintenance of a patient's oxygen levels prevents secondary hypertension and the development of cor pulmonale. Patients are often considered for oxygen at an earlier stage than would usually be recommended for patients with COPD for example.

Pulmonary rehabilitation

Although not yet extensively studied as distinct group, rehabilitation may help in maintaining the fitness of patients with a DPLD and they may benefit from contact with other patients.

Transplantation

This is a last resort for end-stage disease although there are problems with availability of organs and the fact that in the connective tissue disorders the outcome of transplantation is not as good as in other diseases. Patients may also have concomitant disease which precludes transplantation.

Prognosis

For many patients with DPLD the disease is progressive, leading to end-stage disease and eventually death. Unfortunately there are currently few available treatments, and treatment is frequently more trial and error rather than having a good body of evidence behind it. Treatments often only result in temporary improvement or slower progression of the disease and individual response is not predictable. Other possible causes of symptoms such as increasing dyspnoea should be considered in treatment options (Box 1).

Nursing Care

The nursing role in caring for patients with a DPLD is essentially that of good palliative care.

- Information. The patient and their carers should be fully informed of both the diagnosis and prognosis although the prognosis of many of these diseases is poor
- Monitoring. Of response to treatment and also for side-effects of medication. Azathioproine and other cytotoxic treatments will require regular blood tests to monitor renal function
- Symptom control especially for cough and breathlessness:
  - Cough may be treated with codeine, or pholcodine, but patients need to be aware of side-effects such as constipation
  - Morphine may help both breathlessness and cough in the later stages of the disease but again there are side effects
- Panic and anxiety are commonplace with any lung disease that causes breathlessness. Lorazepam 0.5mg used sublingually (unlicensed use in UK) may dissipate the effects of anxiety and is rapidly absorbed by the mucous membranes
- Oxygen therapy. Hypoxaemia and type 1 respiratory failure may mean oxygen is necessary. Patients with DPLD typically do not retain carbon dioxide and therefore can tolerate high flow rates which may be necessary as the condition deteriorates. Oxygen saturations should be monitored regularly and changes of flow rates made appropriately
- Prophylaxis for corticosteroid therapy—bisphosphonates and calcium vitamin D supplementation should be considered
- Benefits advice and use of the DS1500 for terminal disease may help to alleviate some of the financial problems encountered in terminal disease
- Transplant. For those patients considered for transplantation, many physical, psychological, social, and emotional issues may arise which need handling sensitively
- End of life decisions should be discussed with the patient and carers as decisions on preferred place of death and required support will need to be discussed. If the patients' general practice has signed up to the gold standard for palliative care these patents are appropriate for inclusion on the register.

Alternative Causes of Dysponea

- Superimposed infection
- Muscle weakness/osteoporosis due to steroid therapy
- Pulmonary embolism
- Lung cancer
- Atherosclerotic vascular disease.

The nurses' role

The diagnosis of DPLD is often distressing for the patients and in general there is little hope of cure with a bleak prognosis. Symptoms, particularly shortness of breath and cough, are distressing for patients.

Key points

- A diverse group of illnesses with a varied aetiology, treatment and prognosis
- Presenting symptoms are often progressive breathlessness on exertion and cough which is often non productive
- Diagnosis is dependent on history, clinical findings, X-ray/HRCT, blood results and histology
- Lung function usually gives a restrictive pattern although in a patient who also smokes there may also be obstruction
- Treatments include corticosteroids, cytotoxic agents and oxygen.

Lung cancer

Epidemiology

Incidence
- Lung cancer is the most common cancer in the UK, and the most common cause of cancer death
- Each year there are approximately 35,000 new cases
- Average length of survival from diagnosis is 6–9 months
- Only 25% of patients are alive at 12 months
- The number of men affected is falling, but the number of women is rising
- More women die of lung cancer than breast cancer
- It mostly affects people in their 60s and 70s, the median age at death is 72 years.

Causes
- 90% is smoking related
- Stopping smoking decreases the risk, but the risk remains higher than for people who have never smoked
- Passive smokers have a higher risk
- Some evidence shows that the risk of lung cancer is higher in people exposed to asbestos, arsenic, and heavy metals.

Risk factors
- All current and ex-smokers
- Patients with chronic obstructive pulmonary disease (COPD)
- People who have been exposed to asbestos
- People with a previous history of cancer, especially head and neck
- People who have been exposed to radon.

Types of lung cancer

There are two main types of lung cancer:

Non-small cell lung cancer (NSCLC)

NSCLC is classified further into histological type:
- Squamous cell lung cancer—the commonest type
- Adenocarcinoma
- Large cell
- Bronchial alveolar cell (BAC)—the least common.

NSCLC accounts for 75–80% of all lung cancers. Only 15–20% of patients with NSCLC are potentially suitable for curative treatment.

For patients with advanced disease chemotherapy is offered with response rates ranging from 20–40% and median survival is about 8–10 months.

Small cell lung cancer (SCLC)

This accounts for 20–25% of all lung cancers. It has usually spread by the time of diagnosis. There is frequently a secondary spread to the bone, liver, adrenals, and head. Surgery is usually not appropriate.

SCLC is usually sensitive to chemotherapy and radiotherapy. Untreated extensive small cell lung cancer is rapidly progressive, and survival is about 6 weeks.

Presenting symptoms and referral guidelines

The National Institute for Health and Clinical Excellence (NICE) has produced referral guidelines for patients with a suspected cancer. The following are for suspected lung cancer.

Refer a patient who presents with symptoms suggestive of lung cancer to a team specializing in the management of lung cancer.

Immediate referral

- Signs of superior vena caval obstruction: swelling of the face, neck, and arms
- Stridor (noisy or 'hard' breathing).

Urgent referral:

- Persistent haemoptysis (in smokers or ex-smokers aged 40 years and older)
- A chest X-ray suggestive of lung cancer
- A normal chest X-ray where there is a high suspicion of lung cancer
- A history of asbestos exposure and recent onset of chest pain, short-ness of breath or unexplained systemic symptoms, where a chest X-ray indicates pleural effusion, pleural mass or any suspicious abnormality.

Urgent chest X-ray

- Haemoptysis
- Unexplained or persistent (longer than 3 weeks): (p.31)
  - Chest and/or shoulder pain
  - Breathlessness
  - Weight loss
  - Chest signs
  - Hoarseness
  - Finger clubbing
  - Cervical or supraclavicular lymphadenopathy
  - Cough
  - Features suggestive of secondaries from a lung cancer (e.g. brain, bone, liver, skin)
- Underlying chronic respiratory problems with unexplained changes in symptoms.

Further information
http://www.nice.org.uk

Investigations (📖 p.75)

Chest X-ray
This is usually abnormal by the time the patient has symptoms. A normal chest X-ray does not exclude lung cancer.

Blood tests
Full blood count, liver function tests (lactate dehydrogenase [LDH] can be raised in lung cancer), urea and electrolytes, and calcium.

Spirometry
Used to assess respiratory function and eligibility for radical treatment.

Pleural aspiration
If the chest X-ray shows it and/or the patient has clinical signs of a pleural effusion.

Fine needle aspiration
If the supraclavicular or cervical nodes are enlarged.

CT scan of the chest and abdomen
This allows small/equivocal changes on a chest X-ray to be shown in more depth. It shows the position and size of tumours more precisely, and helps assess whether the patient is appropriate for bronchoscopy. A CT scan can help to target tumours for bronchoscopy, and it demonstrates enlarged lymph nodes and any invasion by the tumour into the chest wall and mediastinum.

Diagnostic procedures

Further diagnostic and staging procedures may be inappropriate if the patient is too frail, has advanced disease or comorbidity, or does not wish to pursue further investigations or treatment.

Fibreoptic bronchoscopy

This is a method of obtaining a diagnosis through washings, brushings and/or biopsy. Transbronchial needle aspiration of the lymph nodes can be performed to aid staging. Tumour position at bronchoscopy may aid operative decisions.

Positron emission tomography (PET) scanning

PET scanning uses low-dose radioactive glucose solution to 'label' radioactive tissues, such as tumours. These show as a 'hot spot' on the scan. This improves the rate of detection of local and secondary spread from the tumour. All patients who are being referred for radical treatment should have had a PET scan as part of their staging.

Bone scan

This is indicated if there is any evidence of secondary spread to the bones. If the patient has bony pain, pathological fracture or hypercalcaemia; for example

CT head

This is indicated if there is any evidence of secondary spread to the head. The patient has persistent vomiting and/or nausea, dizziness, headaches, numbness or loss of mobility, blurred vision, fits, personality change or unexplained confusion; for example

CT or ultrasound guided biopsy

This may be a biopsy of the tumour, or a biopsy of enlarged lymph nodes, especially in the neck.

Mediastinoscopy

This is a small invasive procedure done under general anaesthetic, where a biopsy is taken of enlarged mediastinal lymph nodes to determine whether they are inflammatory or malignant. A biopsy of lymph nodes which are not enlarged but have shown up 'hot' on a PET scan can also be performed.

Medical or surgical thorascopy

This may be required to determine whether a pleural effusion contains malignant or inflammatory cells. If malignant cells are identified then the patient is not eligible for surgery.

Staging

The stage of lung cancer is a term used to describe the tumour's size, position and any secondary disease. Staging for small cell lung cancer and non-small cell lung cancer is different.

Small cell lung cancer

This is divided into two stages:

- Limited disease—the cancer can only be seen in one lung, with or without a pleural effusion, and with or without supraclavicular lymph nodes
- Extensive disease—the cancer has spread outside of the lung to other parts of the body.

Non-small cell lung cancer

NCSLC is classified using the TNM staging system (see Figure 12.1).

Extent of primary tumour (T)

Tx	Primary tumour cannot be assesed, or tumour proven by presence of malignant cells in sputum or bronchial washings but not visualized by imaging or bronchoscopy
T0	No evidence of primary tumour
Tis	Carcinoma in situ
T1	Tumour <3cm surrounded by lung or visceral pleura, without bronchoscopic evidence of invasion more proximal than the lobar bronchus
T2	Tumour >3cm, or in main bronchus, >2cm distal t o carina or invading visceral pleura or associated with atelectasis or obstructive pneumonitis that extends to the hilar region, but does not involve whole lung
T3	Tumour of any size which invades chest wall, diaphragm, parietal pericardium, mediastinal pleura, or tumour in main bronchus < 2cm distal to carina, or associated atelectasis or obstructive pneumonitis of the entire lung
T4	Tumour of any size invading: mediastinum, heart, great vessels, trachea, oesophagus, carina, vertebral body, or separate nodules in the ipsilateral lobe as primary tumour, or malignant pleural or pericardial effusion

Regional lymph nodes (N)

Nx	Cannot be assessed
N0	No regional lymph node metastasis
N1	Ipsilateral peribronchial and/or ipsilateral hilar nodes and intra-pulmonary nodes involved by direct extension of tumour
N2	Ipsilateral mediastinal and/or subcarinal nodes
N3	Contralateral mediastinal, hilar nodes, or any scalene or supra-clavicular nodes

Distant metastasis (M)

Mx	Cannot be assessed
M0	No distant metastasis
M1	Distant metastasis present, including separate nodules in different lobes

Fig. 12.1 TNM staging of lung cancer (American Joint Committee on Cancer and the Union Internationale Contre le Cancer).

Reproduced from Chapman S, Robinson G, Stradling J, and West S, Oxford Handbook of Respiratory Medicine, 2005, Chapter 18, TNM Staging of Lung Cancer, 144–145 with permission from Oxford University Press.

Multidisciplinary teams (MDT)

The care of all patients with a working diagnosis of lung cancer should be discussed at a lung cancer MDT meeting. MDT's are especially appropriate for the management of lung cancer, as input from many different health professionals is needed. The MDT can reduce delays in the cross-referral between specialists.

The MDT team should include a chest physician, radiologist, thoracic surgeon, pathologist, oncologist, lung cancer nurse specialist, and palliative care specialist.

Breaking bad news

Most patients want two things:
- A certain amount of information (the right amount). All patients diagnosed with lung cancer should be offered information, both verbal and written, on all aspects of their diagnosis, treatment, and care. This information should be tailored to the individual requirements of the patient—audio and videotaped formats can be considered
- The opportunity to talk and think about their situation. When breaking bad news it is important that trust is maintained between the patient and doctor. This reduces uncertainty, prevents inappropriate hope, allows appropriate adjustment, and prevents a conspiracy of silence that destroys family communication and prevents mutual support
- Treatment options and plans should be discussed with the patient, and decisions on treatment and care should be made jointly. Treatment plans must be tailored around the patient's needs, their wish to be involved, and their capacity to make decisions.

Performance status

Treatment for lung cancer is often determined by the performance status of a patient. Performance status is an attempt to quantify a patient's general well-being. It is a measure of how well a patient is able to perform ordinary tasks and carry out daily activities.

---

0 = Fully active, able to carry on all pre-disease performance without restriction

1 = Restricted in physically strenuous activity but ambulatory and able to carry out work of a light or sedentary nature, e.g. light house work, office work

2 = Ambulatory and capable of all self-care but unable to carry out any work activities. Up and about more than 50% of waking hours

3 = Capable of only limited self-care, confined to bed or chair more than 50% of waking hours

4 = Completely disabled. Cannot carry on any self-care. Totally confined to bed or chair.

Fig. 12.2 ECOG performance status

As published in Am. J. Clin. Oncol.: Oken M.M., Creech, R.H., Tormey, D.C., Horton, J., Davis, T.E., McFadden, E.T., Carbone, P.P. (1982) Toxicity and response criteria of the Eastern Cooperative Oncology Group. *Am J Clin Oncol* **5**: 649–655 Reproduced with permission from the Eastern Operative Oncology Group, Robert Comis M.D., Group Chair.

Treatment options: small cell lung cancer (SCLC)

Surgery

Limited SCLC may benefit from surgical resection, if there is no evidence of secondary disease. This is very rare, and patients should have a head CT and bone scan prior to a decision. Patients having surgery should also be considered for postoperative chemotherapy and/or radiotherapy, especially if the diagnosis of lung cancer is made from the surgery.

Chemotherapy

Combination chemotherapy is used for limited and extensive stage SCLC.

- Give three times weekly, 4–6 cycles depending on response
- Different regimes are selected depending on performance status
- Patients are carefully assessed; if there are no signs of a response to treatment based on the chest X-ray or CT scan, or if the patient is not coping with the side-effects of treatment, they are switched to second line therapies or the treatment is discontinued
- 80–90% of patients respond in limited disease; 60–80% in extensive disease
- Chemotherapy may increase survival to 14 months in limited disease.

Concurrent chemoradiation

Concurrent chemoradiation is used for patients with a good performance status with limited SCLC. Combination chemotherapy is given as above with concurrent radiotherapy commencing with cycle 2 of the chemotherapy regime. This is followed by 10 fractions of prophylactic cranial irradiation (PCI).

Radiotherapy

- Patients with limited disease, who are reasonably fit and obtain a partial or good response, should go on to have consolidation radiotherapy to their chest
- Prophylactic cranial radiotherapy is advised at completion of chemotherapy. This improves survival by about 5.4%
- Patients often find that radiotherapy gives them more side effects than the chemotherapy. They can become extremely 'washed out' by the time it is completed
- Chemotherapy is given first to patients with extensive disease or a poor performance status. If there is a good response, palliative radiotherapy may be given on an individual patient basis.

Treatment options: non-small cell lung cancer

Surgery

The aim of surgery in a patient with NSCLC is to completely excise the tumour, with minimal effect on their respiratory function. The type of surgery, as with the other treatments, depends on the staging of the lung cancer.

- Stage 1 and 2 tumours are usually amenable to surgery. This has a high chance of cure in stage 1 (70% in 1a) and a reasonable chance in stage 2
- In stage 3 tumours, surgery alone is unlikely to be curative, but adjuvant chemotherapy (after surgical treatment) or radiotherapy can improve survival rates
- Stage 3b and 4 are inoperable.

Types of surgery

- Lobectomy or bilobectomy—for localized tumours
- Pneumonectomy—for tumour involving more than one or two lobes
- A radical lobectomy or a pneumonectomy—if hilar nodes are involved with the tumour
- Wedge resection—removes only the tumour, with minimal surrounding lung tissue
- Sleeve resections involving a lobectomy, and the removal of a section of bronchus affected by the tumour—this may avoid a pneumonectomy
- Chest wall resection—if there has been limited local tumour invasion with a 5cm margin.

Chemotherapy

- Adjuvant (postoperative)chemotherapy is now offered to patients with a good performance status (0–2) with stage 1b–2 disease
- Is considered in patients with stage 3 to stage 4 disease, whose performance status is 0–2, even if they are asymptomatic from their cancer
- 40% of patients respond temporarily to chemotherapy
- Chemotherapy results in improvements in quality of life and symptom control, compared to best supportive care
- Combination chemotherapy (using more than one drug) is better than single-agent chemotherapy
- Commonly used drugs are gemcitabine or vinorelbine with a platinum-based drug, usually given for four cycles
- Patients are carefully assessed. If there are no signs of response to treatment based on a chest X-ray or a CT scan, or if they are not coping with the side-effects of the treatment, they are prescribed second-line therapies or treatment is discontinued
- Patients with limited disease who are reasonably fit and obtain a partial or good response, should go on to have consolidation radiotherapy to their chest disease
- If patients relapse more than 6 months after their initial chemotherapy has finished, they can be rechallenged with the same chemotherapy.

Radiotherapy

May be given to patients for:
- Curative intent (high dose or radical)
- Palliative control (high dose)
- Symptom relief (low dose).

Curative intent
- CHART (continuous hyperfractionated accelerated radiotherapy) is high-dose radiotherapy. It involves small radiation doses 3 times a day for 12 days. Patients are often admitted to hospital for this treatment. It is not available in all UK centres
- Conventional radical radiotherapy is given once a day for twenty days
- Side effects are dysphagia, fatigue and 'flu-like' symptoms. Patients should be warned that any breathlessness and cough may become temporarily worse after their treatment.

High dose palliative radiotherapy
- Given to patients with symptomatic disease who have a good performance status
- Given to patients who have no evidence of secondary disease
These regimes vary throughout the UK.

Low dose radiotherapy
- Given for symptom relief in patients unable to tolerate high doses
- Symptoms include pain, haemoptysis, breathlessness or cough.

Urgent radiotherapy
- Given in combination with oral steroids for the relief of superior vena cava obstruction, or spinal cord compression.

Palliative care

Palliative care is defined as the total care of patients whose disease is not responsive to curative treatment. It aims to provide the best quality of life for patients, their carers and their families. It includes controlling pain and other physical symptoms, as well as caring for the psychological, social and spiritual problems.

Supportive and palliative care of the lung cancer patient should be provided by general and specialist palliative care practitioners.

Patients who may benefit from specialist palliative care services should be identified and referred without delay. This works well when a member of the lung cancer multidisciplinary team (MDT) is from a specialist palliative care provider.

Breathlessness

Breathlessness is an uncomfortable awareness of breathing. Breathlessness can be present in up to 70% of patients with lung cancer in the last few weeks before death, and is severe in 25% of patients in their last week of life.

Signs and symptoms
- Increased respiratory rate
- Tachycardia
- Fatigue
- Peripheral cyanosis
- Reduced mobility
- Reduced ability to perform daily activities
- Mouth breathing.

Interventions
- If reversal of the cause of breathlessness is inadequate or impossible, then palliative management is needed. Non-drug interventions based on psychosocial support, breathing control and coping strategies should be considered
- Breathlessness is frightening to the patient, their family and staff. Reassurance and explanation are vital parts of the treatment, whatever the cause
- Modification of lifestyle, breathing retraining and relaxation may be beneficial if instituted early enough
- Consider referral to a physiotherapist
- A table fan directed onto the face often eases breathlessness
- Good mouth care is important if there is persistent mouth breathing
- Oxygen may help acute breathlessness, but it should be used alongside other measures and its use reviewed regularly
- Long-term oxygen therapy for chronic respiratory illness should only be instigated by respiratory physicians
- Many patients requiring palliation for breathlessness will not benefit from oxygen therapy.

Drugs to consider

- All drugs for the symptomatic relief of breathlessness are respiratory sedatives. When prescribed, their use should be monitored carefully. In the context of distressing breathlessness in the terminal stages of illness, the benefits usually outweigh the risks
- Opioids—give oral morphine (normal release) 2.5mg starting dose for all who are breathless, if opioid naive or elderly. Gradually titrate dose according to response, or until unacceptable side-effects occur. If the patient is already taking a strong opioid for analgesia, contact the specialist palliative care team for advice
- Benzodiazepines—lorazepam 0.5mg–1mg (unlicensed use in UK) sublingually may give rapid relief during panic attacks
- For longer-term management consider oral diazepam 2mg bd/od. Midazolam 2.5mg initially subcutaneously may benefit patients who cannot tolerate oral/sublingual route
- Breathlessness management techniques are set out in the following booklets and CD/DVD's produced by Cancerbackup (2006), The Roy Castle Foundation (2005) and Macmillan Cancer Support (2003).

Further information:

Lung Cancer: A Practical Guide to Breathlessness. From the Roy Castle LC Foundation http://www.roycastle.org.

Take a Breather. This video/dvd demonstrates practical techniques to help people with lung cancer cope with breathlessness.

Contact http://www.roycastle.org or 0800 358 7200.

Breathlessness

Contact http://www.cancerbackup.org.uk or 020 7739 2280.

Relax and Breathe. This CD helps people learn to manage breathlessness. Contact http://www.macmillan.org.uk or 0808 808 2020.

Pain

Definition
Pain is an unpleasant sensation caused by noxious stimulation of the sensory nerve endings. It is a subjective feeling with an individual response to the cause. It is a personal experience with physical, psychological, social and spiritual dimensions.

Signs and symptoms
- Local tenderness, swelling, inflammation and/or guarding of affected area
- Restlessness, irritability, disturbed sleep, reduced functioning, inability to focus the mind
- Calling out, or crying
- Reduced appetite
- Reduced interaction with other people
- Depression
- Acute pain—signs of sympathetic overactivity (such as increased blood pressure).

Interventions
- Establish a relationship with the patient
- Assess the individual including:
  - Nature of pain
  - Location of pain
  - History of pain
  - Frequency and duration of pain
- Consider possible reasons for the pain—local progression or secondary disease or other pathology which may be occurring
- Review present analgesics or instigate analgesic ladder (see below) and discuss with the medical team
- Further investigation and anti cancer treatment may be needed
- Consider the use of complimentary therapies if the patient wishes.

Analgesic ladder

Step 1
- Non-steroidal anti-inflammatory drugs (NSAIDs)
- Paracetamol +/– adjuvant analgesics, and aspirin.

Step 2
- Paracetamol plus:
  - Codeine (e.g. co-codamol)
  - Dihydrocodeine (e.g. co-dydramol)
  - +/– adjuvant analgesics.

Step 3
- Strong opioids e.g.
- Morphine
- Diamorphine
- +/– adjuvant analgesics.

The analgesic ladder progresses logically from a non-opioid via a weak opioid to a strong opioid. Start at the bottom of the ladder and work up as necessary. Use the drugs at their optimal dose regularly, i.e. by the mouth, by the clock, by the ladder.

Paracetamol has a different analgesic effect from opioids and may provide additional benefit for patients taking strong opioids.

If the pain is difficult to control, discuss with the patient and medical team and refer to the specialist palliative care team.

What if opioids don't work?

Is the dose high enough?

If there is a partial response, or an inadequate duration of pain relief (that is, if the pain returns in less than 4 h for oral morphine or under 12 h for modified release morphine), increase the dose by 30–50% increments rather than shorten the interval between doses. Remember to check that the prn dose (as required) prescribed is still adequate.

Is the drug being absorbed?

If there is uncontrolled vomiting or dysphagia, consider alternative routes of delivery (e.g. subcutaneous, rectal, intravenous, transdermal).

Is pain breaking through with movement or painful procedures?

Identify and minimize provoking factors. Consider additional doses of morphine, consider NSAIDs. Discuss with specialist palliative care team.

Are co-analgesics required?

Please see below for indications.

Nerve blocks

In 5–10% of cases, some kind of nerve block will help (e.g. coeliac plexus block in pancreatic pain). Discuss with specialist palliative care or pain clinic colleagues.

Co-analgesics

Many of these are unlicensed use.

• NSAIDs. Common indications for use—bone pain, musculoskeletal pain, liver capsule pain, pelvic pain
• Corticosteroids. Common indications for use—raised intracranial pressure, nerve or spinal cord compression, liver capsule pain
• Anticonvulsants. Common indications for use—neuropathic pain
• Antidepressants. Common indications for use—neuropathic pain and useful if patient is also depressed
• Muscle relaxants. Common indications for use—painful muscle spasms
• Anxiolytics. Common indications for use—anxiety which can increase pain.

Further information:
The Protocol for the Provision of Lung Cancer Nurse Specialist Support and Follow Up for Patients with Lung Cancer. Available at http://www.yorkshire-cancer-net.org.uk/html/publications/clinical_lung.

Role of the lung cancer nurse specialist

All cancer units or centres should have one or more trained lung cancer nurse specialist. They will see patients before and after diagnosis, provide continuing support, and facilitate communication between the secondary care team (including the MDT, the GP, the community team, and the patient). Their role includes helping patients to access advice and support whenever they need it.

Emotional support

Coping and living with lung cancer can be a challenge. In addition to the medical issues, people with lung cancer deal with emotional issues such as uncertainty, guilt, loss, and fear.

There is often a huge sense of guilt if people have been smokers; frequently this is what will have prevented them seeking advice about their symptoms.

The emotional and psychological burden of lung cancer should be considered as important as the physical symptoms, and support should be offered.

Support groups and patient networks can be helpful for people when they feel alone or upset. Cancer support groups can enable people with lung cancer to share experiences of living with the disease with others in a similar position.

Patient support networks

http://www.cancerbackup.org.uk contains over 4500 pages of accurate, up to date information on all aspects of cancer. Allows you to send questions to specialist cancer nurses.

http://www.britishlungfoundation.com help and support for people with lung disease and breathlessness.

http://www.roycastle.org gives information about lung cancer, treatments, and research. Has a database of all lung cancer nurse specialists in the UK.

http://lchelp.org a website for people with lung cancer, their families and friends.

http://www.lungcancersurvivors.org caters for the needs of lung cancer patients, and may be a good support for newly diagnosed patients. Much of the factual information comes from the American Cancer Society.

http://www.ncrn.org.uk a database of all national cancer research trials.

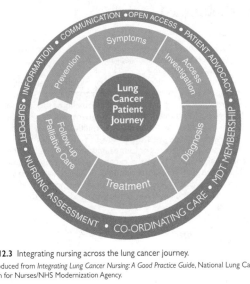

Fig. 12.3 Integrating nursing across the lung cancer journey.

Reproduced from *Integrating Lung Cancer Nursing: A Good Practice Guide*, National Lung Cancer Forum for Nurses/NHS Modernization Agency.

Further information

http://www.modern.nhs.uk/cancer/lung

http://www.nlcfn.co.uk

Mesothelioma 1

Introduction

The word 'mesothelioma' appeared in print in 1931 accredited to Klemperer and Rabin, yet a consensus acknowledging it as a primary neoplasm was not reached until the 1960s.

Mesothelioma is a fatal malignant disease of mesothelial elements within tissues. Principally it affects the pleura and peritoneum but can also occur in the pericardial pleura and testis. Whilst mesothelioma is not lung cancer, it usually involves the thoracic cavity and patients with the disease are therefore often managed by the lung cancer multidisciplinary team.

Pleural mesothelioma causes the pleura to thicken. This thickening of the pleura might begin to press onto the lungs or attach itself to the inside of the chest wall. In either case the expansion of the lung becomes progressively restricted by the tumour. A pleural effusion commonly occurs and sometimes several litres can collect between the two layers of the pleura; this affects the lungs' ability to expand and causes the person to feel breathless.

The peritoneum also has two layers: the inner (visceral) layer which is next to the abdominal organs, and the outer (parietal) layer which lines the abdominal wall.

Peritoneal mesothelioma causes the peritoneum to thicken and often causes ascites.

Incidence

The incidence of mesothelioma in the UK has been increasing rapidly since the late 1960s when the mesothelioma register, which offered a system for recording cases, first began. Currently in the UK approximately 2000 people a year are diagnosed with mesothelioma, and there is approximately one case of peritoneal mesothelioma to every twelve cases of pleural mesothelioma. It is predicted there will continue to be an annual increase in the number of mesothelioma victims. The peak in numbers is expected to be around 1950–2450 deaths per year, and this will occur around 2011–2015.

Causes

Currently it is accepted that around 80% of people who develop mesothelioma have had occupational or environmental exposure to asbestos.

It can take many years after being exposed to asbestos for mesothelioma to occur. The length of time taken is referred to as the latency period. This is rarely less than 15 years and often exceeds 60 years.

Symptoms

Pleural and peritoneal mesothelioma can both cause general symptoms such as sweating, fatigue, loss of appetite, and weight loss. Pleural mesothelioma typically causes patients to feel breathless and/or experience chest pain.

Breathlessness may be due to a combination of factors. The pleura being thickened can act like a rind around the lung, restricting its movement and preventing the lung from expanding. A pleural effusion may also accumulate in the space between the two layers of the pleura, again restricting lung expansion.

Histological diagnosis

In planning treatment for this disease, especially where clinical trials are involved, it is vital that an accurate diagnosis be achieved. It is sometimes possible to make a cytological diagnosis through fluid drained from the pleural effusion. However, in most cases a definitive diagnosis can only be made following a pleural biopsy.

There are three cell types: epithelioid, sarcomatoid and mixed or biphasic. There is a clear survival benefit associated with the epithelial type.

Staging

When diagnosing cancer it is necessary to know the type of cancer (e.g. mesothelioma) and also the extent (stage) of the disease. The stage describes the size and position of the cancer and whether or not there is evidence that it has spread to nearby tissues or to other, more distant, sites. Staging can be helpful in assessing prognosis, in making recommendations for treatment and in assessing and comparing the results of treatment.

Mesothelioma is a difficult cancer to stage. Radiological techniques, chest X-ray and CT of the chest and upper abdomen are often used in the first instance, followed if necessary by PET or a surgical staging procedure.

There are different systems available for staging mesothelioma, none of which are used universally. The most commonly used system, based on TNM assessment, is the International Mesothelioma Interest Group (IMIG) staging system:

STAGE 1 Disease limited to the pleura only on one side of the chest.

STAGE 2 Disease limited to the pleura on one side of the chest but the cancer cells have extended from the pleura into the underlying lung tissue or muscle of the diaphragm.

STAGE 3 The cancer has either spread beyond the pleura to glands in the chest and/or has advanced deeper into the tissues surrounding the pleura.

STAGE 4 The cancer has spread to distant organs or tissues or invaded deeply into tissues close to the pleura, e.g. across the diaphragm into the abdomen, into the pleura of the opposite lung or into the spine or heart muscle.

Mesothelioma 2

Survival

Most patients diagnosed with mesothelioma die within 18 months, with the range in median survival reported as being 4–18 months depending on which paper is read. Sadly this dismal prognosis is also accompanied in many cases by a range of physical symptoms, particularly chest pain and breathlessness, that are difficult to palliate.

Treatment

The treatment of mesothelioma will depend on a number of things including the type of mesothelioma, how advanced the disease is, the general health and fitness of the patient and their personal preferences.

There are various treatments that may be recommended for mesothelioma. These include active symptom control, radiotherapy, chemotherapy, and surgery. A patient may have just one of these types of treatments or a combination of them. All treatment modalities are considered palliative.

Benefits and compensation for mesothelioma patients

People disabled by disease or injury caused by work are entitled to specific, occupationally related benefits as well as benefits targeted at disabled people in general. Additionally, mesothelioma patients may claim a lump-sum compensation payment from the state and they may also sue employers for negligent exposure to asbestos.

Although mesothelioma is almost exclusively caused by exposure to asbestos and is a fatal disease, a significant number of mesothelioma patients fail to claim the benefits and compensation to which they are entitled.

Patients with cancer often lack the information and skills necessary to access benefits they are entitled to but recommendations state there should be a level of support available appropriate to their needs that signposts to services outside the healthcare environment where necessary. Mesothelioma UK is a useful service to signpost mesothelioma patients and carers to; they provide impartial, up to date information for patients, carers and healthcare professional.

Nursing care

Nursing care of the patient with mesothelioma consists of best supportive care in line with the best palliative care provision (📖 p.290, 336, 52). Alongside support patients may need information, especially with regard to compensation issues

Further reading

Cancer Research UK 2005

Website http://www.cancerresearchuk.org

Clayson H (2003) Suffering in mesothelioma: concepts and contexts. *European Journal of Palliative Care* 11(5), 251–255.

Darlison L and Whitston A Benefits and compensation for mesothelioma patients. *British Journal Of Cancer Management* 2006, 2(3), pp16–18.

Klemperer P and Rabin CB Primary neoplasms of the pleura. A report of five cases. *Arch Pathol* 1931, 11, 385–412.

McElvenny DM, Darnton AJ, Price MJ, Hodgson JT Mesothelioma mortality in Great Britain from 1968 to 2001. *Occup Med (Lond)*. 2005, 55(2), 79–87.

National Institute of Clinical Excellence 2004. *Improving Supportive and Palliative Care for Adults with Cancer. The Manual.* http://www.nice.org.

Peto J, Hodgson J, McElvenny D Darnton A and Price M. The expected burden of mesothelioma mortality in Great retain from 2002 to 2050. *British Journal of Cancer* 2005, 92, 587–593.

Stewart D Edwards J, Smythe R Waller D O'Byrne K Malignant pleural mesothelioma—an update. *International Journal of Environmental Health* 2004, 10(1), pp 26–39.

Useful addresses

Mesothelioma UK
National Macmillan Mesothelioma Resource Centre

The University Hospitals of Leicester
Management Offices
Groby Road
Leicester LE39QP

Obstructive sleep apnoea

What is it?

'Apnoea' literally translated means absence of breath, or in other words, stopping breathing. Obstructive sleep apnoea (OSA) describes a condition where there are frequent pauses in breathing during sleep. This is linked to excessive snoring. The condition varies between individuals, so that at one end of the spectrum there may be trivial snoring, through to recurrent complete obstruction at the other end of the spectrum where the person cannot breathe and sleep at the same time.

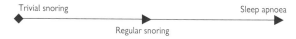

Fig. 13.1 Snoring continuum

What is the cause?

Sleep apnoea occurs when the muscles of the soft palate, the uvula, tongue and tonsils, relax during sleep which narrows the airway and can close it off. This stops the breathing for a brief period of time, cutting off the oxygen supply to the body and allowing levels of carbon dioxide to build up. As the carbon dioxide level builds up the brain will recognize this as potentially dangerous and will wake the person up: this reopens the airways and restarts breathing. The more frequently that this happens during the night the worse the level of severity of the disorder and the more that sleep is disturbed.

Prevalence

The prevalence of OSA is estimated to be around 4% of the population. It is quite a common disorder, although this figure may be an underestimate as many people may not seek treatment. Prevalence figures also vary according to the chosen threshold for defining a significant sleep abnormality and symptoms.

- OSA is more common in men than women, due to differing fat deposition around the neck
- OSA prevalence figures rise with obesity levels so are likely to become higher in the UK in the future
- OSA is the third most common serious respiratory problem after asthma and COPD.

Signs and symptoms

Many people will experience apnoea during sleep; however for a positive diagnosis of the disorder to be made there are a number of daytime and night-time symptoms.

Daytime
- Excessive daytime sleepiness (EDS)
- Tiredness/fatigue
- Falling asleep
- Memory loss
- Difficulty concentrating
- Impaired performance at work or school
- Headaches
- Nausea in the morning
- Heartburn
- Depression.

Night-time
- Snoring
- Gaps in breathing—often noticed by a partner
- Waking up gasping or choking
- Insomnia—not always in getting to sleep but due to sleep disturbance
- Bed-wetting
- Sweating
- Reduced libido or impotence.

Diagnosis

History
A good history will often point towards the diagnosis of OSA. Some of the important things to look for are:
- Onset and duration of symptoms
- Body weight change
- Lifestyle habits, such as diet, smoking, exercise, alcohol, and drug use
- Quantity and quality of sleep
- Collar size.

Systems review
- General
- Heart, eyes, ears, nose, and throat
- Endocrine
- Lungs
- Genitourinary
- Gastrointestinal
- Musculoskeletal
- Neurological
- Psychiatric.

Past medical history
- Hospitalizations
- Surgery
- Trauma
- Comorbid conditions:
  - Diabetes
  - Hypertension
  - Congestive heart failure
  - Arrhythmias
  - Cardiovascular disease
  - Hypothyroidism
  - Depression
  - Gastroesophageal reflux
  - Asthma
  - Nocturnal cardiac ischaemia.

Medications
- Current prescription items
- Over the counter medications (OTC)
- Previous sleep treatments or sedatives taken to help sleep.

Family history
- OSA
- Diabetes
- Hypertension
- Hypothyroid
- Coronary artery disease
- Cerebral vascular accident (CVA)
- Depression.

Psychosocial history
- Depression
- Mental illness
- Cognitive disturbance
- Coping strategies.

Occupation
If OSA is suspected any patient operating machinery or driving is at risk until diagnosis has been confirmed and treatment established. Advice will need to be given about continuing to work.

Physical examination (📖 p.31)
- Vital signs:
  - Blood pressure—OSA is a leading cause of hypertension
  - Pulse
  - Respirations
  - Pulse oximetry—may show type 1 respiratory failure or type 11 if there is also COPD (📖 p.75)
- Height, weight and BMI:
  - OSA more likely in the obese
- Head and neck examination:
  - Upper airway obstruction
  - Polyps
  - Septal deviation
  - Mucosal congestion
  - Enlarged tonsils
  - Small jaw (micrognathia)
  - Large tongue
  - Turbinate hypertrophy
  - Thyroid enlargement
- Neck size
  - >16 women
  - >17 men.

Diagnostic procedures
- Sleep questionnaire:
  - The Epworth Sleepiness Scale is often used and is a validated tool for assistance in diagnosis. A score >9 is considered abnormally sleepy (Figure 13.2)
- Polysomnography:
  - A method of recording body measurements during sleep. This is usually carried out in a sleep laboratory and looks at length of sleep, quality of sleep, breathing, body position and heart rate
- Overnight oximetry:
  - Records the amount of oxygen in the blood at any time and can often be carried out in the patients own home by a sensor worn on the index finger.

Differential diagnosis

There are other conditions that mimic the signs and symptoms of OSA and these should be excluded:
- Narcolepsy
- Marfan's syndrome
- Acromegaly
- Asthma
- COPD
- Congestive heart failure (CHF)
- Depression and panic attacks
- Gastro-oesophageal reflux
- Idiopathic daytime hypersomnolence
- Inadequate sleep time
- Anaemia
- Fibromyalgia
- Restless leg syndrome
- Sleep-associated seizures.

Epworth Sleepiness Scale

Name.....................Hospital number..............Date............

Your age (Yrs)............Your sex (Male =M / Female = F)............

- How likely are you to doze off or fall asleep in the situations described in the box below, in contrast to feeling just tired?
- This refers to tour usual way of life in recent times
- Even if you haven't done some of these things recently try to work out how they would have affected you
- Use the following scale to choose the <u>most appropriate number</u> for each situation

0 = would <u>never</u> doze   2 = Moderate chance of dozing

1 = <u>Slight</u> chance of dozing   4 = <u>High</u> chance of dozing

Situation	**Chance of Dozing**
Sitting and reading	☐
Watching TV	☐
Sitting, inactive in a public place (e.g. a theatre or meeting)	☐
As a passenger in a car for an hour without a break	☐
Lying down to rest in the afternoon when circumstances permit	☐
Sitting and talking to someone	☐
Sitting quietly after a lunch without alcohol	☐
In a car, while stopped for a few minutes in the traffic	☐
Thank you for your cooperation Total Score	☐

Fig. 13.2 The Epworth Sleepiness Scale.
Adapted from Johns MW (1991), *Sleep* 14(6): 540–5.

Treatment

OSA is not a life-threatening condition in itself, but it can lead to cardiac problems due to oxygen deprivation and the heart having to work harder. It does however have a huge effect on quality of life. There is also the potential for an undiagnosed or untreated patient to be at an increased risk of having a road traffic accident due to sleepiness at the wheel. OSA patients are often advised not to drive until they have been successfully treated, and this has enormous implications for anyone who makes their living from driving and may increase the reluctance of people to come forward for diagnosis.

Weight loss

Losing weight has obvious benefits for OSA and can result in improvements or even a disappearance of the problem. Patients should also be encouraged to take regular exercise.

Position change

Snoring is often more pronounced when people sleep on their backs so a change in sleeping position may lead to improvements by reducing snoring and improving breathing.

Reducing alcohol and cigarette consumption

Alcohol can lead to an increase in snoring and a tendency for people to sleep on their backs. If alcohol consumption is reduced especially prior to retiring improvements may be made in breathing. Cigarette consumption is also thought to reduce muscle tone.

Continuous positive airway pressure therapy

Continuous positive airway pressure therapy (CPAP) delivers a continuous flow of air into the airways, essentially to splint them open and ensure that they don't close. This is a long-term treatment, and some patients may be unable or unwilling to tolerate a close-fitting mask over their face overnight and may find the machine noisy.

Oral appliances

Oral appliances are made on an individual basis and serve to alter the structure of the mouth so that snoring is less likely. This is not as effective a treatment as CPAP but may be easier to tolerate. The only downside may be excessive salivation and some discomfort taking the device out in the morning.

Surgery

There are various surgical interventions seeking to move the jaw forward, enlarge the airways or remove part of the soft palate and tonsils (uvulopalatopharyngoplasty). These procedures may not be effective and CPAP may still be necessary.

Medication

There has been some attempt to prevent the loss of tone in the pharyngeal area using mainly serotonergic agents although there is currently little evidence for their use.

Nursing care

Despite its prevalence OSA is not a well known about or understood condition and the nurse will have an important role in explaining the disorder. For people who operate machinery or drive for a living there are potential work implications. A diagnosis of OSA means that the driver has to inform the DVLA, who will then send a questionnaire. If this indicates daytime sleepiness the license will be revoked. Class 2 drivers may be advised to seek alternative employment. Driving can be restarted when the sleepiness has been resolved but in the case of Class 2 licence-holders this has to be verified by a specialist clinic.

Patients commenced on CPAP will often require the treatment for life and non-use of the machine even for one night can mean a return of symptoms. Patients will need support to accept the use of the machine, although in many cases the benefits of treatment far outweigh the disadvantages of using a machine overnight.

There are also implications for lifestyle changes such as weight loss and this will need to be handled sensitively.

Further information

http://www.euoropean-lung-founation.org produce a patient fact sheet.
http://www.sleep-apnoea-trust.org is a patients' association.

Oxygen therapy

Introduction

Oxygen is a colourless, odourless, tasteless gas, which constitutes approximately 21% of atmospheric air. Oxygen therapy is the administration of supplementary oxygen to achieve a higher inspiration of oxygen than is achieved when breathing air. Oxygen therapy aims to correct hypoxaemia (PaO_2 <7.3kPa) (p.75) and reduce the work of breathing.

Regardless of where the patient is, oxygen should be regarded as a drug. It is essential that oxygen is prescribed in detail including flow rate, percentage required and how it is to be administered (cannula or mask).

It is an expensive therapy and only hypoxic patients will benefit clinically. Careful assessment is essential to ensure appropriate and safe prescribing. The assessment process will ensure that oxygen is given to the correct patients via the appropriate devices at the correct flow rate. **Warning:** inappropriate prescribing and administration of oxygen in COPD patients can cause respiratory depression.

Recent data reveals that approximately 75,000 patients in England are currently receiving home oxygen therapy. Appropriate prescribing of domiciliary oxygen encourages independent living for as long as possible; with support from health professionals, patients can lead a relatively normal lifestyle.

A new integrated service for the provision of domiciliary oxygen therapy in England has been introduced. This means there is a wider range of oxygen services available for patients. Nurses need to be aware of these services and to understand which patients can benefit, in order to initiate the assessment process.

The following chapter will outline both the acute and the domiciliary use of oxygen therapy. It will provide nurses with an understanding of the methods of oxygen delivery, why oxygen is being delivered, and an understanding of the needs of the patients receiving it.

Clinical indicators of hypoxaemia

Definitions
- Hypoxaemia is a reduction of the oxygen concentration in the arterial blood
- Hypoxia is a deficiency of oxygen in the tissues.

Clinical indicators (📖 p.31)
- Central cyanosis
- Peripheral oedema
- Raised jugular venous pressure
- Reduced mental alertness
- Polycythaemia (increase in red blood cells due to hypoxaemia)
- SaO_2 less than or equal to 92% at rest breathing air.

Some causes of hypoxaemia:
- Asthma
- Pneumonia
- Pneumothorax
- Sleep disorders
- Bronchiectasis
- Hypoventilation
- COPD
- Pulmonary embolism
- Pulmonary fibrosis
- Pneumonia.

Remember—not all breathless patients are hypoxic and not all hypoxic patients are breathless.[1] Hypoxia can result in death if not treated appropriately; excessive oxygen used in some patients can also be dangerous.

COPD patients may retain carbon dioxide. If oxygen is delivered inappropriately to these patients their CO_2 levels may continue to rise, and they may develop respiratory acidosis (fall in pH <7.35) (📖 p.494) which can be fatal. It is essential that all patients receive appropriate assessment to determine the level of oxygen required to be clinically beneficial.

Whilst some patients may be hypoxic during an acute admission/exacerbation, this does not indicate chronic hypoxaemia. It is recommended that patients be assessed for oxygen therapy during a period of stability (5 weeks post-exacerbation). Pulse oximetry can be used to select patients who will require further assessment. A $SaO_2 \leq 92\%$ at rest on air will require further testing.

Oxygen can be prescribed for:
- Acute management of hypoxaemia
- Chronic management of hypoxaemia including:
  - Long-term oxygen therapy (LTOT)
  - Short-burst therapy
  - Ambulatory therapy (continuous or pulse-dosed flow).

Oxygen delivery systems include:
- Oxygen concentrators
- Oxygen cylinders
- Portable cylinders
- Wall-mounted piped oxygen in acute hospital settings
- Liquid oxygen.

1. Bruera E, de Stoutz N, Velasco-Leiva A *et al.* (1993) Effects of oxygen on dyspnoea in hypoxaemic terminal-cancer patients *Lancet* **342**(8862), 13–14.

Acute oxygen therapy

Oxygen is used in acute respiratory disease. Examples include:
- Emergency situations such as cardiac or respiratory arrest
- Asthma and COPD exacerbations
- Pulmonary embolism
- Pneumothorax
- Pneumonia
- Pleural effusion.

It is imperative to provide optimal oxygen therapy to the acutely breathless patient, and for the majority of patients the major risk to survival is giving too little oxygen. This can lead to:
- Cardiac arrhythmias
- Tissue damage
- Renal damage
- Cerebral damage.

Even patients with COPD who experience an exacerbation are more at risk of death from hypoxaemia than from hypercapnia. Those COPD patients with a hypoxic drive, who have a reduced sensitivity to circulating blood CO_2 (📖 p.249) should have arterial blood gases (ABG) performed to determine whether they fall into this category (📖 p.75). Until the results of ABG are established, patients known to have COPD and requiring oxygen therapy should initially be given controlled oxygen to maintain saturations of between 88 and 92% and closely monitored.

Factors affecting the amount of oxygen received
- The system used to deliver the oxygen
- The breathing pattern of the patient, including depth and rate
- The flow rate set at the outlet port.

Oxygen delivery devices: high-flow devices

The importance of using the right device and flow rate cannot be over-emphasized. Different concentrations of oxygen are administered according to clinical need, and this affects which device is used. Apart from in an emergency situation, such as cardiac or respiratory arrest, the concentration of oxygen used should be prescribed and written on the patient's drug chart. The prescription and device used will depend on:

• Clinical presentation of the patient
• Pulse oximetry or ABG results
• The patient's age—very young and very old patients tend not to tolerate masks well
• For patients who can only mouth-breathe, face masks rather than nasal cannulae should be used.

High-flow devices

High-flow devices provide fixed or controlled oxygen concentrations. Fixed-performance devices—such as Venturi systems—are used on patients who require low concentrations of oxygen. Knowing the exact fractional inspired oxygen (FiO_2) level and keeping this constant is important, especially in patients with COPD (📖 p.249).

Venturi systems are available as individual colour-coded barrels that are attached to a suitable mask. The barrel used depends on the oxygen required, and ranges from 24–60%. Venturi devices have a plastic body with a small jet hole through their middle. The body of the Venturi also has holes through which air can pass. As the oxygen from the outlet port is driven through the jet hole its velocity increases, the surrounding pressure drops, and it draws in room air through the holes in the body of the device. The room air mixes with the 100% oxygen being driven through the jet, and dilutes it to the concentration written on the side of the Venturi barrel.

This concentration is kept constant regardless of the flow rate, because if the flow rate at the outlet port is increased, so too is its velocity at the jet. As this happens, the pressure around the jet drops, drawing in more room air, and maintaining the dilution. The drawing in of room air and its addition to the oxygen flow increases the overall flow to the patient. This is why it is called a high-flow device. The flow delivered is much more than the patient requires for breathing each minute.

This high flow also helps to flush out expired CO_2 from the Venturi mask so that rebreathing of CO_2 does not occur.

The minimum flow rate required to deliver the concentration of oxygen is written on the Venturi barrel.

Patients who are very breathless may be more comfortable and better oxygenated if the flow rate is set higher than is recommended on the barrel. This will not cause harm to the patient as the fraction of inspired oxygen remains the same, but the increased flow rate will exceed the patient's peak inspiratory flow rate.

Oxygen delivery devices: low-flow devices 1

Low-flow devices provide variable or uncontrolled oxygen concentrations. There are a number of devices available such as medium concentration (or simple) masks, non-rebreathing masks, and nasal cannulae.

Medium concentration masks

With this type of mask, the concentration of oxygen delivered depends on the patient's breathing rate and depth. Each breath is diluted by air drawn in from the atmosphere, dependent on the patient's breathing pattern.

The average adult patient has a peak inspiratory flow rate that is greater than the range of settings on the flow meter at the outlet port, usually up to 15 L/min. Every breath in inhales more gas than is flowing from the oxygen flow meter, so the balance is sucked in from the atmosphere: 100% oxygen from the outlet port is diluted with 21% oxygen from the air sucked in through the holes in and around the mask. It is important to remember that no mask is 100% airtight. If the flow of oxygen is set too low at the outlet port (below 5 L for example), there is insufficient flow to flush out from the mask all of the CO_2 that the patient expires with each breath. This may result in the patient re-breathing some of the accumulated CO2 from the mask. If the flow of oxygen is too high—in an attempt to flush out the CO_2—this could result in a FiO_2 too high for hypercapnic COPD patients. This makes these masks unsuitable for patients with type 2 respiratory failure (p.494).

The normal flow rate of oxygen is 6–10 L/min and provides a concentration of between 40–60%.

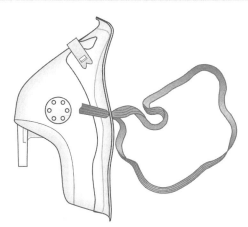

Fig. 14.1 Medium concentration mask. Figure courtesy of Intersurgical.

Oxygen delivery devices: low-flow devices 2

Non-rebreathable devices

It is unlikely that the FiO_2 will increase if the flow rate is increased above 10 L per minute using a medium concentration mask. A re-breathing mask should be considered if a higher FiO_2 is desired.

Non-rebreathe device

On inhalation, the one-way inspiratory valve opens, directing air from a reservoir bag into the mask (see Figure 14.2). On exhalation, gas exits the mask through the one-way expiratory valve and enters the atmosphere. The patient breathes air only from the bag. This delivers the highest possible oxygen concentration (60–80%) quickly. Nurses should be aware that high oxygen flow rates are required to ensure that the bag is inflated during inspiration. The mask needs to be fitted tightly to ensure a high delivery of oxygen. Some patients might find this uncomfortable or may feel claustrophobic when using this device.

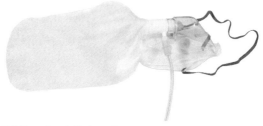

Fig. 14.2 Non-rebreathable device. Figure courtesy of Intersurgical.

Nasal cannulae

Nasal cannulae tend to be less claustrophobic than a mask, and are often preferred by patients (see Figure 14.3). It is also easier to eat and drink with nasal cannulae. They can be used so that patients can continue to receive oxygen whilst having nebulized drug therapies (💷 p.391). As they are low-flow devices the exact FiO_2 is unknown.

Nasal cannulae are suitable for patients with type 1 respiratory failure, but can be used in patients with type 2 respiratory failure only if the accurate prescription of oxygen is not necessary. They are usually used at a flow rate of 1–4 L/min and can deliver an oxygen concentration of between 22–35%. If the flow rate is increased to 6 L/min or more, the mucous membranes of the nose may become dry, with little additional improvement in FiO_2. This lack of improvement is because at 6 L/min the oropharynx and nasopharynx are already full, so there is no appreciable increase in FiO_2.

Patients must have patent nasal passages, and the nasal cannulae must be correctly fitted if they are to benefit from the device. Patients who are mouth breathers can still benefit from nasal prongs, as the airflow in the oropharynx will pull oxygen from the nasopharynx, but the FiO_2 may be lower than if they were nose-breathing.

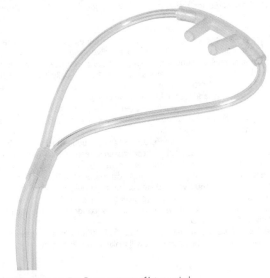

Fig. 14.3 Nasal canullae. Figure courtesy of Intersurgical.

Humidification of acute oxygen therapy

Oxygen can dry the mucous membranes of the upper airway. This can lead to sticky chest secretions, which are difficult to expectorate. If oxygen is to be administered for more than a short period, humidification should be considered, particularly if the concentration of oxygen administered is high—over 35% or at a rate of 4 L/min or above.

There are several points to consider when humidifying oxygen. These include the risk of encouraging bacterial growth, as humidification provides a moist environment. Sterile water needs to be used to minimize bacterial contamination. The water should be changed daily if sterile packs are not used; the bottles should be changed according to the manufacturers' instructions and local infection control guidelines.

Cold water systems are generally used for humidification of oxygen as they are inexpensive and easy to operate on a short-term basis. They have been found to be fairly inefficient.

Heated water systems—where the oxygen is bubbled across a heated water reservoir—are available. These systems seem to be much more efficient, but there is a risk of mucosal overheating or burning, and excess condensation in the oxygen tubing which can reduce the flow of oxygen.

With both cold and heated systems, nurses should be aware that the humidification alters the oxygen concentration provided by a Venturi mask (Figure 14.4), as the water vapour may condense in the jet hole, thereby altering the FiO_2.

Nurses should explain to patients that humidification may make their faces damp, and that the equipment will make a bubbling sound.

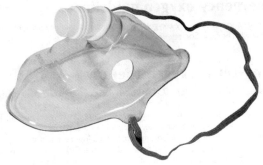

Fig. 14.4 Venturi mask. Figure courtesy of Intersurgical.

Emergency oxygen guidelines

Guidelines for emergency oxygen use in adult patients are available from the British Thoracic Society, www.brit - thoracic.org.uk

Long-term oxygen therapy

The weight of evidence for LTOT has been demonstrated in COPD patients. In this group, chronic hypoxaemia causes constriction of the pulmonary blood vessels leading to increased pressure (pulmonary hypertension). This puts a strain on the right ventricle, which will eventually fail.

Landmark studies[2,3] have demonstrated that if low-concentration oxygen therapy is administered to patients with severe COPD for a minimum of 15 h/day, three-year mortality rates reduce from 66% to 45%. Recent Cochrane reviews confirm these findings.

Indications for LTOT include the following conditions with chronic hypoxaemia:

• COPD
• Severe chronic asthma
• Interstitial lung disease
• Cystic fibrosis
• Bronchiectasis
• Pulmonary vascular disease
• Primary pulmonary hypertension
• Pulmonary malignancy
• Chronic heart failure.

Patients with severe COPD (FEV_1 <30% predicted) (📖 p.75) should be routinely (twice-yearly) screened for chronic hypoxaemia. NICE also recommend consideration for assessment in moderate airflow (FEV_1 30–49%). This should be done during a period of stability (5 weeks post-exacerbation). Pulse oximetry can be used to identify these patients. During a period of stability, a patient who has a $SaO_2 \leq 92\%$ at rest breathing air will require referral. Patients should usually have rested for 30 min before readings are taken.

Smoking cessation advice and assistance should always be offered prior to assessment for oxygen therapy, and patients should have stopped smoking prior to oxygen being prescribed (📖 p.541).

2. MRC Working Party (1981) Long-term domiciliary oxygen therapy in chronic hypoxic cor pulmonale complicating chronic bronchitis and emphysema. *Lancet* 681–686.

3. Nocturnal Oxygen Therapy Trial Group (1980) Continous or nocturnal oxygen therapy in hypoxemic chronic obstructive lung disease. *Annals of Internal Medicine* **93(3)**, 391–398.

Pulse oximetry

A pulse oximeter is a safe and simple medical device used to measure the percentage of haemoglobin (Hb) saturation in tissue capilliaries.

Oxygen molecules are carried around the body by Hb on red blood cells. The oxygen molecules bind to the haemoglobin as blood passes the alveoli. As one molecule binds, it allows for the next molecule to bind up to a total of four molecules on each haemoglobin. Oxygen is then transported around the body and deposited in the tissues. The oxygen saturation (SaO_2) is a measure of how much oxygen the blood is carrying, as a percentage of the maximum it could carry. This is often referred to as the 'sats' reading.

How does the pulse oximeter work?

It is a safe, non-invasive and painless procedure. A finger probe is the most common method, however, ear probes and small pads can also be used. The probe emits wavelengths of light through the nail bed, and calculates the absorption of light by oxygenated blood to produce a SaO_2 reading. This is usually accurate to within + or −2%:

Readings can be inaccurate or misleading if:
• Nail varnish is worn or there are tattoos on the nails
• Peripheral vasoconstriction or vascular disease is present
• The sensor is badly positioned or soiled
• There is repeated shaking or shivering
• If cardiac arrythmias are present
• The patient smokes a cigarette within 4 h of the test
• Following carbon monoxide poisoning.

Table 14.1 Use of pulse oximetry

Pulse oximetry is useful for:	It is not useful for:
Identifying patients for LTOT assessment	Being used alone to assess for LTOT, as it gives no indication of hypercapnia and its responses to oxygen
Identifying de-saturation during/after exercise	
Overnight monitoring of nocturnal desaturation	

Table 14.2 SpO_2 levels

Levels	SpO2%
Normal	95–99
Mild hypoxia	90–94
Moderate hypoxia	84–89
Severe hypoxia	<80

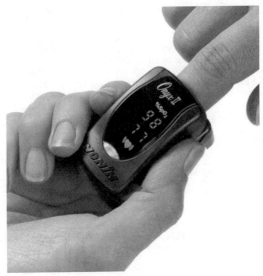

Fig. 14.5 Picture of finger probe. Reproduced with permission from Nonin Medical Inc.

Assessment for LTOT by respiratory team

- Assess during period of stability (5 weeks post-exacerbation)
- Confirm diagnosis (plus severity, if COPD)
- Maximize pharmacological therapies
- Two blood gas measurements, not less than 3 weeks apart
- Smoking cessation advice if applicable.

Table 14.3 Criteria for prescribing LTOT

Arterial oxygen (PaO$_2$) <7.3kPa when clinically stable

Or

PaO$_2$ of 7.3–8kPa plus one or more of the following:
- Secondary polycythaemia
- Peripheral oedema
- Pulmonary hypertension
- Nocturnal hypoxaemia (SaO$_2$ <90% for more than 30% of time)[4]

The BTS COPD guidelines recommend a starting flow rate of 2 L/min via nasal cannula or 24% controlled facemask, aiming for a PaO$_2$ of at least 8.0kPa.

24–28% oxygen significantly increases haemoglobin saturation without risking further under-ventilation and a rising PaCO$_2$, which can cause coma and death. Repeated blood gases are required to assess that a PaO$_2$ of 8.0kPa has been achieved, and to assess the PaCO$_2$ and pH response to the oxygen.

Patients with an unacceptable rise in PaCO$_2$ or acidosis will not be suitable for long-term therapy. This can often be upsetting for a patient, who may require support and counselling. Some hospitals issue warning cards to these patients to alert staff to the risk of CO$_2$ retention in future admissions. Some patients may require higher flow rates to correct hypoxaemia. A PaO$_2$ of 8.0kPa should be aimed for.

LTOT should be prescribed for a minimum of 15 h in 24 h, most of these hours being during sleep. The remaining hours can be utilized to suit the patient's lifestyle. Greater benefits have been demonstrated in those patients' using more than 20 hours per day.[5]

Patients with borderline blood gases should be reassessed after 3 months.

Patients with neuromuscular disease or scoliosis can develop dangerous rises in PaCO$_2$ with LTOT, and should be referred to a physician with a clinical interest.

Nocturnal hypoxaemia

Assessment indicated in:
- COPD patients reporting morning headaches
- Persistent oedema or polycythaemia, despite LTOT
- Neuromuscular conditions
- Sleep apnoea.

Assessment will be as above for LTOT. Patients with neuromuscular conditions or sleep apnoea should be assessed by a consultant with a special interest, as they may require non-invasive ventilation alongside LTOT.

4. Nocturnal Oxygen Therapy Trial Group (1980) Continuous or nocturnal oxygen therapy in hypoxemic chronic obstructive lung disease. *Annals of Internal Medicine* **93(3)**, 391–398.

5. British Thoracic Society (2006). *Clinical component for the home oxygen service in England and Wales.* http://www.brit.thoracic.org.uk.

Short-burst oxygen therapy

Used for episodic breathlessness not relieved by other treatments in:
• Severe COPD
• Interstitial lung disease
• Heart failure
• Palliative care.

This is usually given for 10–20 minutes at a time to relieve dyspnoea. There is no adequate evidence to support its use—it should only be prescribed if there is improvement in breathlessness or exercise tolerance. Check for other causes of breathlessness and refer for LTOT if PaO_2 is less than 7.3kPa.

Uses
• Pre- and post-exercise
• Control of breathlessness at rest
• Used in palliative care
• After exercise in patients with COPD, to bridge the gap until full LTOT assessment is carried out.

Cylinders are usually provided for short burst therapy.

If a concentrator is provided, patients should be identified for early assessment as they may be a CO_2 retainer.

Review
• Review should be by a GP or hospital specialist
• Therapy should be reviewed at least once a year to check if continued use is needed
• If clinical deterioration occurs repeat blood gases—LTOT assessment may be required.

Ambulatory oxygen

Portable oxygen is for use outside the home during exercise and activities of daily living. The aim is to increase exercise capacity, reduce breathlessness and improve quality of life.

Indications:

- COPD
- Severe chronic asthma
- Interstitial lung disease
- Cystic fibrosis
- Pulmonary vascular disease
- Primary pulmonary hypertension.

Candidates for ambulatory O_2 will be on LTOT, or demonstrate a fall in SaO_2 of 4% to a value of less than 90%.

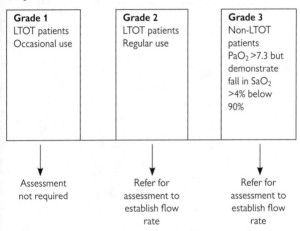

Grade 1	Grade 2	Grade 3
LTOT patients Occasional use	LTOT patients Regular use	Non-LTOT patients PaO_2 >7.3 but demonstrate fall in SaO_2 >4% below 90%
↓	↓	↓
Assessment not required	Refer for assessment to establish flow rate	Refer for assessment to establish flow rate

Assessment aims to establish the required flow rate to correct exercise induced fall in SaO_2 and hours required per day. Assessment may be a 6-minute walking test or shuttle walk test (📖 p.75). SaO_2 can be recorded during the test to establish required flow rate to maintain SaO_2 above 90%. Borg or visual analogue score tools can be used to measure resting/end exercise dyspnoea.

Oxygen equipment

Oxygen concentrators

This is an electrical device used to produce oxygen from room air. Air is drawn in through filters that remove dust and small particles. It is then passed through cylindrical chambers filled with zeolite (a fine blue powder with an affinity for nitrogen and CO_2). Oxygen is then passed into a compressor, pumped through a flow meter and out of an outlet to the patient. Waste gases are pumped back into the room.

Up to 50 foot of tubing can be attached to enable patients to mobilize around the home. One machine can provide flows rates of 0.5–4 L/min. However, new machines are now available that provide flow rates up to 15 L/min. If these new machines are not available two or three machines can be joined to achieve higher flow rates. Special arrangements can be made to provide smaller flow rates, i.e. less than 0.5 L/min.

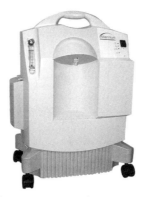

Fig. 14.6 Example of an oxygen concentrator. Image courtesy of Air Products PLC. Air Products PLC retains all copyright and moral rights in the image.

Oxygen cylinders

These contain pressurized oxygen, so care needs to be taken with storage, carrying and use of the product. Due to their size (71cm) and weight (15kg), they are not suitable for moving around the house and are designed for short-burst therapy. They can provide a flow rate of 0.5–15 L/min.

A 2122-L cylinder will last approximately 17 h 41 min at 2 L/min. A gauge indicates the volume of oxygen left, and a flow rate selector is present at the top of the cylinder.

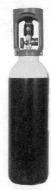

Fig. 14.7 Example of an oxygen cylinder. Image courtesy of Air Products PLC. Air Products PLC retains all copyright and moral rights in the image.

Ambulatory cylinders

Portable cylinders are ideal for going out. Their weight (3.2kg) and height (53cm) make them ideal for carrying; oxygen suppliers will provide a carrying bag, and sometimes a trolley. They will last approximately 3 h 35 min on 2 L/min. Smaller (43cm), lightweight (2.1kg) cylinders are available which last 2 h 34 min. Suppliers will decide on the most appropriate device to suit the patient's needs.

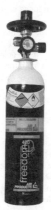

Fig. 14.8 Example of an ambulatory cylinder. Image courtesy of Air Products PLC. Air Products PLC retains all copyright and moral rights in the image.

Conserver devices

Conserver devices can increase the duration of an oxygen cylinder by around three times its original volume. The battery-operated device is triggered by the patient's inspiratory flow and releases a precise amount of oxygen during inspiration. They are attached to the outside of the portable unit. Not all patients maintain their saturations whilst using these devices so care should be taken.

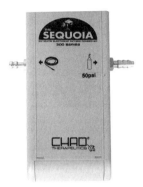

Fig. 14.9 Example of an oxygen conserver. Image courtesy of Air Products PLC. Air Products PLC retains all copyright and moral rights in the image.

Liquid oxygen
- Cryogenic liquid oxygen is produced in air separation units using low temperatures to liquefy the gas
- Liquid oxygen is far more condensed than its gaseous form, therefore small portable units can contain up to 8 h of oxygen when used at 2 L/min
- Large reservoirs of liquid oxygen are delivered to the patient's home
- Patients fill their portable units from this reservoir to go out
- This form of delivery is advantageous to those patients on higher flow rates of oxygen
- Some units have integral conserver devices increasing the longevity of the portable units.

Humidification
- Humidification is available to attach to the concentrators
- They are best used for those patients on 4 or more L/min as the machines are not under pressure, and the lower flow rates will not humidify the water
- Patients are required to clean and change the humidifier daily, using boiled cooled water or distilled water to refill.

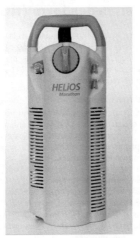

Fig. 14.10 A liquid oxygen container. Image courtesy of Air Products PLC. Air Products PLC retains all copyright and moral rights in the image.

Home oxygen order form (HOOF)

A new integrated home oxygen service was introduced in February 2006. The aim of the service was to improve quality of life, increase choice and improve cost-efficiency. There are ten regions across England and Wales, each with a single dedicated oxygen supplier, providing an integrated service. To access details on local providers and HOOF forms see http://www.primarycarecontracting.nhs.uk

How the service has changed

All patients for LTOT are formally assessed and need to sign a consent form. The clinician requests a service rather than specific equipment and it is the contractor's responsibility to communicate with the patient and decide upon an appropriate device. Only one prescription (HOOF form) is needed for the duration of treatment.

All modalities of delivery are available—concentrators, cylinders, ambulatory cylinders plus conserver devices and liquid oxygen. Emergency deliveries are possible within 4 h and next day hospital discharge arrangements can be made. Holiday delivery of oxygen is also available.

All funding is now allocated to PCT unified budgets rather than shared between discretionary and non-discretionary budgets, and there are fixed prices per day.

Note: patients requiring oxygen for palliation in breathlessness do not require a formal assessment; GPs will also prescribe for this group.

How to prescribe

- Two forms are required. The HOOF and the HOCF (home oxygen consent form)
- The patient signs the HOCF to give consent for their personal details to be given to the supplier
- The HOOF needs to be completed in full, including the flow rate, hours per/day required and method of administration e.g. nasal cannula or % mask
- Once fully completed, the HOOF form is faxed to the local supplier. An automatic fax receipt will be returned. Copies of the prescription should be forwarded to the PCT or common services agencies, GP, the trust clinical oxygen lead and a copy kept in the patient's notes
- The patient is given a copy of the consent form and the original is filed in the patient's notes
- Once a HOOF has been completed, there will be no further prescriptions required unless the patient's oxygen needs change.

Delivery details

- **Standard deliveries** are made within three working days. All equipment is delivered to the patients address as shown on the HOOF
- **Hospital discharge** section ensures that oxygen will be delivered within 24 h of notification of the discharge
- **Emergency oxygen** may be necessary when the patients' needs are urgent but not requiring hospital admission. The emergency section will ensure the patient receives oxygen within 4 h and the charge to the PCT is higher for this service.

Holiday oxygen

Patients can access http://www.homeoxygen.nhs.uk for information regarding holiday deliveries.

The patient should:

- Give at least 2 weeks notice to the supplier
- Ensure the holiday site is in agreement about the delivery and storage of oxygen
- Check with health professionals that they are fit to travel
- Provide full details of holiday arrangements to the person completing the HOOF
- Ensure that any equipment taken with them from home is taken back with them
- Ensure that equipment delivered to the holiday destination by the contractors is left there.

If the patient is travelling outside their local suppliers' area, the supplier will arrange with the appropriate contractor regarding delivery.

In Scotland and Northern Ireland, pharmacies continue to provide a cylinder service. Supply arrangements are extended to Scotland and Northern Ireland for those who wish to travel from England and Wales.

If patients are to travel from Scotland or Northern Ireland to England or Wales they should arrange oxygen supply before their travel, as they will require a HOOF.

Follow-up care

- Within 4 weeks of starting LTOT—education, oximetry
- After 3 months—repeat arterial blood gases, on and off O_2
- After 6 months—home visit, education, oximetry
- After 12 months—repeat arterial blood gases
- If SaO_2 <92% on oxygen, further assessment is required (patient may require higher flow rate)
- If SaO_2 >92% on air repeat 4 weeks later—if still above 92% refer back to team (patient may no longer require LTOT).

Education includes:
- Reason for LTOT, time required and compliance
- Check patient is able to use equipment, and is aware of the role of the supplier
- Correct use of cannula/mask
- Nose, mouth, eye and ear care
- Smoking cessation if applicable, or warning of dangers
- Need and principles of ambulatory oxygen
- Need for humidification
- Travel—is patient aware of arrangements?
- Contact numbers for troubleshooting/support (supplier and nurse).

All LTOT patients should be followed up 6-monthly at home with measurement of SaO_2 at home on air and on LTOT.

Advice for patients

- Patients using oxygen should not use oil-based lubricants up or around the nose whilst using oxygen. KY jelly is a recommended alternative
- Patients on LTOT may experience oral thrush and require treatment as necessary
- Patients on high-flow masks can experience dry eyes—artificial tears can help
- Soft skin around the ears can break down with oxygen tubing pressure. E-Z wraps (foam wraps) can alleviate the pressure.

Discharge from acute care

Whilst hypoxia during an acute admission is not an indication for long-term oxygen therapy, it may in some cases be necessary to discharge a patient home on oxygen following an acute phase. This may be due to unsafe PaO_2 readings on air or palliation. This hypoxic period may be temporary and it is therefore essential that these patients receive follow-up and are assessed when stable (5 weeks post-exacerbation), to determine future oxygen requirements. If saturation readings have corrected themselves (>92% on air), post-exacerbation, oxygen may no longer be required and the patient will require an explanation to help them understand this. If levels do not correct themselves and the patient is on optimal therapies the pathway for formal assessment should be followed. This will ensure that the patient is receiving the appropriate flow rate to correct hypoxia.

Patient support groups

These groups are run by patients. They provide support and information for–patients and families living with respiratory disease. Patients can contact the British Lung Foundation for details of their nearest group. Head office 020 7688 5555 or visit the website on http://www.lunguk.org.

To download a copy of a HOOF and a HOCF please go to http://www.primarycarecontracting.nhs.uk.

Pharmacology

Introduction

Pharmacology is the study of the actions, mechanisms, uses, and adverse effects of a drug. A drug is any natural or synthetic substance that changes the physiological state of a living organism. In respiratory medicine drugs are used for the prevention, diagnosis, and treatment of a disease.

Drugs are intended to benefit the patient, but with any drug there is always a risk of adverse effects. The benefits of giving the drug should always outweigh the risks of adverse events.

An appropriate knowledge and understanding of pharmacology is vital for safe prescribing. As more nurses qualify as prescribers, an understanding of how the drugs work, what constitutes an adverse reaction and when to stop a drug is essential. The Nurses and Midwives Council (NMC) Code of Conduct (2002) for all nurses states:

> You are personally accountable for your practice. This means you are answerable for your actions and omissions, regardless of advice or directions from another professional.

This has implications for life-long learning, as new drugs, delivery devices and techniques are being introduced frequently. Employers and patients will expect nurses, especially those working in specialized roles, to be aware of new developments, and have an up-to-date knowledge of new drugs coming onto the market.

This chapter will discuss respiratory drugs in common use. Later chapters will discuss drugs used for specific respiratory conditions.

Basic pharmacology

Drug names and classification

A drug can have a number of names and belong to many classes. The generic name of a drug is the nonproprietary name as listed in national pharmacopeias or the chemical name. All drugs available on prescription or sold over the counter have a generic name; it may vary from country to country.

Newly patented drugs usually have one generic name, such as beclometasone, and one brand name such as Becotide®. Once the patent expires, the drug can be marketed under a variety of brand names, such as Beclazone® but the generic name remains the same.

Routes of administration

Drugs may act locally (topically) or systemically. Systemic drugs have to enter the vascular and lymphatic systems for delivery to body tissues; oral corticosteroids for example. The oral route is probably the least predictable route of administration, owing to metabolism of the liver, chemical breakdown, and the possible binding to food. Some topical drugs also have systemic effects, especially if given in large doses over a long period of time.

Pharmacokinetics

Pharmacokinetics considers the movement of drugs within the body and the way in which the body affects drugs over time. Once a drug has been administered, either topically or systemically, it will undergo four processes:

- Absorption
- Distribution
- Metabolism
- Excretion.

The composition of the drug has an influence on where the drug is absorbed, where it is distributed to, and how effectively it is metabolized and excreted. Other factors that can affect this process include:

- The dose of drug given
- The patient's condition
- Dosing schedule
- Route of administration.

Absorption

Generally, unless a drug is absorbed into the body in sufficient amounts, it will not work. The pharmaceutical industry aims to devise the right formulation for the drug to be absorbed and to stay at the site long enough to be effective.

Drugs that are absorbed systemically must cross at least one cell before they can reach the circulation. This is generally done by passive diffusion—movement from an area of high concentration to an area of low concentration. The rate and extent of drug absorption across a cell membrane depends on:

The lipid solubility of a drug

Cell membranes are composed of a double layer of phospholipids, arranged so that the hydrophilic (water-loving) positively charged heads face outwards and the lipophilic (lipid-loving) tails face inwards. Lipid-soluble drugs will pass through cell membranes more easily than water-soluble drugs. The more lipid-soluble the drug is, the easier it is absorbed from the small intestine after oral administration.

Surface area for absorption

The larger the surface area available for absorption, the quicker absorption will occur. The small intestine has a very large surface area for absorption. If a patient has a condition—such as inflammatory bowel disease—that reduces this area, the absorption rate, and therefore the effect of the drug, may be reduced.

Gastric motility

Most absorption from oral medication takes place in the small intestine. Drugs taken orally disintegrate in the stomach, and are emptied into the intestine with the gastric contents; except those specially formulated to pass into the intestine e.g. enteric coated preparations.

Anything that affects gastric motility and emptying will alter the rate of absorption. Food in the stomach after a meal will slow gastric emptying. If drugs are taken with food the absorption and effect of the drugs may be delayed. This is why when the patient takes their medication is important.

Some drugs are prescribed to take with food. This may be to prevent local side-effects such as irritation of the stomach lining by using food as a barrier.

First-pass metabolism

Some drugs are absorbed from the small intestine directly into the liver via the hepatic portal vein. The drugs are then partially or fully metabolized by the liver. The amount of the drug entering the circulation is either reduced or completely negated.

Blood flow

Blood flow to the site of administration will affect the absorption rate. Some areas of the body, such as the muscles, have variable blood flow and absorption from intramuscular injections may vary.

Common routes of drug administration

- Intravenously
- Intramuscularly
- Subcutaneously
- Orally
- Topically
- Transdermally
- Inhaled
- Via mucous membranes: rectally, vaginally, buccally.

Distribution

Once the drug has been absorbed it is transported around the body. This is known as distribution. There are a number of factors that influence the distribution of drugs around the body:

- Blood flow
- Plasma protein binding
- Barriers to distribution
- Storage sites.

Blood flow

Depending on how the drug is administered, the blood flow to the site of administration will affect the rate of absorption. Organs such as the heart, liver, and kidneys are highly vascular, and will acquire drugs quickly. Skin, bones, fat, and muscles have a reduced vascularity and receive drugs at a slower rate. The patient's level of activity and tissue temperature may also affect drug distribution.

Plasma protein binding

In the circulation, a drug can be 'bound' to circulating plasma proteins, usually albumin, or 'free' in an unbound state. If a drug is bound it is thought to be ineffective, as only a free drug can cross plasma membranes and have a pharmacological effect. As free molecules leave the circulation, drug molecules are released from plasma proteins to re-establish a ratio between the bound and the free molecules. Plasma proteins will bind to many drugs and these drugs compete for binding sites on the plasma protein. If one drug displaces another there may be serious consequences. Some drugs are highly protein-bound and have a narrow therapeutic index (theophylline for example). A narrow therapeutic index means that the concentration of the drug needed to have an effect is close to that which may be inneffectual or cause toxicity.

Barriers to distribution

- The placental barrier—this permits the passage of lipid-soluble, non-ionised compounds from mother to foetus, and prevents the entrance of substances that are poorly lipid-soluble
- The blood–brain barrier—capillaries of the central nervous system are different from those in other parts of the body. This constrains the passage of lipid-insoluble drugs.

Storage sites

Fat tissue acts as a storage site for lipid-soluble drugs and drugs that are stored there remain for some time. Calcium-containing structures such as teeth and bone can accumulate drugs that are bound to calcium.

Metabolism

Drug metabolism is the first stage of drug clearance. It describes the process of altering the chemical composition of the drug. It is also called 'biotransformation'.

Most drug metabolism happens in the liver, where hepatic enzymes catalyse various reactions. Metabolism of drugs also occurs in the kidneys, intestinal mucosa, the lungs, plasma, and placenta.

Metabolism occurs in two phases:

- **Phase one:** These reactions try to biotransform the drug to a more ionized metabolite. This process results in oxidation, reduction or hydrolysis of a drug
- **Phase two:** Phase two metabolites which are not sufficiently ionised to be excreted by the kidneys are made more water-liking (hydrophillic) by conjugation (synthetic) reactions, with compounds provided by the liver. The resulting conjugates are then more readily excreted by the kidneys.

With some drugs, especially those given repeatedly, the drug metabolism becomes more effective due to enzyme induction. This results in larger doses of the drug being required in order to produce the same effect. This is known as drug tolerance.

Various factors affect a patient's ability to metabolize drugs. These include:

- Genetic differences—the enzyme systems controlling drug metabolism are genetically determined
- Age—first-pass metabolism may be reduced in older people, resulting in increased bioavailability. Also, the delayed production and elimination of metabolites may prolong drug action, resulting in reduced drug doses being required
- Disease processes—liver disease will affect metabolism. Reduced hepatic blood flow as a result of heart failure or shock may also reduce the metabolism of drugs.

Excretion

Drugs are excreted in the kidneys, in bile, in saliva, the lungs, and in breast milk.

Kidneys

Most drugs are excreted by the kidneys. This only applies to free drugs and not to drugs bound to plasma proteins. Several factors may affect the rate at which a drug is excreted by the kidneys. These include:
• The presence of kidney disease
• Altered renal blood flow
• The pH of the urine
• The concentration of the drug in plasma
• The molecular weight of the drug.

Bile

Some drugs are secreted by the liver into bile. These then enter the duodenum via the common bile duct and move into the small intestine. Some drugs are reabsorbed into the bloodstream and return to the liver. The drug then undergoes further metabolism, is secreted back into the bile and ultimately excreted in faeces.

Lungs

Anaesthetic gases and small amounts of alcohol undergo pulmonary excretion and are exhaled.

Breast milk

Drugs may pass from maternal blood into breast milk. The amount of drug may be small, but a breastfed baby may be affected as it has less ability to metabolize and excrete drugs.

Half-life

Half-life is the time taken for the concentration of drug in the blood to fall by half its original value. The process of metabolism and excretion determines a drug's half-life. Standard dosage intervals are based on half-life calculations. This is considered when setting up a dosage regime which produces stable drug concentrations, keeping the level of drug below toxic levels but above the minimum effective level.

Occasionally an effective plasma drug level must be reached quickly, and a larger dose of drug than usual is given. This is called a loading dose. Once the required plasma level is reached the normal dose is given. This dose is continued at regular intervals to maintain a stable plasma level and is known as a maintenance dose.

Pharmacodynamics

Pharmacodynamics considers the effects of the drug on the body and the mode of drug action. For drugs to be effective, they must reach cells through the processes of absorption and distribution. Once at the site of action, drugs work in either a specific or non-specific manner.

Specific mechanisms

• Interactions with receptors on the cell membrane.

Drugs frequently interact with receptors to form a drug–receptor complex. To allow a drug to interact with a receptor, the drug molecule has to be able to 'lock' onto a receptor site to form a drug–receptor complex. Some drugs will combine with more than one type of receptor (Figure 15.1):

- • A drug that has an affinity for a receptor, and that once bound to the receptor can cause a response, is called an agonist
- • Drugs that bind to receptors and do not cause a response are called antagonists. Antagonists reduce the likelihood of another drug or chemical binding and reduce or block further drug activity
- • Antagonists may be competitive, when they compete with an agonist for receptor sites and inhibit the action of the agonist
- • Drug receptor binding may be reversible and the response to the drug is reduced once the drug leaves the receptor site

• Interference with ion passage through the cell membrane:

- • Ion channels are selective pores in the cell membrane that allow the movement of ions in and out of the cell
- • Some drugs block these channels, which then interferes with ion transport and cause an altered response

• Enzyme inhibition or stimulation:

- • Some drugs interact with enzymes. Drugs often resemble a natural substrate and compete with the natural substrate for the enzyme

• Incorporation into macromolecules. Some drugs can be taken up by a larger molecule and will interfere with the normal function of that molecule

• Interference with metabolic processes of microorganisms. Some drugs interfere with metabolic processes that are very specific or unique to microorganisms and kill or inhibit activity of the microorganism.

Non-specific mechanisms

• Chemical alteration of the cellular environment. Drugs may not alter specific cell function, but because they change the chemical environment surrounding the cell, cellular responses or changes occur

• Physical alteration of the cellular environment. Drugs may not alter specific cell function, but because they change the physical as opposed to the chemical environment around the cell, cellular responses or changes occur.

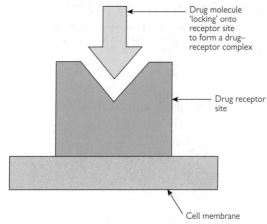

Fig. 15.1 Drug–receptor complex

Adverse drug reactions (ADRs)

Many drugs can cause unwanted effects. The severity and frequency of these will vary from drug to drug and from person to person. Terms that are used to describe drug effects include:

- Adverse reaction
- Side-effect
- Toxic effect
- Drug allergy or hypersensitivity.

Many factors determine an individual's clinical response to a drug. These include:

- Age
- Body weight
- Pregnancy and lactation
- Nutritional status
- Food/drug interactions
- Disease processes
- Mental and emotional factors
- Genetic and ethnic factors.

There are two types of drug reactions: common predictable ADRs and rare, unpredictable ADRs.

Common predictable ADRs or Type A reactions

These are due to the pharmacological or physiological actions of a drug. They are caused by an excessive or inadequate response to a drug. They are often dose-related and can be managed by adjusting the dose of the drug.

Rare unpredictable ADRs or Type B reactions

These are idiosyncratic in nature and are unrelated to the dose of the drug. They cannot be predicted from a drug's known pharmacology. While they are not as common as Type A reactions, the effect of a Type B reaction can be very serious, causing an anaphylactic, life-threatening reaction.

Reporting ADRs

All prescribers have a responsibility to report a potential ADR to the proper authorities. In the UK, the Commission on Human Medicines collect data and reports of ADRs. This can be done via the Yellow Card system, either on their website or on the yellow reporting cards at the back of the *British National Formulary* (BNF).

Table 15.1 Points to consider when prescribing drugs

Points to consider	Factors
Patient factors	• Age • Sex • Weight • Renal and liver function • Hypersensitivity • Contraindications • Functional state • Concordance factors • Genetic factors • Pregnant or breastfeeding
Drug/dose selection	• Appropriate drug choice • Appropriate dose selected • Dose adjusted if required for patient factors
Dose administration	• Route of administration • Absorption properties • Bioavailability • Speed of effect • Timing of dose • Functional state of patient
Pharmacokinetic factors	• Absorption across membranes • Distribution around circulation • Volume of distribution • Half-life • Protein binding • Renal and hepatic function • Drug–drug interactions
Pharmacodynamic factors	• Genetic factors • Drug–drug interactions • Drug–receptor affinity and selection
Adverse drug reactions	• Predictable and unpredictable • Reported to CHM
Patient outcome	• Drug has desired effect • Drug is efficacious • Minimal side-effects • No ADRs

Further reading and information

Beckwith S and Franklin P. Oxford Handbook of Nurse Prescribing. http://www.oup.com

Yellow card reporting www.yellowcard.gov.uk

Short- and long-acting inhaled β_2 agonists

β_2 agonists are commonly used for rapid relief of symptoms in both asthma and COPD. They are available in either short- or long-acting formulations, but the mode of action is similar for both classes.

β_2 agonists act upon the β_2 receptors in the airways, causing the relaxation of bronchial smooth muscle (p.13). When the β_2 agonist attaches to the receptor, the subunit splits off and leads to the production of cyclic adenosine monophosphate (cAMP). This mediates the β_2 agonist effects of the drug.

β_2 agonists are classified according to the onset and duration of action.

Short-acting β_2 agonists (salbutamol and terbutaline)

Short acting β_2 agonists have a rapid onset of action, usually within 5–15 min and last approximately 4 h. They are recommended for use on an 'as required' basis for wheeze, cough, breathlessness, and chest tightness in asthma and mild COPD. They are used in high doses in worsening and acute asthma and for moderate and severe COPD.

Stimulation of β receptors in other areas, such as the heart and skeletal muscle, can cause side-effects of palpitations, cardiac arrhythmia and tremor.

Short-acting inhaled β_2 agonists are available in a number of preparations:
- Pressurised meter dose inhaler (pMDI) (salbutamol)
- Dry powder inhaler (DPI) (salbutamol and terbutaline)
- Nebulizer solution (salbutamol and terbutaline).

Long-acting β_2 agonists (salmeterol and formoterol)

Long-acting β_2 agonists have a 12 h duration of action. This is due to exceptional receptor binding. Salmeterol has an effect within 30 min, whereas formoterol has a faster onset of action. In asthma, they provide good symptom relief, reduce acute exacerbations, and improve quality of life when added to inhaled corticosteroids. They should not be used in asthma unless the patient is also on an inhaled corticosteroid. COPD studies have shown that they improve lung function and reduce hyperinflation, so they are used before inhaled corticosteroids. This results in a reduction in breathlessness, better exercise tolerance, and a sustained improvement in quality of life. In asthma they are effective against nocturnal respiratory symptoms. They should be considered in patients who:
- Have symptoms that are not controlled by regular short-acting β_2 agonists
- Have two or more exacerbations of COPD a year as they may help to reduce exacerbation rates
- Have asthma symptoms despite being on an inhaled corticosteroid.

Long-acting β_2 agonists are available in a pMDI (salmeterol) and in a DPI (salmeterol and formoterol).

Side-effects of β_2 agonists

As β_2 agonists are selective, the side-effects are dose-related. These include:
- Fine muscular tremor
- Tachycardia
- Headaches

- Muscle cramps.

Interactions
- Salbutamol possibly reduces the plasma concentration of digoxin
- Increased risk of hypokalaemia when high doses of β_2 agonists are administered with corticosteroids, diuretics or theophyllines.

Oral β_2 agonist bronchodilators

Inhaled bronchodilators should be used wherever possible, as they have a more rapid mode of action and are less likely to cause side-effects. Oral bronchodilators have a limited use and are mainly prescribed for people who are unable or unwilling to use any form of inhaled therapy. They are available in tablet and syrup preparations.

There are some controlled-release formulations which may be useful for asthmatic patients to prevent nocturnal dyspnoea. These include:
• Modified release salbutamol.

They are formulated in such a way that the drug is released in a controlled fashion over an extended period of time. They are usually given on a twice-daily basis, or once daily in the evening, for prevention of nocturnal symptoms.

Bambuterol

Bambuterol is rarely prescribed today. However, many patients may have been prescribed it for many years and be reluctant to discontinue it. It is a once-daily oral preparation that has bronchodilator effects after metabolism. One dose of bambuterol provides enough terbutaline to last 24 h. Once-daily dosing is possible as bambuterol is an active precursor of terbutaline. It is transformed over an extended period in the liver, the blood and the lungs to terbutaline, which produces bronchodilation.

Such a long duration of action means that it can be taken once daily to relieve nocturnal symptoms, as well as providing relief of daytime symptoms. However, it cannot be used as a substitute for conventional β_2 agonists, as it does not give acute symptomatic relief.

Antimuscarinic (anticholinergic) bronchodilators

Antimuscarinics are competitive antagonists of muscarinic acetylcholine receptors. They block the vagal control of bronchial smooth muscle tone in response to irritants and reduce bronchoconstriction. Three muscarinic-receptor subtypes—M1, M2 and M3 have been identified in the lung. Each offers a distinct site for influencing cholinergic activity:

- M1 receptor—facilitation of ganglionic transmission and enhancing cholinergic reflex in airways
- M2—autoinhibitory effect on acetylcholine release
- M3—stimulation of bronchoconstriction and mucus secretion.

They have two mechanisms of action:

- Reduction of reflex bronchoconstriction
- Reduction of mucous secretions.

As antimuscarinics only affect the vagally mediated element of broncho-constriction, they are not the first choice bronchodilator in asthma. Their main use is in COPD.

Short-acting antimuscarinic (ipratropium bromide)

This drug reaches its maximum effect within 30–60 mins and acts for between 3–6 h. Whilst it has a slower onset of action than β_2 agonists, it is equally effective in achieving symptom relief.

Long-acting anticholinergic (tiotropium)

Tiotropium is the first once-daily bronchodilator. It is a muscarinic receptor antagonist. Although it does not display selectivity for specific muscarinic receptors, on inhalation it acts mainly on M3 muscarinic receptors located in the airways to produce smooth muscle relaxation, thus producing a bronchodilatory effect.

In studies, tiotropium improved lung function, reduced breathlessness, reduced the number of exacerbations, and helped reduce the decline in health status associated with increasing exacerbations.

Side-effects

Side-effects are rare but include:

- Dry mouth
- Urinary retention
- Constipation.

Interactions

They do not usually apply to inhaled therapy.

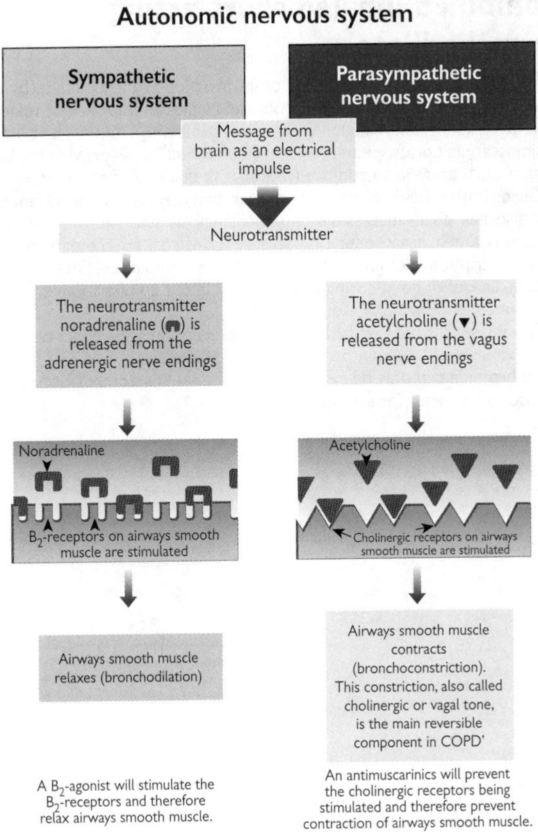

Autonomic nervous system

Fig. 15.2 β and cholinergic pathways.
Reproduced with permission from Boehringer Ingelheim.

Combined inhaled short-acting bronchodilators

As β_2 agonists and antimuscarinic drugs produce bronchodilation by different mechanisms, it is logical to combine inhaled therapy. A combination of a quick-acting, short-acting β_2 agonist (salbutamol) and a short-acting antimuscarinic (ipratropium bromide) (Combivent®), can provide the benefits of both drugs in an additive fashion, with quick relief of symptoms.

Giving both drugs in a combined preparation may offer some advantages but also has disadvantages. For a patient who is stabilised on the exact dosage regimen, it can offer simplicity, reduced cost for the patient (only one prescription see) and potentially enhance compliance. Disadvantages include lack of optimal dosing of salbutamol in this combination limited by the fourtimes a day dosage of ipratropium.

Combivent® is only available in nebulizer solution. Peak effect occurs at approximately 30–60 min post-dose and lasts between 4–6 h. As ipratropium bromide can only be given four times a day, the combination cannot be used as fequently as salbutamol alone.

Methylxanthines (theophyllines)

Theophyllines have been used in patients with asthma and COPD for over 50 years. In the UK today theophyllines are third or fourth line therapy.

They appear to work by inhibiting phosphodiesterase, thereby preventing the breakdown of cAMP. The amount of cAMP within the bronchial smooth muscle cells is therefore increased, which causes bronchodilation in a similar way to β_2 agonists.

Theophyllines are metabolized in the liver, and there is considerable variation in half-life between individuals. This has important implications because there is a small therapeutic window. Theophyllines produce only small amounts of bronchodilation in COPD, and tend to be most effective in the higher parts of the therapeutic range (blood levels of 10–20mg/litre). Other effects that have been reported are anti-inflammatory actions, and improvements in respiratory muscle strength. Factors that alter theophylline clearance include:

Increased clearance
- Smoking (patients who stop smoking may need their theophylline dose decreasing to avoid side-effects)
- Alcohol
- Drugs (e.g. rifampicin)
- Childhood.

Decreased clearance
- Pneumonia
- Liver disease
- Drugs (e.g. cimetidine, clarithromycin)
- Old age.

It is preferable to give theophyllines in a slow-release form, and to monitor levels regularly.

Side-effects

There is considerable potential for side-effects, especially with long-term use. Recognized side-effects include:
- Arrhythmias
- Headaches
- Insomnia
- Gastrointestinal symptoms
- Hypokalaemia (which may potentiate resulting from other therapy including β_2 agonists and steroids)
- Convulsions.

Inhaled corticosteroids (ICS)

Corticosteroids are anti-inflammatory agents. They are used for the management of reversible and irreversible airway disease. They have been shown to reduce both the morbidity and mortality of asthma, and are the cornerstone of management for all but the mildest forms of asthma. Their role in treating COPD is less clear.

When the corticosteroid is inhaled, the molecules pass through the cell membrane of the airway epithelial cells. Once in the cytoplasm, they conjugate with the corticosteroid receptors, and the resulting steroid/steroid receptor complex moves to the nucleus, where it binds to many sites to alter the transcription of genes. The overall effect is to suppress the inflammatory process.

The main functions of ICS are:
• To reduce eosinophils—T-cells and mast cells in the airways
• To inhibit the late bronchoconstrictor response caused by allergen exposure
• To suppress the inflammatory cell influx, cytokine production and oedema.

The advantage of ICS is that they deliver the drug directly to the airways. This means that lower doses of the drug can be given. They are most effective when they are used over an extended period of time.

ICS in asthma and COPD

ICS in asthma

Corticosteroids have been shown to influence all aspects of the inflammatory process. ICS works by altering the production of many genes that are involved in the inflammatory process, influencing the synthesis of inflammatory proteins and cytokines (🕮 p.145). They have the ability to treat the disease rather than modify the symptoms.

Actions of corticosteroids

- Reduce mucus production by goblet cells
- Restore epithelial cell growth
- Inhibit inflammatory cell recruitment to the airways
- Reduce the number of mast cells in the airways
- Reduce bronchial hyper-reactivity
- Increase the number of β_2 adrenoreceptors.

ICS in COPD

Although COPD is primarily a chronic inflammatory airway disease it has a different underlying pathology to asthma. Its response to drug treatment varies.

In the late 1990s, four large-scale randomized controlled studies assessing the long-term role of ICS in the management of COPD were undertaken. These trials looked at the rate of decline in lung function over time. All the studies found that ICS given in reasonably large doses did not alter the natural course of the disease. It was concluded that ICS were of no benefit in mild COPD (🕮 p.249).

Some benefits of ICS were noted; chiefly a reduction in exacerbation rates. It is currently recommended that patients with moderate or severe COPD are prescribed high doses of ICS. Prescribers should note that ICS as a single preparation is not currently licensed for use in COPD in the UK. It is only licensed when given as part of a combination therapy with a long-acting β_2.

Side-effects of ICS

ICS are absorbed via the oropharynx, lungs and gut. Absorption which bypasses the gut, and does not undergo first-pass metabolism in the liver, has a greater chance of causing systemic side-effects. The dose–response curves for systemic adverse effects and beneficial effects are different (see Figure 15.3).

At low doses of ICS, predominantly prescribed in asthma, there is good clinical efficacy with minimal side-effects. As the dose increases, for example in more severe asthma or in COPD, there is an increasing risk of adverse effects, with minimal improvement in clinical efficacy. It can be difficult to determine the optimal dose of ICS; this varies for many reasons including:

- The potency of the ICS
- The delivery device used
- The calibre of the patient's airway
- The severity of asthma.

Local side-effects

- Oropharyngeal infection such as *candida albicans*
- Vocal cord problems such as hoarseness and occasionally vocal cord paralysis
- Nebulized corticosteroids are associated with skin thinning under the mask.

Systemic side-effects

- Higher doses of ICS for prolonged periods have the potential to induce adrenal suppression
- Bone mineral density may be reduced following long-term high-dose ICS
- There is a small risk of glaucoma and cataracts with prolonged high doses of ICS.

Interactions

Interactions do not generally occur.

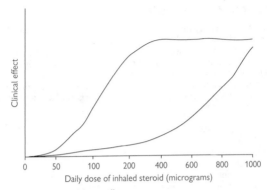

Blue line = Adverse effects
Black line = Clinical benefit

Fig. 15.3 Schematic dose–response curves for beneficial and adverse effects of ICS

Choice of ICS

There are various considerations to take into account when prescribing an ICS. These include the:
- Type of patient
- Severity of the disease
- Inhaler device needed
- Dose of ICS required
- Therapeutic:side-effect ratio
- Cost implications.

Types of ICS

There are five types of ICS currently on the market, in both aerosol and dry powder formulations:
- Beclometasone diproprionate
- Budesonide
- Ciclesonide
- Fluticasone propionate
- Mometasone furoate.

The dose of ICS varies depending on the preparation and inhalation system used.

Oral corticosteroids

Although oral steroids can be very effective in controlling symptoms, these drugs are associated with very significant side-effects. They are used during acute exacerbations of asthma, COPD, and bronchiectasis, and very occasionally as maintenance treatment for all three diseases. They are also sometimes used for the maintenace of interstitial lung disease.

In these situations, the benefits of high-dose systemic oral corticosteroids are judged against the potential risk of side-effects. The list of known side-effects include:

• Weight gain
• Thinning of the skin
• Hypertension
• Glucose intolerance
• Fluid retention
• Immunosuppression
• Mood changes such as depression or hypermania
• Gastrointestinal disturbance
• Myopathy
• Cataracts
• Osteoporosis
• Growth suppression
• Adrenal gland suppression.

Patients should be told about the possibility of side-effects before starting oral corticosteroids, particularly when the treatment is expected to be lengthy. Patients should also be supplied with a steroid warning card when they collect their prescription. These cards advise patients about potential side-effects, and about how and when to stop the treatment. Patients are advised to show the card to other health professionals they come into contact with, so it is known that they are on steroids.

Dosage regimen

Systemic corticosteroids should be used at the lowest effective dose and for the shortest possible time in order to avoid adverse events (📖 p.259).

Those patients who are on maintenance steroids should be monitored and treated for osteoporosis. Any patient requiring several short courses or maintenance oral steroids should be referred for specialist assessment and supervision.

Adrenal suppression

Prolonged treatment with high doses of corticosteroids may result in adrenal suppression and acute adrenal crisis. Situations, which could potentially trigger acute adrenal crisis, include:

- Trauma
- Surgery
- Infection
- Rapid reduction in dosage.

Presenting symptoms are typically vague and may include anorexia, abdominal pain, weight loss, tiredness, headache, nausea, vomiting, decreased level of consciousness, hypoglycaemia, and seizures.

Respiratory specialist advice should be sought for advice on weaning patients who have been treated with oral steroids for a prolonged period of time.

Special precautions

There is an increased risk of hypokalaemia when corticosteroids are given with high doses of β_2 agonists and theophyllines. When administered in prolonged or repeated courses during pregnancy, systemic corticosteroids increase the risk of intrauterine growth restriction.

Traces of prednisolone have been found in small amounts in the breast milk of women treated with the drug.

Interactions

High-dose corticosteroids impair the immune response to live vaccines.

Combined inhaled corticosteroids and long-acting bronchodilators (ICS/LABA)

Combined inhaled corticosteroids and long-acting bronchodilators are available in one inhaler device. There are currently three long-acting β-agonist/ICS combinations available in the UK: Symbicort® (budesonide and formoterol), Seretide® (fluticasone and salmeterol) and Fostair® (beclometasone and formoterol). Symbicort® and Seretide® have been licensed for use in both asthma and COPD, Fostair® is currently only licensed for use in asthma.

Studies have indicated that there are benefits from using combination therapy in both asthma and COPD. These include:
- Reduction in exacerbation rates
- Improvements in symptoms
- Improvements in lung function
- Improvements in health status
  The ICS/LABA combination offers advantages. These include:
- Patient convenience
- Greater treatment adherence
- Preventing asthmatic patients using LABA's as monotherapy
- Cost savings to health providers—combination therapy is cheaper
- Cost savings for patients—only one prescription fee to pay
- Combination medication is recommended for patients who are on step three and above on the BTS/SIGN asthma guidelines (📖 p.147), and for patients with COPD with an FEV_1 of less than 50% predicted, who experience two or more exacerbations a year (📖 p.249)
- The disadvantage of using a combined inhaler is that you cannot titrate the doses independently without changing the product the patient is familiar with
- Symbicort is licensed at step 3 of the guidelines as both a reliever and a preventer, known as SMART therapy.

Side-effects and interactions

As for LABAs and ICS

Leukotriene receptor agonists (LTRAs)

LTRAs are anti-inflammatories used in the management of asthma. Unlike ICS, which act on a variety of sites within the inflammatory cascade, LTRAs block the effect of cysteinyl leukotrienes in the airways. Leukotrienes are implicated as a cause of bronchoconstriction in asthma. They can also cause airway wall oedema and attract eosinophil inflammation in the airways.

About 20–40% of the asthmatic population have asthma modulated by leukotrienes. Clinical practice suggests a 4–6 week trial of LTRAs. If there is no improvement in symptoms after this period they should be stopped.

One of the advantages of LTRAs is that they can be given in oral form in either a tablet or granules. There are two drugs currently available:
• Montelukast
• Zafirlukast.

With the exception of exercise-induced asthma , neither drug is licensed for use alone. They are ineffective in an acute attack of asthma.

Effects of LTRAs

LTRAs:
• Cause an increase in peak flow measurements and FEV_1
• Reduce β_2 agonist use
• Improve symptom scores in moderate to severe asthma
• Improve exercise-induced asthma symptoms
• Provide an additive effect for patients with uncontrolled asthma, despite being on high-dose ICS
• May reduce the risk of acute exacerbations of asthma.

LTRAs in allergic rhinitis

LTRAs are effective treatments for allergic rhinitis, either used as a single agent or combined with an oral antihistamine. They should be considered for people who have moderate or severe persistant allergic rhinitis with accompanying asthma (📖 p.145). Only montelukast currently has a licence in the UK for allergic rhinitis.

Adverse effects of LTRAs

LTRAs are generally well tolerated. Common adverse effects include:
- Headache
- Nausea and vomiting
- Gastrointestinal upset
- Skin rashes.

Rare adverse effects are:
- Abnormalities of liver function tests
- Churg–Strauss syndrome, characterized by systemic vasculitis with eosinophilia and asthma. It occurs more often in women than men.

No studies have been undertaken in pregnancy; the recommendations are to use the LTRAs only if the potential benefit outweighs the risk. They are contraindicated in breastfeeding women.

Interactions
- Plasma concentrations of zafirlukast are increased by aspirin and decreased by erythromycin, terfenadine and theophylline
- Zafirlukast enhances the anticoagulant effect of warfarin
- Plasma concentrations of montelukast are reduced by primidone, rifampicin and phenobarbital.

Cromones

Cromones are anti-inflammatory drugs, licensed for use in asthma. There are two cromones currently available on prescription: sodium cromoglicate and nedocromil sodium. Sodium cromoglicate was the first non-steroidal anti-inflammatory drug to be introduced for the treatment of asthma.

The mode of action of both drugs is not completely understood. They are thought to inhibit sensitized mast cell degranulation, which occurs after exposure to specific allergens, and are effective against both the early and late responses to allergens, reducing airway hyper-responsiveness to some degree. However, their anti-inflammatory properties are less potent than those of ICS.

They may be of benefit in asthma with an allergic basis, or for exercise-induced symptoms, but in practice, it is difficult to predict who will benefit. A 4–6 week trial is advised to assess clinical response. They need to be given four times daily to be effective, and offer no value in the treatment of acute attacks of asthma.

Side-effects

An unpleasant taste.

Contraindications and interactions

None.

Anti-IgE monoclonal antibody (omalizumab)

Omalizumab is a novel development in the management of patients with IgE-mediated asthma. It is a recombinant humanized monoclonal anti-IgE antibody that selectively binds IgE. This inhibits free IgE from binding to the high-affinity IgE receptor on the surface of the mast cells and basophils, decreasing the allergic response.

It is licensed for use as additional therapy in adults and adolescents (over 12) with:

- Proven IgE-mediated sensitivity to inhaled allergens
- Severe persistent allergic asthma which cannot be controlled adequately with high-dose ICS together with a LABA
- Documented frequent exacerbations of asthma
- Reduced lung function (FEV$_1$ <80% of predicted)
- Frequent day and night symptoms.

Dosing regimen

The dose of omalizumab is based on pre-treatment IgE serum level (range is >30 and <700 IU/ml) and maximum body weight <150kg.

Administration

Omalizumab is administered by subcutaneous injection every 2–4 weeks, depending on the dose required. Treatment effectiveness should be reviewed by a clinician at 16 weeks. Treatment is continued if there is a subjective or objective improvement in asthma control.

Side-effects include

- Headache
- Injection site reactions.

Special precautions

- Should not be used in pregnancy unless clearly needed
- Breastfeeding is contraindicated.

Interactions

- No formal drug interaction studies have been undertaken.

Mucolytics

Mucolytic drugs are mucus-controlling agents. They act directly on mucus, altering its molecular composition and breaking down sticky, thick secretions, making it easier to expectorate. They are generally used in individuals with COPD, and occasionally in bronchiectasis.

Mucolytics can be considered for either chronic or acute management of COPD.

Chronic management

There are two drugs currently available in the UK: carbocisteine and mecysteine. Clinical trials have suggested benefits such as:

- Reductions in exacerbations
- Reduction in days with illness
- Improvement of symptoms.

They should be considered in patients with chronic productive cough and continued in patients who have an improvement in their symptoms.

Dosing regimen

- Carbocisteine: initially 750mg 3 times daily for 2 weeks, followed by 750mg twice daily
- Mecysteine: 200mg 4 times daily for 2 days, then 200mg 3 times daily for 6 weeks, then 200mg twice daily.

Acute management

Erdosteine has recently been licensed as an adjunct to standard care for the symptomatic treatment of acute exacerbations of COPD. It also modulates mucus production and viscosity, and increases mucociliary transport, thereby improving expectoration.

Co-administration of erdosteine with an antibiotic such as amoxicillin results in higher concentrations of antibiotic in the sputum, leading to earlier and more pronounced treatment of infection.

Dosage regimen

- Erdosteire: 300mg twice daily.

Contraindications of mucolytics

- Should be used with caution in those with a history of peptic ulceration
- Pregnancy.

Inhaler devices

Inhalation is the preferred route of administration for asthma and COPD therapies, because fewer systemic side-effects are produced by inhaled compared with oral therapy. Drugs go directly to the airways where they are needed. Large amounts of the drug are not removed by the enzymes in the liver, as the drugs do not have to pass through the digestive system. Lower doses of drugs can be used when administered through an inhaler compared to oral preparations, and the risk of side-effects is reduced (see Table 15.2, p. 411).

With the exception of xanthines and LTRAs which are given orally, and omalizumab which is given subcutaneously, all other therapies are available in inhaled form.

Basic principles

The dose of drug released from the inhaler travels through the mouth to the oropharynx, down the bronchi and into the lungs to reach the target site. Ideally, all of the drug would reach the intended site, but even in the best cases, much of the dose never reaches it (see Figure 15.4). There are many reasons for this, but the most important factors are the aerosol particle size, airway geometry, the efficiency of the inhaler device and the technique used.

Particle size

- Particle size is measured in millionths of a metre, known as micrometres (previously measured in microns)
- Deposition within the respiratory system depends on the size of the particles
- To achieve maximum effect, the medication needs to pass through the larger airways to the smaller airways deeper within the lung
- If the particle size is too large (>6 micrometres) they are deposited in the oropharynx and mouth
- If the particle size is too small (<2 micrometres) they are deposited in the peripheral airways and alveoli or may be exhaled without being deposited in the lungs
- Optimal particle size needs to be between 2–5 micrometres to have a therapeutic effect

Airway geometry

- The route the inhaled drug must follow to reach the lungs is through a series of bends and branches (bifurcations) where the main airway splits into two or more smaller air passageways
- These bifurcations happen many times before the airway eventually end at the alveoli
- The medication particles must be carried in the airflow without impaction on the large airway walls; the more that is impacted, the less that is carried to the smaller airways.

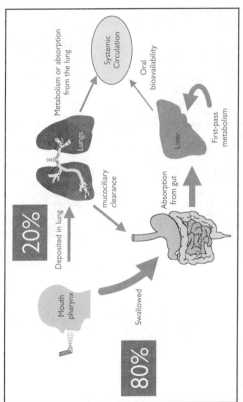

Fig. 15.4 Fate of inhaled drugs

Reproduced with the kind permission of J Bell/Canday Medical Ltd

Inspiratory flow

Airspeed is an important influence on how well an aerosol travels into the lung. Aerosol dose and particle size from different types of device may not change significantly, but no matter how fast the patient inhales, if the inhalation is the wrong speed, little of the aerosol produced will reach the target site in the lungs.

General principles

- Putting an inhaler device in or near the mouth affects how easily air can be inhaled
- An inhaler that allows air to travel with little difficulty will have little effect on the speed of inhalation, and will be found to have a low resistance
- Those inhalers that prevent air from moving easily will have a large effect on the speed of inhalation, and have a high resistance
- It is not possible to differentiate between high- and low-resistance inhalers just by looking at them
- The route air follows when travelling through an inhaler will determine its internal resistance
- Internal resistance will also be affected by airway resistance—caused by bronchoconstriction, found in asthma and COPD
- The speed of inhalation can be increased when a resistance is present, by putting additional effort into breathing in, but the higher the resistance experienced, the greater the effort needed to overcome it
- Individuals have their own personal maximum inspiratory flow for a resistance they encounter
- This depends on the strength of their respiratory muscles, the effort that is comfortable when inhaling, and is reduced if there is fatigue or exhaustion.

Types of inhaled therapy

There are four types of inhaled therapy currently available:
• Pressurized aerosol inhalers
• Dry powder inhalers
• Nebulized systems
• Fine mist inhaler (Respimat®).
All four systems will be discussed in detail.

There are many things that should be considered when selecting an inhaler device for a person with asthma and COPD. These include:
• Choosing a device the patient finds easy to use
• The age of the patient and their ability to use the device appropriately
• A device that fits in with the patient's needs
• The use of multiple medications
• Costs and reimbursement
• Drug administration time
• Convenience and durability
• Patient preference.

Patient factors

Acceptance of the device by the patient is critical to its successful use. If a patient has problems learning to use one device, it is worth trying a different one. Regular and frequent checks of technique are essential for acceptance and understanding of the device.

The health professional's role in matching the device to the patient is critical, and the patient must have a key role in the choice. Therapy for asthma and COPD is often changed or adjusted because symptoms do not improve, or become worse. Before any change in dose or therapy class is considered, inhaler technique should be reviewed in case the patient is not using the device correctly.

Table 15.2 Comparison of oral versus inhaled therapies

Feature	Inhaled therapy	Oral therapy
Dose	Low	High
Speed of onset	Rapid	Slow
Side-effects	Few	Some
Administration	Requires instruction	Easy
Site of action	Direct access	Indirect access

Pressurized metered dose inhalers

The pressurized metered dose inhaler (pMDI) is still the most widely prescribed inhaler device in the UK, and is used by over 75% of patients. Because of the need to coordinate actuation with inspiration, the patient needs careful instruction to ensure correct use. Speed of inhalation is important, and aerosol inhalers require slow inhalation so that small particles of the drug carried in the aerosol reach the smaller airways.

The drug is suspended in a propellant, consisting of either chlorofluro-carbon (CFC) or hydrofluoroalkane (HFA).

CFC v. HFA

Following the signing of the Montreal protocol on reducing the use of chorofluorocarbons worldwide, pMDIs containing CFCs are being withdrawn. The production, importation, and use of CFCs have been stopped in most developed countries because of the effect on the ozone layer. Most HFA pMDIs have a one-to-one equivalence with their CFC-containing counterparts and can be replaced dose for dose. Where such an HFA is not available, dose adjustments will be necessary.

Advantages of pMDIs
- If used properly, a pMDI is at least as effective as any other form of delivery and is much cheaper
- Most drug classes come in a pMDI
- They are small and portable.

Disadvantages of pMDIs
- Difficulty in coordinating actuation with inhalation
- Deposition of drug at the back of the mouth and throat
- Even with good technique, only about 10% of a metered dose reaches the lower airways where it is needed
- The chilling effects of the propellant (cold freon effect) impacting on the oropharynx may stop the patient inhaling.

- **Inhaler technique with pMDI**
- Shake inhaler and breathe out
- Remove lid
- Close lips and teeth around mouthpiece
- At the start of inspiration, press the canister down and continue to inhale slowly and deeply
- Remove device from mouth and close lips
- Hold breath for 10 s, or as long as is comfortable
- If a second dose is required, wait 30–60 s and repeat before replacing the cover.

Points to consider

pMDIs are often misused, with the most common fault being a failure to inhale at the appropriate rate at the same time the device is actuated. Some patients do not have enough strength in their fingers to depress the pMDI canister. Fitting the right size Haleraid® to the device may assist the patient to actuate the device.

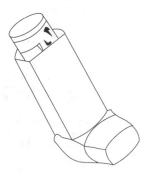

Fig. 15.5 Example of pMDI

Spacer devices

Problems of coordinating actuating the pMDI and inhaling the drug can be overcome by using a spacer device. The spacer device reduces the speed of the aerosol and subsequent impaction on the oropharynx. A spacer device also allows more time for the propellant to evaporate, allowing a larger proportion of the drug particles to be inhaled and deposited in the lungs, while reducing the proportion absorbed into the body (which is usually the cause of unwanted effects).

Spacer devices are particularly useful for patients:
• With poor inhaler technique
• Requiring high doses of drugs
• Who are prone to oral candidiasis.

There are two types of spacer available: large and small volume spacers. The large volume spacers (LVS) (Volumatic, Nebuhaler) are made of plastic and can hold approximately 750mls of air. The small volume spacers (SVS) (Aerochamber Plus, Able spacer) are also made of plastic. There is one SVS (Nebuchamber) which is made of metal. They can hold between 145–250mls. Both LVS and SVS have a valve system which prevents exhalation of the drug through the mouthpiece.

The dose may be reduced by accumulation of electrostatic charge so that the drug is absorbed onto the plastic. This can be avoided by periodic washing of the device in soapy water or detergent. Patients should be advised to let the spacer air dry, and not to dry it with a towel. The devices may be fitted with a mask, which can aid administration of medication to people who are unable to grip the mouthpiece. Where a mask is fitted to a spacer device, the inhaler may need to be tilted to help the valve fall open.

Compared with pMDI alone, lung deposition is generally thought either increased or unchanged by using spacers. Factors such as inhalation technique and the amount of electrostatic charge present in the spacer are likely to account for this.

Advantages of spacers:
• More effective treatment with fewer side-effects—because of better pattern of deposition
• Problems of poor inhaler technique largely overcome—but spacers need to be used properly too
• Easily used by children and the elderly—except those with weak or arthritic hands
• May be as effective as a nebulizer in the treatment of acute attacks—but light, cheap, maintenance-free, portable, and available on prescription
• Useful for treatment for first attacks of wheezing in patients who have not used inhalers before
• Useful for administration of bronchodilator when testing reversibility in the surgery to establish the diagnosis of asthma
• Reduced prescribing costs by basing treatment on cheaper pMDIs.

Disadvantages
- Bulkier and less portable than pMDI alone
- Require cleaning to reduce electrostatic charge
- Not suitable for all types of pMDI canister.

Inhaler technique
- Remove the cap from the mouthpiece of the inhaler and shake the inhaler
- Insert the inhaler mouthpiece into the hole in the end of the spacer
- Put lips and teeth around the spacer mouthpiece (not in front of it and do not bite it), and seal lips around the spacer mouthpiece
- Press down on the canister in the inhaler to spray one puff of inhaler into the spacer
- EITHER breathe in slowly and deeply, then hold your breath for 10 s or as long as is comfortably possible
- Breathe out, then breathe in deeply again through the mouthpiece of the spacer and hold the breath. You should take two deep-held breaths from the spacer for each puff from the inhaler
- OR take five breaths in and out (tidal breathing), keeping lips and teeth around mouthpiece
- If a second dose is required, wait 30 s, shake the inhaler again, then repeat as above.

Points to consider
- The dose should be inhaled within 10 s, as settling of the drug reduces deposition
- Single rather than multiple actuations should be used, as the latter will reduce the drug available for inhalation
- The right spacer should be used with the appropriate inhaler
- When masks are used they should be closely applied, as a gap of more than 1cm between mask and face will greatly diminish drug deposition
- Child masks should be used in children to reduce peripheral deposition
- Spacers are important in treating acute severe asthma and are as effective as nebulizers for administering β_2 agonist medication
- Patients prescribed any spacer device for the first time, or switched to a different device should be monitored frequently for the emergence of or worsening of symptoms.

Breath actuated pMDIs

There are two types of breath-actuated devices currently available on prescription: the Easibreathe and Autohaler devices. A vacuum-operated trigger mechanism actuates the device when the patient inhales. Like the pMDI, a slow inspiration is required.

Advantages of breath actuated devices

- The technique is simple to teach
- There is no need for coordination of actuation and inhalation when using these devices
- The Easibreathe device has an extension tube provided to lessen the risk of oropharangeal deposition.

Disadvantages

- These devices are bulkier than unadapted pMDIs
- They are only available to deliver salbutamol and beclometasone
- Some of these devices produce a click on inspiration, which may inhibit full inhalation.

Inhaler technique

- Prime the device if using the Autohaler
- Shake the device and exhale
- Close lips and teeth around mouthpiece
- Inhale deeply and slowly
- Remove the device from the mouth and close lips
- Hold breath for 10 s
- Close cap of Easibreathe device—this action primes the inhaler
- With the Autohaler, push the lever back down
- If a second dose is required, wait 60 s and repeat.

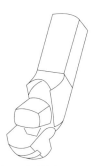

Fig. 15.6 Example of a breath-actuated inhaler

Table 15.3 Example of drugs available in aerosol devices

Device	Manufacturer	Drug available
AeroBec® Autohaler	3M	Beclometasone
Airomir® pMDI and Autohaler® Breathe-actuated device	IVAX	Salbutamol
Alvesco® pMDI	Altana	Ciclesonide
Atimos Modulite® pMDI	Trinity-Chiesi	Formoterol
Clenil Modulite® pMDI	Trinity-Chiesi	Beclometasone
Easi-Breathe® Breathe-actuated device	IVAX	Salbutamol Beclometasone
Evohaler® pMDI	A&H	Salbutamol Fluticasone Salmeterol Combined fluticasone and Salmeterol
Generic preperations		Salbutamol Salmeterol Ipratropium bromide Beclometasone
Pulmicort® pMDI	AstraZeneca	Budesonide
Qvar® pMDI, Autohaler and Easi-Breathe	IVAX	Beclometasone

Table 15.4 Drug available in soft mist device

Device	Manufacture	Drug available
Fostair pMDI	Trinity Chiesi	Combined beclometasone and formoterol
Spirivia Respimat®	Boehringer Ingelheim	Tiotropium

Dry powder inhalers

Dry powder inhalers (DPIs) were designed to overcome issues related to coordination and difficulties in the use of pMDIs. They consist of a drug in powder form, either contained in a multidose inhaler or in a capsule, which needs to be loaded into the inhaler device.

All the devices are breath actuated, with turbulent airflow from inspiration through the device, providing the power to create an aerosol of drug particles. Unlike aerosol inhalers, DPIs rely on the airflow through the device to create the aerosol cloud; they need harder, faster inhalation to produce better deposition. There are several types of DPIs available (see Table 15.5).

Advantages of DPIs
- Small and portable
- Short preparation and administration time
- Easy to use and teach
- Decreased coordination requirements
- No CFC propellants
- Count of remaining doses available.

Disadvantages of DPIs
- Limited range of drugs available in each device
- Possible reaction to carrier substance (lactose/glucose)
- Increased inspiratory flow rates required for some devices to generate small enough particles to penetrate the airways
- Some devices need to be loaded prior to use
- Sometimes patients complain that they are not certain if they have taken a dose; devices may be discarded well before they are empty
- The dry powder can make some patients cough
- Those with arthritis in the hands may find some of these devices difficult to use.

Inhaler technique
- Follow manufacturer's instructions for loading the device
- Breathe out
- Place lips and teeth firmly around the mouthpiece
- Breathe rapidly and deeply
- Repeat as above for second inhalation.

Points to consider
- Patients should be advised not to breathe out through the device in case the powder is blown out before inspiration
- Some DPIs can be affected by humidity; the device should be kept in dry surroundings
- Extreme heat may also affect the DPI device.

Fig. 15.7 Example of a DPI

Table 15.5 Examples of dry powder devices and drugs available

Device	Manufacture	Drug available
Turbohaler®	AstraZeneca	Terbutaline Budesonide Formoterol Combined budesonide and formoterol
Accuhaler®	A&H	Salbutamol Fluticasone Salmeterol Combined fluticasone and salmeterol
Clickhaler®	Celltech	Salbutamol Beclometasone
Diskhaler®	A&H	Fluticasone
Pulvinal®	Trinity Chiesi	Salbutamol Beclometasone
Cyclohaler®		Salbutamol Beclometasone Budesonide
Easyhaler®		Salbutamol Beclometasone Budesonide
Foradil® Device	Novartis	Formoterol
Novolizer®	Viatris	Budesonide
Twisthaler®	Schering-Plough	Mometasone furoate
Aerohaler®	Boehringer Ingelheim	Ipratropium bromide
HandiHaler®	Boehringer Ingelheim	Tiotropium
Spinhaler®	Rhone-Poulenc Rorer	Sodium cromoglicate

Nebulized therapy 1

A nebulizer is a device that turns an aqueous solution of a drug into a mist of fine particles, which are then inhaled into the lungs. The aim of nebulizer therapy is to deliver a therapeutic dose of the drug within a short delivery time. This is usually less than 10 min.

A nebulizer is most beneficial when:
- Large doses of drug are required
- Patients are too unwell or are unable to coordinate inhaler devices
- Drugs are unavailable in inhaled form.

Indications for use

- To deliver bronchodilators to treat acute exacerbations of asthma or COPD
- To deliver bronchodilators on a regular basis to patients with severe asthma or COPD who have been shown to benefit from regular treatment
- To deliver an antibiotic to patients with bronchiectasis or cystic fibrosis
- To deliver prophylactic medication such as corticosteroids to patients unable to use any other form of inhaled therapy.

Types of nebulizers

There are two types of nebulizer generally available, jet and ultrasonic.

Jet nebulizers

Jet nebulizers are most commonly used; and consist of a nebulizer chamber attached to a mask or mouthpiece. Nebulizers are driven by compressed air generated by an electrical pump (compressor), or driven by compressed air or oxygen from a cylinder. A conventional 2 L/4 L cylinder does not generate the power necessary to reduce the particle size of the inhaled drug. High-pressure oxygen pipelines can be used. A flow of gas is passed through a precisely engineered narrow hole known as a Venturi.

Gas passes through the Venturi at high pressure, creating a negative pressure around it. This sucks the liquid for nebulization up the feed tube into the stream of gas where it is atomized into large particles of between 15 and 500 micrometres. These particles are then impacted against the nebulizer baffle to form small, respirable particles which pass out of the chamber to the patient. Any remaining large particles are trapped against the baffle and drop back into the liquid for re-nebulization.

The proportion of a nebulizer solution that reaches the lungs depends on the type of nebulizer used. It can be as high as 30%, but is more often around 10%. The deposition rate depends on:
- Drug particle size—particles of 1–5 micrometers are deposited in the airways, and are suitable for patients with asthma and COPD
- The characteristics of the chamber
- The output speed of the compressed gas
- The viscosity of the solution—antibiotic solutions are usually more viscous
- If two drugs are given together, they should be well mixed beforehand and not left to stand, or the less viscous will be preferentially nebulized first

- Fill volume (minimum 2.5ml, maximum varies—refer to manufacturers' instructions).

Using a jet nebulizer

The technique has a dramatic effect on drug delivery, so the correct procedure should be followed. The following factors are important

- Driving gas—in acute asthma, oxygen should be used as the driving gas, but only if an appropriate source is available. In all other situations air should be used
- Diluents and fill volumes—all nebulizer chambers leave a residual volume of between 0.5–1.0ml
- Flow rates—gas flow rates influence both nebulization time and the size of the droplets being dispersed. An increased flow rate means that although nebulization time is shorter, the size of the droplets is smaller. The flow rate should be set at 8 L/min
- Delivery time—the nebulizer will never run dry because of the residual volume. Up to 80% of the total dose is administered within the first five minutes of delivery, depending on the type of drug and nebulizer. Compliance reduces with longer administration time, and the nebulizer chamber should be tapped when spluttering occurs
- Patient position—if possible, the patient should be sitting upright. Ensure that the mask fits properly and encourage the patient to breathe normally. Discourage talking whilst using the nebulizer, as this reduces the efficiency of the drug delivery.

Nebulized therapy 2

Ultrasonic nebulizers

Aerosol particles are produced by the rapid vibration of a piezo crystal.

The crystal vibrates in response to electrical current from a battery. These vibrations are transmitted through the drug solution causing particles to break off from the surface. Large particles impact against the baffle. A valve opens as the patient inhales, drawing air through the nebulizer to carry the smaller, respirable particles to the airways.

Advantages of ultrasonic nebulizers
- Small and portable
- Can be run off batteries or car cigarette lighters
- Almost silent in use.

Disadvantages
- They are not as efficient at nebulizing drug suspensions, such as corticosteroids
- They are expensive
- They can become warm in use
- They are recommended for occasional rather than long-term use.

Nebulizer care

Jet nebulizers
- Nebulizer chambers are for single patient use and must be disposed of on discharge from hospital
- If antibiotics have been used the nebulizer should be disposed off after the course, and every 24 h in patients with cystic fibrosis
- Patients on long-term nebulized therapy should be issued with a durable nebulizer which should be replaced annually
- The durable nebulizer should be rinsed after use and air-dried
- Once a week, the durable nebulizer and mouthpiece should be boiled for 5 min in water and a drop of liquid detergent
- Patients with non-durable nebulizers should also rinse after each use, but replace the chamber every three months
- The filters in the compressor should be changed according to the manufacturer's instructions
- The compressor should be placed on a hard surface when in use
- Patients' should be provided with spare fuses and filters to minimize the risk that they will be left without a useable machine.

Jet and ultrasonic
- All nebulizers should be serviced annually
- Patients should be advised to ask for medical assistance if they do not get their usual relief of symptoms from their nebulizer.

Implications of nebulized therapy
- Current evidence suggests that there is little difference in the effectiveness of nebulizers and alternative inhaler devices
- Nebulized drugs are much more expensive than either pMDIs or DPIs
- Nebulizers can be cumbersome, expensive, noisy, and treatment can take a long time. All these factors can tie the patient to the home

- Advantages include not needing to be able to co-ordinate the inhaler device with breathing technique, so they can be used by patients of all ages.

Table 15.6 Nebulized therapies available

Drug type	Drug name/strenth	Comment
β agonist	Salbutamol unit dose vial (UDV) 2.5–5mg in 2.5ml Terbutaline UDV 5mg in 2ml	
Anticholinergic	Ipratropium bromide UDV 250mcg in 1ml UDV 500mcg in 2ml	Use of mouthpiece preferable to mask to reduce damage to eye
Combination products*	Combivent® UDV ipratropium bromide 500mcg/salbutamol 2.5mg Duovent® UDV fenoterol 1.25mg/ipratropium bromide 500mcg	Use of mouthpiece preferable to mask to reduce damage to eye
Corticosteroids	Budesonide UDV 500mcg in 2ml Respule 1mg in 2ml Fluticasone UDV 500mcg in 2ml UDV 2mg in 2ml	Use of mouthpiece preferable to mask to reduce deposition of drug around mouth, face and eyes

* Giving 60m drugs in a combined preparation may offer some advantages but also has disadvantages (see page 412).

Further information

http://www.bnf.org
For images of all inhaler devices see *mims for nurses*.

Inspiratory flow meters

As the majority of respiratory medication is inhaled, optimum inhaler technique is an important factor in the management of the disease. Assessing inspiratory flow is an opportunity to educate and review inhaler use.

Assessing inspiration can also:
- Determine whether or not a patient can obtain sufficient inspiratory flow for a device, a significant step towards optimizing treatment
- Reveal a patient's inability to use a particular device
- Alert health professionals to a likely reason why a patient may not have responded to a particular treatment.

Benefits of inspiratory flow meters

- Recognition of suboptimal inhalation is more difficult than many perceive; experienced respiratory professionals now recognize that a visual observation of technique may be inaccurate without an objective test
- Patients can be shown exactly how much they need to modify their technique
- Encouraging a patient to either slow down or speed up their inhalation is easier when there is a gauge to measure progress.

Types of flow meters

In-check dial® (Clement Clarke)

This is the most commonly available meter. It is a hand-held mechanical flow measurement device, providing objective assessment of inspiratory flow through up to six selectable resistances—simulating commonly prescribed inhaler designs. There are different In-check dials® and not all models will simulate all available inhalers in the UK.

It measures inspiratory flow rates in the range of 15 to 120l/min, with an accuracy of +/– 10% or 10 L/min (whichever is the greatest). It is the only device available to assess both pMDI and DPI technique. Manufacturer's instructions for cleaning should be followed.

2Tone Trainer® (Canday Medical LTD)

This is a medical device that helps people who use pMDI inhalers learn to inhale at the correct speed. It has a similar appearance to a pMDI, but does not contain a pressurized aerosol canister.

This device provides audible feedback on how fast air is being inhaled. There is a different tone depending on whether inhalation is too fast, slow or just right. The lower tone is triggered when the airflow reaches 30 L/min or more, and the patient is inhaling correctly.

Only when airflow is greater than 60 L/min (too high for pMDI) does the second tone start, and the patient should be advised to breathe more slowly. If no tone is heard, the patient is inhaling too slowly and should be advised to breathe faster. The device is for single patient use only.

Aerosol Inhalation Monitor® *(AIM) (Vitalograph)*

This is a machine that checks patient's ability to use an MDI. It has a visual display indicating the patient's ability to:

- Inhale at correct speed
- Coordinate aerosol firing with inhalation
- Cease inhalation after firing of aerosol
- Breath-hold after inhalation.

The manufacturer's instructions for cleaning should be followed.

Placebo devices

When demonstrating an inhaler to a patient, the nurse should use a device that contains no active drug. This is known as a placebo device. Placebo inhaler devices, spacers and inspiratory flow meters are designed for single patient use because of the potential risk of cross-infection. Each Trust and health care organization must assess the potential risk of infection if they are used for multiple patients. There needs to be a balance between the risks of cross-infection, against not checking or teaching a patient how to use an inhaler. There are some steps that can be taken to minimize the risk. These include:

• Washing hands before and after handling inhalers, spacers and inspiratory flow meters
• Reminding patients to bring their own inhaler device to review appointments
• Inhaler devices and spacer devices that can be washed should be soaked for one hour in hypochlorite solution 1000 parts per million and dried thoroughly before further use
• Disposable single-use mouthpieces are available for use on some dry powder inhalers
• Inspiratory flow meters should be used and cleaned as per manufacturer's In-check dial® instructions
• Disposable mouthpieces with one-way inspiratory valves should always be used.

Currently there is little evidence of cross-infection from placebo inhaler devices or lung function equipment, but certain infections are a cause of concern, and single use devices should be used. These include:

• Acquired immune deficiency syndrome (AIDS)
• Hepatitis B and C
• *Methicillin-resistant Staphylococcus aureus* (MRSA)
• Tuberculosis
• Rhinovirus and other upper respiratory tract infections
• *Burkholderia cepacia*

The Medicines and Healthcare Products Regulatory Agency (MHRA) has statutory functions and responsibilities to safeguard public health and safety. Medical devices are regulated under the Medical Devices Agency.

Further information

HPSS (2004) *Controls Assurance Standard: Decontamination of reusable medical devices.* http://www.dhsspsni.gov.uk

Medical Devices Agency (2001) *Devices in practice.* http://www.mhra.gov.uk

MHRA (2003) *Decontamination of community equipment.* http://www.mhra.gov.uk

Pleural effusion

Definition

The pleural space is the area between the lungs and the chest wall; it is lined by the visceral and parietal pleura. This space contains pleural fluid to allow the lungs to expand and contract (📖 p.13).

If the fluid in this space builds up to over 100 mls on one side, the patient is deemed to have a pleural effusion.

Pleural effusion is a very common presentation for a variety of different pathologies.

Aetiology

There is a regular turnover of pleural fluid oozing out of the parietal pleura in a healthy person, because of the relatively high pressure in the parietal capillaries.

This fluid is usually reabsorbed through the visceral pleura as the pulmonary capillaries are at a lower pressure. The amount of pleural fluid is held in balance by hydrostatic pressure in the capillaries forcing fluid out, and oncotic pressure due to the serum proteins retaining or reabsorbing fluid.

If the protein content of serum falls, then hydrostatic pressure exceeds oncotic pressure, and excess fluid will accumulate in the pleural space. For example, in nephrotic syndrome, left ventricular failure or liver failure. As the effusion will have a low protein content it will be known as a transudate.

If the capillaries are 'leaky', excess protein and cells escape into the pleural space. As the protein content of the pleural fluid rises, oncotic pressure is also raised, resulting in more fluid being drawn out, in inflammation for example. This effusion is rich in protein and will be an exudate.

Reasons for transudate and exudate effusions are listed in Table 16.1.

Clinical features (📖 p.31)

The main clinical feature of a pleural effusion is breathlessness; the degree of breathlessness corresponds to the size of the effusion. Other symptoms such as cough are rarer; this tends to be non-productive and resolves once the effusion has drained.

Other symptoms such as pain and weight loss are usually indicative of an underlying disease process, such as a malignancy. Symptoms such as fever, sweats, weight loss, and anorexia are suggestive of an infection or empyema.

Findings on examination include reduced chest wall movement, dullness to percussion, reduced breath sounds, decreased vocal fremitus and resonance on the side affected.

A good history may reveal occupational exposure to aid diagnosis, such as asbestos exposure. It is important to ascertain the onset of symptoms, and past medical history.

Table 16.1 Some differential diagnoses for pleural effusions

Transudates	Exudates
Left ventricular failure	Parapneumonic effusion
Pulmonary embolism (10–20%)	Pulmonary embolism (80–90%)
Malignancy (5%)	Malignancy (95%)
Cirrhotic liver disease	Rheumatoid arthritis
Nephrotic syndrome	Mesothelioma
Peritoneal dialysis	Empyema
Atelectasis	Tuberculosis
Hypothyroidism	Infection
Myxoedema	Autoimmune disease
Ascites	Drug-induced Radiotherapy

450 CHAPTER 16 Pleural effusion

Investigations (📖 p.75)

Investigations will confirm the clinical suspicion of an effusion, and help diagnosis.

Chest X-ray

A chest X-ray is the most useful investigation; it will confirm the extent and distribution of the excess fluid. Any underlying pathology may be discernable on the chest X-ray, such as pleural plaques, bone destruction or cardiomegaly. Care on interpretation of the X-ray is important if the patient is supine, as only a diffuse haze over the affected hemi-thorax may be seen.

Ultrasound

An ultrasound is useful to confirm the presence of an effusion; it may be the investigation of choice, for example in pregnancy when X-ray exposure is not advisable.

CT thorax

A CT of the thorax enables the pleura and mediastinum to be viewed in greater detail, and allows for a pleural biopsy to be undertaken under CT guidance. Using CT-guided needle biopsies has increased the diagnostic yield rate to around 90%; a blind biopsy of the pleura is rarely undertaken because of the poor yield rate.

Pleural aspiration

Undertaking a pleural aspiration is the quickest and easiest way to characterize the effusion. This can be done with a needle and large syringe, and can be both diagnostic and/or therapeutic depending on how much fluid is removed.

The presentation of the fluid should be examined, as a foul-smelling fluid would indicate infection, and pus would indicate an empyema. Bloodstained fluid may indicate malignancy.

If the aspirate has a protein content of less than 30 g/L it is likely to be a transudate, and if the protein is higher than 40 g/L it is likely to be an exudate.

Lactate dehydrogenase (LDH)

A LDH concentration greater than 1000 IU/L strongly suggests an exudate.

Cytology

Cytology can sometimes be helpful, but it is only diagnostic in around 20–45% of pleural effusions.

Other investigations include:

- Full Blood Count (FBC)
- Blood cultures and serology for pneumonia
- Renal and liver function
- Erythrocyte sedimentation rate (ESR)
- C-reactive protein (CRP)
- Immunological tests and rheumatoid factor (RF).

Thoracoscopy

Thoracoscopy can be undertaken surgically—open or in a video-assisted procedure—or medically. Whilst a surgical thoracoscopy involves a general anaesthetic, a medical thoracoscopy is performed under a local anaesthetic.

Both allow the pleural space to be visualized, the space to be drained and biopsies to be taken of the affected site followed by a pleurodesis if deemed necessary. The diagnostic yield from a medical thoracoscopy is around 80–90% so it is a worthwhile procedure as it will, in the majority of cases, give a definitive answer. A pleurodesis introduces a foreign substance into the pleural cavity after the effusion has been drained to prevent a pneumothorax.

Management

The management of a pleural effusion is dependent upon the cause.

For transudates, treatment is directed at the cause. If the effusion is large, then drainage by aspiration may provide symptomatic relief whilst treatment is initiated or increased.

Malignant pleural effusions should be drained if the patient is symptomatic, either by aspiration, chest drain or thoracoscopy. Pleurodesis may be undertaken with the latter two procedures, and should be considered in patients with a good performance status and life expectancy.

A pleurodesis should be undertaken as soon as possible before the fluid becomes loculated, trapping the underlying lung. For a pleurodesis to be successful, the space should be drained dry, and the lung expanded, before a sclerosant agent is used (Table 16.2).

If the patient is on corticosteroids (📖 p.391), these should be discontinued prior to the procedure, as they will inhibit the pleural inflammatory response and development of adhesions.

Table 16.2 Common sclerosant agents

Talc*
Tetracycline
Bleomycin
Doxycycline
Minocycline
Interferon
Interleukins
Cisplatin
Autologous blood

* Whilst talc is the preferred agent, graded talc with the smaller particles removed is preferred, due to a link of talc use and Adult Respiratory Distress syndrome (📖 p.137).

Nursing care

Symptom control

Breathlessness is the main symptom of a pleural effusion, but fear and anxiety about the cause can exacerbate the problem. The nurse will be involved in monitoring the patient's condition and explaining any procedures undertaken.

Care of drains and wound sites

Care of the patient before, during and after any procedure or intervention will be an essential part of nursing care and management. If a surgical procedure is undertaken, then care and management will follow usual pre and post-operative care.

Information and support

When the underlying cause of the effusion is uncertain, it is a worrying time for a patient. When the cause is ascertained, the patient may be faced with major changes in lifestyle, and in the case of malignancy, possibly a shortened life span.

Information and support will be vital at all stages of the patients' journey to help patients deal with their condition and their feelings

Pneumonia

Background

Pneumonia is an inflammation of the lungs. It is usually caused by an infection of the lung tissue by one of many different microorganisms and is a common disease in the UK, affecting 1 in 100 people annually. It is more common in older or very young people. Pneumonia can occur at any time of the year, but it is more common in the autumn and winter.

Most types of pneumonia can be effectively treated with antibiotics, but it can be a serious illness, especially in frail older people, young people and those already ill or immunocompromised. The death rate from pneumonia is estimated to be around 5%.

Origins

Pneumonia is often divided into two main categories reflecting its origins; community-acquired and nosocomial or hospital-acquired pneumonia. Transmission may be by inhalation, aspiration, or haemotagenous.

Community acquired

Community-acquired pneumonia (CAP) is a common condition. It carries a high morbidity and is the sixth leading cause of death in the UK. CAP is predominantly bacterial in origin, caused by Gram-positive cocci. The streptococcus bacteria are the main causative agents, and a single pathogen is identified in 85% of cases.

Around 40% of patients with CAP will require hospital admission, and hospital mortality rates for the disease are estimated at between 5–12%. Around 5–10% of hospitalized patients will require intensive care admission, and these patients have high mortality rates of around 50%. The mortality rate for those patients with CAP treated in the community is around 1%.

Nosocomial (hospital acquired)

Hospital-acquired or nosocomial pneumonia manifests itself at least 48 h after hospital admission. It is quite a significant problem, and carries with it a high morbidity and mortality.

Nosocomial pneumonia may be described as:
- Early nosocomial—appearing within 5 days of hospitalization, usually with Gram-positive cocci, or
- Late nosocomial—appearing more than 5 days after hospitalization, usually with Gram-negative cocci.

Several factors affect the aetiology of nosocomial pneumonia:
- Time of onset after hospitalization
- Stress-induced flora changes
- Antibiotic induced flora changes
- Exposure to contamination with nosocomial pathogens.

Gram-positive and Gram-negative bacteria

Identifying bacteria in the laboratory involves culturing the bacteria on solid media in petri dishes and then examining the growth both visually and by staining the bacteria prior to examination under the microscope. The most common staining is known as Gram's method. Bacteria are stained a deep purple with a mixture of violet dye and iodine which attaches to the magnesium ribonucleate present in some bacteria. If the purple colour cannot be washed out readily with alcohol the bacteria is Gram-positive. Bacteria without magnesium ribonucleate can easily be washed out, hence Gram-negative. This is an important way of distinguishing bacterial types.

Types of pneumonia

Within the two categories of community-acquired and nosocomical pneumonia there are different types of pneumonia dependent on the causative agent:.

Typical pneumonia

There are a range of bacteria that may cause the infection leading to 'typical pneumonia', and these include the common bacterial pneumonias; streptococcus pneumonia, and pneumococcal pneumonia. *Typical pneumonia* is the commonest type of pneumonia. Viruses can also be a source of infection, including influenza (flu).

Infection with a virus and with bacteria can occur in the same patient. For example, *streptococcus pneumoniae* infection is usually secondary to influenza. This is known as secondary infection, and can slow down recovery significantly.

Atypical pneumonia

The causes of atypical pneumonia are less common and include Legionnaire's disease caused by bacterium, and severe acute respiratory syndrome (SARS) caused by a virus (📖 p.137).

Aspiration pneumonia

Aspiration pneumonia is caused by the inhalation of substances such as caustic chemicals, food or vomit into the lungs. Aspiration pneumonia is not infectious.

Immunosuppressed pneumonia

Pneumonia-type symptoms may occur in people who have a weakened immune system following an organ transplant, patients with AIDS, and those taking immunosuppressant drugs. Examples of this are fungal infections such as *pneumocystis carinii*, which is rare in those with a fully functioning immune system.

Symptoms

Symptoms often depend on the amount of lung affected and the type of infection. They include:

- Dry cough initially
- Productive cough with green/yellow or rust coloured sputum—may smell offensive
- Haemoptysis
- Breathlessness—fast and shallow breathing
- Shivering fits
- Pain in the chest
- Discomfort when breathing or coughing
- Fever
- Loss of appetite
- Aches and pains
- Cyanosis
- Acute confusional state—more common in older people
- Herpes.

Severity assessment

Severity assessment is by the CURB or CURB-65 score which is a recognized scoring system used to denote the level of severity of the pneumonia.

Confusion

Urea ≥7mmol/l

Respiratory rate raised ≥30/min

Blood pressure – systolic BP ≤90 and/or diastolic BP ≤60

65   age ≥65

The presence of the four core CURB factors correlates with mortality.

Transmission and risk factors

The microorganisms that cause pneumonia may be present in the body for some time before the illness develops, or they may be spread by droplet infection.

There are several factors that reduce the ability of the body to fight infection:
- Poor general health
- Age—it is more difficult for older and very young people to fight infections
- Smoking
- Excessive alcohol intake
- Heart disease
- Diabetes
- COPD/asthma
- Splenectomy
- Immunosuppression—more difficult for those with AIDS or on chemotherapy.

There are additional risk factors for hospital-acquired pneumonia. These include:
- Reduced cough reflex following surgery or illness
- Invasive ventilation
- Weakened immune system
- Different bacteria than in the community
- Antibiotic-resistant bacteria.

Diagnosis

A diagnosis of pneumonia may be made after carrying out the following procedures:
- History
- Chest examination
- Temperature
- Respiratory rate
- Urea
- Blood pressure
- CXR
- Blood cultures
- Sputum
- Invasive sample collection
- CURB or CURB65 score.

Treatment

Antibiotics

If the pathogen is known or suspected, then antimicrobial therapy guided by local sensitivities should be started. In most cases empirical antibiotic treatment will be required.

Antibiotic choices will be influenced by:

- Community-acquired or nosocomial pneumonia
- Time of onset of the illness after admission (early or late)
- Local resistance patterns
- Severity of the pneumonia
- Underlying disease
- Recent antibiotic treatment.

Empirical therapy, which is *treating in a pragmatic fashion when sensitivities are unknown*, must cover a range of organisms in hospital-acquired pneumonia, including and especially *pseudomonas aeruginosa*.

Investigations

Sputum cultures

Sputum cultures may be useful for patients who have failed to respond to empirical treatment and patients with purulent sputum admitted to hospital that have not commenced antibiotic therapy. Sputum cultures are also recommended for all patients with severe pneumonia. Routine collection of sputum samples is not recommended for community-acquired pneumonia.

Blood cultures

Blood cultures are recommended for all patients with pneumonia, preferably before antibiotics are commenced.

Microbiological investigations help to ascertain the optimal antibiotic for use which can reduce antibiotic resistance, whilst allowing the ongoing monitoring of pathogen trends.

CXR

Can be useful in showing areas of consolidation, the lobar involvement and whether there is any pleural effusion.

CT scan

Not usually recommended unless there is doubt over the diagnosis or if the patient is severely ill or fails to respond to treatment. It may be useful in excluding underlying disease.

Blood tests

These will include full blood count (FBC), renal and liver function tests, metabolic acidosis and C-reactive protein. These may be useful markers of the extent of infection and response to treatment.

Oxygen assessment

Patients admitted to hospital with pneumonia should have oxygenation levels monitored. Those with oxygen saturations <92% or with severe pneumonia should have arterial blood gases measured.

Other investigations

May include:
- Pleural fluid
- Viral and atypical pathogens
- Serological testing.

Additional treatments
- Increased fluid intake
- Painkillers such as paracetamol or NSAIDs if required
- Antiviral drugs for viral infection
- Antifungals for fungal infection
- Intravenous fluids if volume depleted
- Nutrition
- Oxygen therapy. Hypoxia is due to ventilation/perfusion (V/Q) mismatch through the consolidated area of lung. A rising CO_2 may be indicative of the need for assessment of ventilatory support.

Complications

These are more common in older people and can include:
- Pleural effusion
- Breathing difficulties—may need medical intervention, possibly ventilation
- Septicaemia.

Prevention

Antibiotics

People with a weakened immune system may be given preventative antibiotics.

Vaccinations

There are immunizations for some of the infections that can cause pneumonia.

Pneumococcal vaccine

This can prevent pneumonia caused by streptococcus pneumonia. Currently there are two on the market branded as Pneumovax11 and Prevenar. These are recommended to anyone with lung or heart problems—including people over 65 and children—as part of the child immunization programme.

A **Haemophilus influenza type B** *vaccine (Hib vaccine).*

This is given routinely to babies, older people and people with heart, lung or kidney disease, and to those with weakened immune systems.

Nursing care

Whilst bed rest and an antipyretic such as paracetamol are usually sufficient treatments for milder cases of pneumonia, some patients with more severe pneumonia require hospitalization and treatment with intravenous antibiotics. Patients may require oxygen which should be humidified to avoid the drying out of secretions and encouraged with fluids. Physiotherapy may help with the effective removal of secretions and the early mobilization of the patient, although it is of no proven benefit in acute pneumonia.

Care should be taken to avoid the risk of spread of the infection between patients and between patients and staff.

As a preventative measure in the community the nurse should encourage those patents in at risk categories to have annual influenza vaccinations and pneumonia vaccination in accordance with local guidelines.

Further information

Pneumonia guidelines
British Thoracic Society
020 7831 8778
http://www.brit-thoracic.org.uk

Pneumonia best treatments
http://www.besttreatments.co.uk

Pneumonia: British Lung Foundation
http://www.lunguk.org

Prodigy guidelines
http://www.prodigy.nhs.uk

Pneumothorax

Introduction

Definition

A pneumothorax is defined as air in the pleural space. The pleural space is the potential space between the parietal and visceral pleura layers of the lung and thoracic cavity. A pneumothorax may occur in normal lungs (primary pneumothorax) or due to an underlying lung disease (secondary pneumothorax). Pneumothorax can be spontaneous, occur as the result of trauma, or be iatrogenic.

Incidence

Globally the annual incidence of primary pneumothorax is around 18–28 per 100,000 in men and 1.2–6 in women with a male to female ratio of around 5:1. It occurs most commonly in tall thin males aged between 20 and 40 years of age. In the UK reported rates for hospital admissions for both primary and secondary pneumothorax are reported as 16.7/100,000 for men and 5.8/100,000 for women (see suggested reading).

Mortality rates for primary and secondary pneumothorax combined between 1991 and 1995 and sourced in the BTS guidelines for pleural disease 2003 were 1.26 per million in men and 0.62 per million in women

Risk factors

Cigarette smoking is a major risk factor increasing the risk of pneumothorax by a factor of 9 in women and 2 in men.

There have on rare occasions been reported deaths from pneumothorax following bronchoscopic lung biopsy.

Pneumothorax can occasionally be familial.

Pathophysiology

Primary pneumothorax is believed to follow an air leak from apical bullae, although small airway inflammation is also often found and this may be a contributory factor due to increasing airways resistance.

Secondary pneumothorax may be due to underlying diseases such as COPD (in 60% of cases), asthma, interstitial lung disease, necrotizing pneumonia, tuberculosis, cystic fibrosis, Marfan's syndrome, lung cancer, ruptured oesophagus, pulmonary infarction, catamenial pneumothorax, Langerhans' cell histiocytosis, and lymphangioleiomyomatosis.

A pneumothorax may be the first presenting complaint of a patient prior to establishing the underlying disease.

Features

Patients with a pneumothorax commonly present with pleuritic chest pain on the affected side and/or breathlessness. Younger patients often have minimal breathlessness although in secondary pneumothorax breathlessness may be increased.

A pneumothorax will reduce the compliance of the lungs and so the lungs will become stiffer. Because of reduced compliance in the affected lung greater pressure needs to be generated during inspiration to move the same volume of air into the lungs. As a result breathing will become more of an effort and the sensation of breathlessness will be increased. The patient may also have pleuritic chest pain from inflammation of the pleura, generally due to bleeding and heightened by attempts to inflate the affected lung. There is often tachycardia.

When looking at the chest, movement will be unilateral in the presence of a total pneumothorax, and there will be reduced expansion on the affected side.

There will be reduced and quiet breath sounds on the side of the pneumothorax.

A decrease in fremitus occurs because of uncoupling of the chest wall so it no longer transmits the vibration of sound.

Hyper-resonance will be noted on percussion.

Hamman's sign denotes a 'click' sound in time with the heart sounds on auscultation and is due to the movement of the pleural surfaces in a left-sided pneumothorax.

If there is subcutaneous emphysema 'bubbles' or 'crackles' may be felt under the skin of the chest and neck. The patient will appear swollen in the affected area.

Investigations

A chest X-ray is the most useful investigation for suspected pneumothorax. A chest X-ray will show an absence of peripheral lung markings, and a visible lung edge. Supine films may not be as diagnostic and very small pneumothoraces may only show on a lateral chest X-ray.

Pneumothoraces are classified as:
- Small—rim of air <2 cm
- Large—rim of air >2 cm.

A 2 cm rim of air approximately equates to a 50% pneumothorax.

A chest X-ray may also show the underlying respiratory disorder if this has been causative, although this may not be easy to see with a large pneumothorax.

A CT scan may be necessary to differentiate between bullous disease and pneumothorax. It may also be useful in trauma cases where an underlying pneumothorax is suspected, and in diagnoses of underlying respiratory disease, or malignancy.

Blood gases will give the extent of hypoxia and there may be hypercapnia in secondary pneumothorax.

Management

There is a variation in the clinical management of pneumothoraces.

Management depends on the extent of the problem, the size of the pneumothorax, degree of patient symptoms, breathlessness, pain, hypoxia, haemodynamics, and the underlying cause.

Management options

- Aspiration (thoracocentesis)
  - Can be very painful for the patient
  - Is difficult if the patient has an excessive cough
  - Is likely to fail in a large pneumothorax
  - If the first aspiration is unsuccessful one-third of patients will respond to a repeat aspiration
- Chest drainage (tube thoracotostomy)
  - Not necessary for the majority of patients with primary spontaneous pneumothorax
  - Has a significant morbidity and also on occasions mortality, if not performed by an expert and is not required for the majority of patients with primary spontaneous pneumothorax
  - Small drains (10–14F) are adequate in most cases and may be more comfortable for the patient
- Oxygen
  - High flow rates of around 10 L/min needed unless there is CO_2 retention
  - Reduces the partial pressure of nitrogen in the blood and encourages removal of air from the pleural space thus helping resolve the pneumothorax
  - Helps resolve the pneumothorax and may reduce the paitent's anxiety
- Surgery
  - Aims to repair the apical hole or bleb and close the pleural space
  - Can be by Video Assisted Thorascopic Surgery (VATS), open thoracotomy, or mini thoracotomy.

Prognosis

Primary pneumothoraces: 30% recur within 2 years, with smoking increasing the risk of recurrence. After a second pneumothorax recurrence is around 40% and >50% after a third.

In secondary pneumothorax mortality is around 10%.

Recurrence in secondary pneumothorax depends on the underlying problem and increasing age augments the risk.

Nursing care

Nursing care of the patient with a pneumothorax will depend upon the extent of the pneumothorax, patient symptoms and intended treatment options. Patients will need support with treatment of symptoms, through procedures and in the case of secondary pneumothoraces with diagnosis. Patients should also be advised about the risks of flying as ascent to altitude is potentially unsafe. Although generally the advice is to avoid flying for 6 weeks depending upon the extent of the pneumothorax and the treatment some patients may be advised not to fly for up to a year. All patients are advised not to scuba dive. (📖 p.613)

Care of chest drains—practical points

Insertion of a chest drain may be a traumatic procedure for a patient and the patient will need support through the procedure, help with positioning and adequate pain relief prior to the procedure and afterwards.

- Bubbling chest drains should never be clamped because of the risk of tension pneumothorax
- Sometimes when air leaks appear to have ceased clamping of the drain for several hours followed by a chest X-ray may be advocated to detect very slow or intermittent air leaks. Whilst this avoids inappropriate drain removal it requires careful observation of the patient and should be considered only in ward areas with specialist nurses accustomed to the care and management of drains
- Drains should be observed to ensure that they 'swing' with respiration: that is, the fluid level moves up and down as the patient breathes. If there is no 'swing' then the tube should be checked particularly where it enters the skin in case there is a kink in the tube, alternate explanations may be a blocked, clamped or incorrectly positioned drain
- Patients will require advice on keeping the drain below chest level, especially important if they are moving around or going off the ward for procedures
- Depending on the position of the drain careful positioning of the patient to help with sleep and assistance with hygiene needs, especially changing clothing, may be necessary
- Heimlich flutter valves or alternative thoracic vents are sometimes used rather than a chest drain as they allow greater mobilization of the patient and occasionally treatment on an outpatient basis
- Removal of a chest drain should be undertaken by experienced staff according to local procedures.

Suggested reading

Henry M, Arnold T et al. (2003). BTS Guidelines for the management of spontaneous pneumothorax. *Thorax* 58(suppl. 11), ii39–ii52.

Pulmonary embolism

Definition

A pulmonary embolism is a clinically significant obstruction occurring in part of or the entire pulmonary vascular tree. The most common cause is a thrombus from a distant site such as the leg.

Overview

Annually, it is estimated that there are around 60–70 cases of pulmonary embolism (PE) per 100,000 population. 50% of these occur in hospital inpatients or those in institutional care, probably due to immobility. Pulmonary embolism remains the major cause of maternal death in the UK.

It is estimated that the average general hospital will diagnose around 50 cases of PE annually, but this figure may be low, as many are found at post mortem. It is estimated that around 1% of all acute emergency admissions could be due to PE (see suggested further reading)

The in-hospital mortality rate due to PE is estimated to be somewhere between 6–15%.

Aetiology

Most pulmonary emboli originate from detached portions of venous thrombi that have formed in the deep veins of the lower limbs. Other sites where they form include the right side of the heart and the pelvis.

Non-thrombotic emboli, mainly fat, air and amniotic fluid may also occur, but these are rarer.

The factors that predispose individuals to the formation of venous thrombi, and subsequently PE, fall into three broad categories:
- Stasis of blood
- Alterations in the blood coagulation pathway
- Abnormalities of the vessel wall.

It is usual to find at least one predisposing factor in the majority of patients.

Most suspected pulmonary embolis occur as an acute event, although minor or recurrent episodes may present as more insidious cardiorespiratory symptoms.

These risk factors are documented in Table 19.1.

Table 19.1 Risk factors for PE

Category	Causes
Surgery	**Major abdominal/ pelvic surgery**
	Hip/knee surgery
	Intensive care – post operatively
Lower limb	**Fracture**
	Varicose veins
	Stroke/spinal cord injury
Malignant disorders	Abdominal/pelvic
	Metastatic/advanced disease
	Chemotherapy
Cardiorespiratory	Acute myocardial infarction
	Severe respiratory disease
Obstetrics	Pregnancy/puerperium
Miscellaneous	Ageing process
	Previous thrombotic disease
	Immobility for over one week
	Clotting disorders
	Trauma
	Air travel
	Oral oestrogens eg Tamoxifen
	Central venous catheters
	Dehydration
	Smoking
	Obesity
	Family history of thromboembolic disease

Note: Bold print denotes the more common reasons.

Clinical features and assessment

Clinical features

The most common clinical features of a PE include:

- Dyspnoea
- Tachypnoea (>20bpm)
- Pleuritic pain
- Cough
- Haemoptysis
- Leg pain
- Clinical deep vein thrombosis (DVT)
- Sudden collapse (less common).

And in addition what has been described as a 'sense of impending doom'

Whilst the presence of certain clinical features may not determine the diagnosis of PE; if they are absent PE is extremely unlikely. It would appear that dyspnoea and tachypnoea are the most common presentations in around 90% of cases, and that these two symptoms plus pleuritic chest pain are present in 97% of cases. The remainder of cases have either chest X-ray changes or low arterial oxygen tension.

Signs of massive pulmonary embolus include collapse, shock, severe dyspnoea, and right heart failure.

Clinical assessment

An accurate clinical assessment of the patient is important. This should include an accurate history to assess the likelihood of PE, noting the presence of significant risk factors and then careful examination of the patient for signs and symptoms consistent with thromboembolic disease. These findings can then be used to predict the probability of PE.

PE is more likely in patients with features consistent with PE; these are principally breathlessness and/or tachypnoea, with or without chest pain and/or haemoptysis.

Two other predictive factors that should be considered are the absence of another alternative diagnosis, and the presence of a major risk factor. If both of these are present, the probability of a PE is high. If one predictive factor is present the probability is intermediate, if both are absent then the probability is low.

The probability of a PE should always be assessed and documented, as it guides further investigation, and avoids unnecessary investigations. For example d-dimers are unnecessary in a patient with intermediate/high clinical probability as they will require ventilation perfusion scanning (VQ) and/or computerized tomography pulmonary angiography (CTPA.)

Investigations

Investigations for PE include some or all of the following:

Chest X-ray

Chest X-ray changes in PE may be fairly non-specific or indeed absent. Small effusions are seen in around 40% of cases. Other findings may include segmental collapse, prominent central pulmonary arteries (Fleischner sign), raised hemi-diaphragm, absence of vascular markings (Westermark sign) and focal infiltration. The chest X-ray is also useful in excluding other pathologies such as left ventricular failure, pneumothorax, and pneumonia or lung cancer.

ECG

The ECG often changes in PE but it can be non-specific; the most common change is sinus tachycardia, but atrial fibrillation, right-bundle branch block, changes in the ST segment and/or T-wave inversion may also be seen. A large pulmonary emboli may result in signs of right heart strain. Once again the ECG may be useful in excluding or diagnosing other conditions such as pericardial disease or myocardial infarction.

Arterial blood gases

As pulmonary embolism is characterized by a mismatch of the VQ ratio, a physiological shunt, hypoxia and hypocapnia may often be seen, due to hyperventilation. If the embolus is large enough to cause circulatory collapse, a metabolic acidosis may be seen. Arterial blood gases may be normal in the otherwise young and healthy patient.

D-dimers

Plasma d-dimers are a simple blood test with an important role in diagnosing and excluding PE. It relies on the measurement of cross-linked fibrin degradation, or d-dimer. Values are rarely normal (<200) in those with acute embolism. However, d-dimers may also be raised in a number of other conditions, including infection and trauma.

The value of this test is that if the d-dimers are less than 200 then a diagnosis of PE is highly unlikely. A negative test is unhelpful and unnecessary for patients presenting with a high clinical probability of PE.

VQ scan

VQ scanning involves the intravenous injection of a radioisotope and the inhalation of a different radioisotope to compare the ratio of ventilation to perfusion. VQ scanning should normally be performed within 24 h of the onset of symptoms, as many scans revert to normal quite rapidly; with over half doing so within one week. VQ scanning is useful in those presenting with a normal CXR.

Scans are reported within the clinical context of the presentation, and in conjunction with a recent, good-quality chest X-ray. They are reported as low, intermediate or high probability, and these results need to be interpreted alongside clinical findings.

Although a high probability VQ scan correctly identifies pulmonary embolism in the majority of patients with a clinical suspicion of PE, there are limitations. The interpretation may be misleading or difficult in the presence of a number of respiratory diseases including previous PE, COPD, lung fibrosis and proximal lung tumours. Left ventricular failure can also cause localized variations in pulmonary perfusion. In these situations, computerized tomography (CT) scanning with pulmonary angiography is preferable.

CTPA

CTPA has a high sensitivity and specificity for PE, so is regarded as the gold standard for diagnosis. With CT it is possible to identify and define non-invasive pulmonary emboli in the central and the second to fourth division of the pulmonary arteries.

The main drawback is that CTPA fails to detect subsegmental pulmonary emboli due to the small diameter of the vessels, and insufficient enhancement of vessels and thrombi below this level. This disadvantage is also true of VQ scanning and pulmonary angiography.

The clinical significance of subsegmental emboli is doubtful; only 1.6% of patients with subsegmental emboli progress to symptomatic pulmonary embolism within 6–12 weeks. CTPA has other advantages; it can determine the age of the thrombus and of other pathologies that mimic the clinical picture of PE, such as pneumonia, pneumothorax or aortic dissection.

CTPA is quick to perform and rarely necessitates further investigation or imaging; it may provide an alternative diagnosis when PE is excluded. It does, however, need a specialist to report the results.

Management

Anticoagulation is the mainstay of treatment. Unless contraindicated, heparin should be started if there is a high or moderate suspicion of a PE, prior to the results of further investigations.

Standard heparin and low-molecular weight (LMW) heparin are used unless there is a requirement for an early rapid reversal of effect. LMW has the advantages of rapid but predictable anticoagulation, easy subcutaneous administration, set dosage syringes and no requirement for laboratory monitoring. Heparin is continued during the introduction of warfarin, until adequate anticoagulation is achieved, and it may be discontinued once the international normalized ratio (INR) is within the therapeutic range of 2.0–3.0.

If the risk factors for venous thromboembolism are thought to be temporary, for example post surgery, 6 weeks to 3 months of anticoagulant treatment is sufficient to prevent recurrence. The longer the duration of anticoagulant therapy the greater the benefits in terms of reduced embolism, although this has to be balanced against the risks of bleeding. First episodes of PE will usually only require 3–6 months of treatment. In recurrent embolism, lifelong anticoagulation may be necessary.

Other interventions

Thrombolysis (using streptokinase or urokinase), pulmonary embolectomy and inferior vena caval (IVC) filters can be used in the treatment of pulmonary embolus, but are uncommon, and are usually reserved for patients with massive PE (the former two), or recurrent multiple pulmonary emboli (the latter two).

High-flow oxygen

100% oxygen is usually administered to patients suspected of having a PE; care in administration, plus usual oxygen precautions should be adhered to (📖 p.278).

Nursing care

Due to the commonality of PE, nurses may be involved at several levels with patients who have suspected and confirmed PE. Involvement may include:

Clinical assessment

Nurses may be the first line of contact for patients presenting with PE; they require knowledge of the presenting symptoms so that prompt treatment and management can be initiated. In some instances nurses may undertake the clinical assessment and initial investigations.

Outpatient DVT management programmes

Programmes to support patients on an outpatient basis have been established in many areas, and may be nurse run. Ongoing monitoring of patients' INR will be important.

Information and support

Patients with a PE will require information on prescribed medications and on interactions, dosage purpose, time of administration and side-effects. Information on preventative measures and lifestyle changes will also be important for ongoing management.

Further reading

British Thoracic Society. BTS Guidelines for the Management of Suspected Acute Pulmonary Embolism, 2003. The British Thoracic Society Standards of Care Committee, Pulmonary Embolism Guideline Development Group Thorax: 48: 470–484

British Thoracic Society (1997). Suspected acute pulmonary embolism: a practical approach. *Thorax* 52(suppl.), S1–24.

Pulmonary hypertension

Introduction

Pulmonary arterial hypertension (PH) is an often misdiagnosed lung disorder occurring as a primary idiopathic disease or as a complication of a large number of respiratory and cardiac diseases. PH is due primarily to either increased vacular resistence, increased pulmonary blood flow or elevated pulmonary venous pressure. PH can also occur with or without an identifiable cause. It was previously thought to be a rare condition with a relentlessly progressive course and few treatment options. However, it is increasingly recognized in association with other conditions and recent advances have resulted in the development of effective therapies. This has focused attention on making an early and accurate diagnosis. Despite these recent advances it is important to consider that it remains an alarming, incurable disease with a poor prognosis. PH describes a number of devastating diseases causing breathlessness, loss of exercise capacity, and death due to right-sided heart failure. Right-sided heart failure or cor pulmonale is a pathological diagnosis ariisng in many lung diseases but the most commonest cause will be secondary to COPD, accounting for 90% of cases of cor pulmonale. Estimates of pulmonary hypertension in COPD are between 5-40% in severe COPD and clearly corelate with an increased mortality from this disease. (📖 p.249)

Definition

PH is defined as a mean pulmonary artery pressure (MPAP) ≥25 mmHg at rest or 30 mmHg on exercise. The World Health Organisation (WHO) have classified PH and identified five major groups (see Table 20.1). This classification illustrates the importance of identifying the cause of PH in defining treatment. Patients with pulmonary arterial hypertension (PAH), (see Table 20.2), can be improved with selective pulmonary arterial vaso-dilators. However, these same drugs can precipitate pulmonary oedema in patients with pulmonary venous hypertension.

PH is a challenging disease to diagnose, accurately classify and treat. There is often a delay from the onset of symptoms to diagnosis of up to 3 years. It is important that patients who are being treated for more common causes of breathless and who fail to stabilize or improve are investigated for the possible existence of PH. It is rarely picked up in a routine medical examina-tion. Even in its later stages, the signs of the disease can be confused with other conditions affecting the heart and lungs. Thus, much time can pass between the time the symptoms of PH appear and a definite diagnosis is made.

The diagnostic process currently requires invasive investigations and the treatments are effective but often complex. Until the introduction of trans-plantation in the 1980s there was no specific treatment for PH. The last two decades have seen the development of new therapies which have been shown to improve symptoms and survival of patients with PH. Patients with severe disease have a 5-year survival of only 27% with supportive treat-ment, increased to 54% with certain targeted therapies. These treatments are often complicated and their use requires significant expertise.

Table 20.1 WHO classification of PH 2003

Pulmonary arterial hypertension

Pulmonary hypertension with left heart disease*

Pulmonary hypertension with lung disease and/ or hypoxaemia*

Pulmonary hypertension due to thrombotic and/ or embolic disease

Miscellaneous group

*In these instances treatment is best aimed at the underlying disease and usually these
patients do not require specialist assessment.

Table 20.2 Pulmonary arterial hypertension

Idiopathic pulmonary hypertension:
Sporadic
Familial

Related to:
Collagen vascular disease
Portal hypertension
Congenital heart disease
HIV infection
Drugs/ toxins
Persistent pulmonary hypertension of the newborn
PAH with significant venous or capillary involvement

Epidemiology, diagnosis and classification

Epidemiology

PH is rare, with an estimated prevalence of 30–50 cases per million. It has a median survival of 2.8 years from diagnosis. PH is now increasingly recognized in association with other diseases such as systemic sclerosis, congenital heart disease and HIV infection.

Pathophysiology

The characteristic of pulmonary hypertension is an increase in the pulmonary vascular resistance and increased workload placed on the right side of the heart. In PH the typical changes are seen in small arteries with medial smooth muscle hypertrophy, thickening or fibrosis of the intima of the vessels with *in-situ* fibrosis, and in some cases plexiform lesions.

Diagnosis and classification

The non-specific nature of the symptoms and subtle nature of the signs of pulmonary vascular disease often delay diagnosis.

Functional classification

Once PH is diagnosed, the patient is classified according to the functional classification system developed by the New York Heart Association. It is based on patient reports of how much activity they can comfortably undertake.

- Class 1 is assigned to patients with no symptoms of any kind, and for whom ordinary physical activity does not cause fatigue, palpitation, dyspnoea, or angina pain
- Class 2 is assigned to patients who are comfortable at rest but have symptoms with ordinary physical activity
- Class 3 is assigned to patients who are comfortable at rest but have symptoms with less-than-ordinary effort
- Class 4 is assigned to patients who have symptoms at rest.

Clinical features and investigations

Clinical features

The early symptoms of PH—dyspnoea, dizziness and fatigue—are often mild and are common to many other conditions. At rest there are often no symptoms and no apparent signs of illness. PH is often diagnosed only once other conditions have been investigated and ruled out. The non-specific nature of symptoms associated with PH means that the diagnosis cannot be made on symptoms alone. A series of investigations is required to make an initial diagnosis.

The principal symptom of PH is breathlessness because the right heart is unable to generate a sufficient increase in cardiac output on exercise. Initially this may be mild but it is progressive and later may be accompanied by chest pains (frequently similar to angina) and syncope, often on exercise. As right heart failure develops there are the usual symptoms of ankle swelling, abdominal distension and general fatigue.

Investigations

Most patients with significant dyspnoea will seek medical advice and have some investigations performed. Key basic investigations that may alert to the presence of PH include:

- Electrocardiogram: can be normal, common abnormalities range from sinus tachycardia through to overt right ventricular hypertrophy and strain
- Chest X-ray: can be normal, with common abnormalities being prominent pulmonary arteries, peripheral pruning of vessels in PH and cardiomegaly
- Pulmonary function tests: patients may have a mild restrictive or obstructive defect, although the degree of breathlessness is significantly greater than would be expected by the pulmonary function tests alone if the cause was primarily respiratory
- The most common non-invasive investigation suggesting PH is a trans-thoracic echocardiogram (TTE). With TTE an estimate of the systolic pulmonary artery pressure (SPAP) can be derived from the jet of tricuspid regurgitation when present.

If significant PH is suspected the patient should be referred to a specialist centre for further investigation and assessment. Patients with PH due to left-sided heart problems and underlying respiratory disease are most effectively treated by addressing the underlying cause. These patients do not usually require specialist assessment, although there is renewed interest in therapies for PH complicating respiratory diseases. In patients with severe PH seen in association with interstitial lung disease or sarcoidosis, for example, specific pulmonary arterial vasodilators may be of value.

Assessment and key investigations

Further assessment

Once referred to a specialist centre the aims are:
- Confirm or exclude diagnosis of PH
- Assess disease severity
- Establish disease aetiology
- Institute management plan with patient education and agreement.

Key investigations

When a patient is referred with suspected PH, invasive investigation (right heart catheterization) is usually required to both establish the diagnosis and provide important prognostic information. A vasodilator challenge is usually performed to assess the vasoreactivity of the pulmonary circulation. Further investigations are shown in Table 20.3.

The initial assessment encompasses a number of non-invasive investigations. Most importantly the patient is able to meet members of the multidisciplinary team including medical, nursing and allied staff. It gives an ideal opportunity to provide the patient and their family/friends with information about the disease and to try and answer a number of concerns the patient may have regarding their diagnosis.

Clinical investigations

Respiratory: (📖 p. 108)
- Arterial blood gases in room air
- Lung function including FEV_1, FVC, total lung capacity (TLC), single breath helium dilution volume (VA), total lung carbon monoxide transfer factor (TLCO), carbon monoxide transfer factor (KCO)
- Nocturnal oxygen saturation monitoring.

Cardiology:
- ECG
- Submaximal exercise test (6-minute walk or shuttle walk test)
- Cardiac catheterization (including right heart catheterization with saturations and haemodynamics, and acute pulmonary vasoreactivity study as appropriate).

Blood investigations include:
- Routine biochemistry and haematology
- Thrombophilia screen
- Thyroid function
- Autoimmune screening
- Hepatitis serology
- Serum angiotensin-converting enzyme
- HIV.

Table 20.3 Imaging investigations recommended in the assessment of pulmonary hypertension

Investigation	Comments
Chest x-ray	May show increase in cardiac chambers, increased pulmonary artery size, hypoperfused areas of lung and evidence of parenchymal lung disease
High-resolution CT scan	May show parenchymal lung disease, mosaic perfusion (a sign of pulmonary vascular embolism or thrombosis but for which there are other causes such as air trapping), and features of pulmonary venous hypertension
CT pulmonary angiography	Used to look for enlargement of pulmonary arteries and filling defects in the arteries. Detects enlarged bronchial circulation
Ventilation perfusion scanning	More sensitive for chronic pulmonary thromboembolism than CTPA but not helpful when there is underlying parenchymal lung disease
Selective pulmonary angiography by direct injection of the pulmonary arteries	Gold standard for delineating chronic pulmonary thromboembolism but may be superseded by MR angiography or multislice CT
Echocardiography	Screening tool of choice for pulmonary hypertension. Detects cardiac disease (congenital, myocardial, valvular, intracavity clot or tumour)
Cardiac magnetic resonance	Best examination for visualizing the right ventricle. Helpful in delineating congenital heart defects and the pulmonary circulation
Abdominal ultrasound	Used for investigation of liver disease and suspected portal hypertension

Treatment

If an underlying disease or condition can be found, treatment of this disease or condition should be part of overall PH care. There is currently no cure for PH, but advances in understanding how the disease develops means that there are now treatments available which have helped to improve prognosis for patients with this disease.

Treatment of patients with PH should ideally be instituted in a specialist centre. They have experience with the initiation and continued use and monitoring of targeted drug treatments and the infrastructure necessary for patient education and support. Many of the drug therapies used in the treatment of PH are complex and very expensive. They also have expertise in patient selection for, and the timing of, surgical interventions. The treatment of these patients is challenging but often rewarding.

Central to the management of any chronic disease, particularly a condition that is rapidly progressive, is the involvement of the patient. A clear explanation of the pathophysiology of pulmonary vascular disease aids the patient's understanding as to why they get breathless and in what situations they are most likely to blackout etc. This helps the patient gain an element of control over their disease.

Standard supportive treatments for PH include warfarin, diuretics, digoxin, and oxygen therapy. Chronic anticoagulation with warfarin is recommended to prevent thrombosis and has been shown, in retrospective studies, to prolong life in patients with PH. Patients with PH are prone to thromboembolism because of sluggish pulmonary blood flow, dilated right heart chambers, venous insufficiency and relative physical inactivity. Maintaining an INR of 2.0–3 is recommended. Other anticoagulants are also used if warfarin is not appropriate. Because hypoxia is a potent pulmonary vasoconstrictor, it is critical to identify and reverse hypoxaemia. Low-flow supplemental oxygen therapy prolongs survival in hypoxemic patients. Diuretics are used to control and manage heart failure in these patients.

Specific targeted therapies used in the treatment of PH

At present these fall into three drug categories:

Endothelin receptor antagonists

Endothelin is implicated in the pathogenesis of PH through actions on the pulmonary vasculature. Endothelin is found to be elevated in patients with PH and levels of endothelin are directly related to disease severity and prognosis. Endothelin receptor antagonists (ERAs) are oral treatments that either block the ETA receptor alone or both the ETA and ETB receptors. They have been shown to improve exercise ability and decrease the rate of clinical worsening in PH patients and improve survival.

Prostacyclin analogues

These will be delivered by continuous intravenous or subcutaneous infusion or via an intermittent nebulizer. To date, oral agents have shown limited effectiveness. These are a potent vasodilator that relaxes the blood vessels in the lungs and slows the process of scarring and cell growth within the lung's blood vessels, which prevents further narrowing. They can also assist in increasing cardiac output and oxygen saturation. They have been shown to improve exercise tolerance and prolong survival in patients with PH. Historically these drugs were used as a bridge to transplantation, but have now emerged as an alternative to transplant. While this group of drugs have a vital role to play in treating this devastating disease, they can be complex to administer and appropriate patient selection is required by experienced PH clinical staff to avoid potential major complications.

Phosphodiesterase 5 inhibitors

They induce relaxation and antiproliferative effects on vascular smooth muscle cells by preventing the reduction in levels of guanosine 35-cyclic monophosphate (cGMP). They are powerful vasodilators. The most commonly used drug in this class in the treatment of PH is sildenafil citrate, marketed under the trade names Viagra® and Revatio®. They work by relaxing smooth muscle in blood vessels throughout the body, which results in an increase in blood flow.

Nursing care and advice

Nursing care of the patient with PH is about responding to patients' symptoms, explaining the disease and the treatments and best supportive care. PH is clearly a disease entity with a poor prognosis and patients and their carers face a bleak prognosis. Simple advice can help in the relief of symptoms.

Advice for patients with pulmonary hypertension

- Avoid high altitude
- Avoid pregnancy
- Conserve energy by planning your day
- Have regular small meals
- Avoid smoking and alcohol
- Ensure good dental hygiene
- Take medciation as prescribed
- Don't be afraid to ask for advice
- Prepare well in advance for travel.

Recommended reading

European Lung Foundation. *Pulmonary arterial hypertension. Lung Factsheets.* http://www.european-lung-foundation.org
Humbert M, Sitbon O, Simonneau G. (2004). Treatment of pulmonary arterial hypertrension. *N Eng J Med* 351, 1425–1436.
Simonneau G, Galie N, Rubin LJ et al. (2004). Clinical classification of pulmonary hypertension. *J Am Coll Cardiol* 43, 5S–12S.

Recommended websites

PH Association http://www.phassociation.org
PHA UK http://www.pha-uk.com

Non-invasive positive pressure ventilation

Background

Non-invasive positive pressure ventilation (NiPPV) is an effective form of ventilatory assistance. It was first used at the beginning of the twentieth century; since then there has been growing interest in its role in treating type 2 (hypercapnic) respiratory failure.

In the last twenty years NiPPV has had an important role in the management of acute exacerbations of COPD, but its use is not limited to those with COPD. Initially, NiPPV was used mainly to support patients with neuromuscular disease, poliomyelitis and pulmonary oedema. Since then many different groups of patients have been found to benefit from NiPPV, including patients requiring bridging pre-transplant, post-surgical respiratory support, and weaning from mechanical ventilation.

NiPPV in the more recent literature is described as Non Invasive Ventilation (NIV) and these terms are used interchangeably in this chapter.

Respiratory failure

Acute respiratory failure is frequently seen in all acute settings. It can be grouped into type 1 (hypoxaemic) and type 2 (hypercapnic). The former is usually managed by oxygen therapy and treatment of the underlying condition. If the type 1 respiratory failure is severe and ventilation is necessary then continuous positive airway pressure (CPAP) is often used, although recent research has shown some benefits in using NIV in the management of hypoxaemia.

Many patients with neuromuscular disease and chronic respiratory illness live day-to-day with chronic respiratory failure; NIV has made a tremendous impact on the overall management of these patients, especially in keeping them out of hospital.

The majority of trials support the use of NIV in the management of hypoxaemic failure where there is hypercapnia, especially in patients presenting with COPD. Hypercapnic failure occurs when a stable $PaCO_2$, either normal or chronically increased, cannot be maintained without extreme dyspnoea or mechanical support.

Patients with hypercapnic respiratory failure may present with the following signs and symptoms:

- Extreme dyspnoea
- Exhaustion
- Drowsy and sleepy
- Central cyanosis
- Hypercapnic flush
- Possible chest pain.

Clinically, these patients may be cardiovascularly stable, but they may have a tachycardia, especially if they are receiving beta-adrenergic receptor agonist therapy—such as Salbutamol. They will be hypoxic on SpO_2 monitoring (usually <90%). Arterial blood gas analysis should be performed on air, or the patient's regular home therapy, however, if the patient is very ill arterial gases may be undertaken with the patient on oxygen and this should be taken into account when looking at the results

It is important to be aware of these signs and symptoms, as they will help you to identify seriously ill respiratory patients quickly.

Ventilators and interfaces

There are several types of ventilator available for use in the acute setting. These vary from large machines that can fully ventilate a patient (those seen on intensive care units) to small portable machines for use in the ward or in domiciliary settings.

The types of machines available are:
- Volume assist–control ventilators deliver set volumes to the patient
- Pressure assist–control ventilators can be positive or negative pressure. Positive pressure ventilators deliver volume or pressure support. Negative pressure ventilators assist inspiration by sucking out the chest wall with expiration occurring through elastic recoil of the lungs
- Bilevel assisted spontaneous breathing ventilators providing pressure support between selected inspiratory and expiratory positive pressures (IPAP and EPAP).

The British Thoracic Society (BTS) Guidelines on NIV suggest that bilevel machines are probably the best machines to deliver NiPPV, as they are easy to use, and relatively cheap to purchase and run.

All settings wishing to provide a comprehensive NIV service should ensure that both pressure and volume control machines are available for the management of complex patients who may respond more efficiently to one modality over the other.

NIV machines used in the management of acute respiratory failure should provide:
- Pressure control
- Pressure capability of up to 30 cm H_2O
- Capacity to support inspiratory flows of at least 60 L/min
- Assist–control and bilevel pressure support modes
- Rate capability of at least 40 breaths/min
- Sensitive flow triggers
- Disconnection alarm.

NIV interfaces are available in many shapes and sizes, but basically are:
- Nasal masks (various facial moulds available)
- Full-face masks
- Nasal pillows.

It is important that all varieties of NIV interface are available for use. For initial management of acute respiratory failure, the full-face mask is the most preferred interface as it assists patients who may mouth breathe when in extreme respiratory distress. This can then be changed to a nasal mask once the patient has settled, if desired, and is ideal as it does not obstruct the patient's vision.

When fitting the interface bear in mind:
- Appropriate sizing
- A good fit for the patient
- Minimal leaks
- No broken areas—if so address the area involved
- Patient compliance—can be gained by a caring approach to application. This may take some time.

Indications for use

According to the BTS Guidelines, there are three levels at which NIV may be used:

- A holding measure to assist ventilation in patients before tracheal intubation would be considered
- A trial with a view to intubation if NIV fails
- As the ceiling of treatment in patients who are not candidates for intubation.

Table 21.1 highlights the key principles involved, and when to consider initiating NIV.

A decision about tracheal intubation, the ceiling of care and resuscitation state should be in place before starting a trial of NIV. This should be clearly documented in the patient's medical notes.

Clinically, the following criteria are indicated for a trial of NIV:

- Patients with an acute exacerbation of COPD or bronchiectasis, presenting with a persisting respiratory acidosis (pH <0.35kPa, and $PaCO_2$ >6.0kPa), despite maximal medical management and oxygen
- Those who have failed to respond to CPAP (postoperatively, pneumonia, post-transplant respiratory failure and cardiogenic pulmonary oedema), on an intensive care unit (ICU) only
- Those with acute-on-chronic respiratory failure due to chest wall deformity or neuromuscular disease
- As an adjunct to weaning in ICU.

Table 21.1 When to use NIV

Patients
- COPD
- Chest wall deformity, neuromuscular disorder, decompensated OSA
- Cardiogenic pulmonary oedema, unresponsive to CPAP

Blood gases
- Respiratory acidosis ($PaCO_2$ >6.0kPa, pH <7.35kPa), which persists despite maximal medical treatment and appropriate controlled oxygen therapy. Note patients with pH <7.25 respond less well and should be managed on a high dependency unit(HDU)/ICU.
- Low A-a oxygen gradient (patients with severe life threatening hypoxaemia are more appropriately managed by tracheal intubation)

Clinical state
- Sick but not moribund
- Able to protect airway
- Conscious and cooperative
- Haemodynamically stable
- No excessive respiratory secretions
- Few comorbidities.

Contraindication excluded
- Facial burns/trauma/recent facial or upper airway surgery
- Vomiting
- Fixed upper airway obstruction
- Undrained pneumothorax

Premorbid state
- Potential for recovery to a quality of life acceptable to the patient
- Patient's wishes considered.

Reproduced with permission from the BTS guidelines on non-invasive ventilation in acute respiratory failure. *Thorax* (2002) 57:192–211.

Contraindications

As more research is being conducted into NIV for the management of acute and chronic respiratory failure, new guidance is likely to be utilized in updated guidelines.

In order for NIV to be successful, the following contraindications should be considered before starting (BTS Guidelines, 2002):

- Facial trauma/burns
- Recent facial, upper airway, or gastrointestinal tract surgery*
- Fixed upper airway obstruction
- Inability to protect airway* low Glasgow Coma Scale (GCS) score
- Life-threatening hypoxaemia*
- Haemodynamic instability*
- Severe comorbidity*
- Impaired consciousness*
- Confusion/agitation*
- Vomiting
- Bowel obstruction*
- Copious respiratory secretions*
- Focal consolidation on chest radiograph*
- Undrained pneumothorax* (should ideally have a drain *in situ*).

*NIPV may be used—despite the contraindications—if it is the ceiling of care.

Nursing care and monitoring

Nursing care and monitoring is essential for delivering a successful NIV service. Patients starting NIV may initially need a lot of reassurance and care to ensure that they will tolerate the intervention and respiratory support. There is greater chance of success in using NIV if there is adequate time to support the patient.

There may be a risk of aspiration, secondary to gastric distension and vomiting. If the NIV is in place for a substantial time there are risks of dehydration, poor nutritional intake and pressure sores on the nasal bridge and chin. If patients are haemodynamically unstable, strict monitoring is essential for the safe delivery of NIV.

These possible complications can be avoided if basic routine care is in place. This includes:

• Regular blood pressure, pulse rate, SpO_2 and respiratory rate observations (anything from 15–60 minutes)
• Repeated blood gas analysis at 1 h post commencement
• Regular removal of face/nasal mask (ideally every hour) to ensure adequate hydration and expectoration
• Possible insertion of a nasogastric tube
• Regular tracheostomy care if delivered via a tracheostomy
• *In situ* nebulizer chamber for bronchodilator therapy
• Regular checks to NiPPV delivery and chest drains.

If patients present with excessive secretions, a referral should be made for regular respiratory physiotherapy, to assist in their removal.

Starting a patient on NIV is relatively simple, if it is done with plenty of time and empathy. Reassurance is important, as success is reliant upon patient compliance. Table 21.2 highlights the important stages for starting a patient on NIV, and Table 21.3 suggests settings for the machine set up.

Table 21.2 How to set up NIV

- Decide on a management plan if trial of NIV fails, after discussion with senior medical staff, and document this in the medical notes.
- Decide where trial of NIV should take place (HDU/ICU or respiratory ward).
- Consider informing ICU.
- Explain NIV to the patient.
- Select a mask to fit the patient, and hold it in place to familiarize the patient.
- Set up the ventilator (Table 20.3 below).
- Attach pulse oximeter.
- Commence NIV, holding the mask in place for the first few minutes.
- Secure the mask in place with straps and headgear.
- Reassess after a few minutes.
- Adjust settings if necessary.
- Add oxygen if SpO_2 <85%.
- Instruct the patient on how to remove the mask and how to summon help.
- Clinical assessment and repeat arterial blood gas analysis at 1–2 hours.
- Adjust settings/oxygen if required.
- Institute alternative management plan if $PaCO_2$ and pH have deteriorated after 1–2 hours of NIV on optimal settings. If there is no improvement, consider continuing with NIV and reassess with repeat arterial blood gas analysis after 4–6 hours. If there is no improvement in $PaCO_2$ and pH by 4–6 hours, institute alternative management plan.

Reproduced with permission from the BTS guidelines on non-invasive ventilation in acute respiratory failure. *Thorax* (2002) 57: 192–211.

Table 21.3 Typical ventilator settings for bilevel pressure support in a patient with acute hypercapnic respiratory failure due to COPD

Mode: spontaneous/timed EPAP 4–5 cm H_2O
IPAP 12–15 cm H_2O (to be increased as tolerated to 20 cm H_2O)
Triggers maximum sensitivity
Back-up rate 15 breaths a minute
Back-up I:E ratio 1:3

Reproduced with permission from the BTS guidelines on non-invasive ventilation in acute respiratory failure. *Thorax* (2002) 57: 192–211.

Service provision

Every establishment is different, and the appropriate environment for the delivery of NIV will therefore differ. Specialist centres may have the expertise to deliver NIV in several clinical areas; whereas more general hospitals may require NIV to be delivered in one designated setting. The type of service delivered depends on:

- Who leads the NIV service—physician, anaesthetist, clinical specialist physiotherapist, consultant nurse or ideally through a multidisciplinary team (MDT)
- The skills of the the nurses staffing the clinical area
- The training available for those initiating and delivering care
- The support available for complications.

Essentially, any member of the clinical team can lead, deliver and manage the service. However, for an effective service to be delivered all members of the team should have an active role. It is essential that nursing staff have a sound understanding and level of competence in the delivery and care of patients on NIV, even if they do not make decisions about the setting up of the machine. There is no reason why specialists such as consultant nurses and physiotherapists cannot manage NIV services.

In many establishments, domicilary NIV is managed and delivered by respiratory physiology departments. This ideal as they are able to see patients either at home or in the clinic, where they can conduct pulmonary investigations and review the need for NIV in one setting.

Summary

NIV is an essential therapeutic modality that should be available in all acute care centres. It has a strong evidence base for its use, especially in acute and acute-on-chronic exacerbations of COPD. Once a clinical assessment of the patient has been conducted and a formal and realistic plan is in place—including establishing the ceiling for treatment—NIV can start.

Services should be staffed by trained and competent clinicians/nurses, in an appropriate and safe environment. So long as the clinicians and nurses delivering NIV follow the protocol and guidance, there is a good chance of success and a comfortable patient experience.

Further reading

Bach JR (2002). *Non-invasive Mechanical Ventilation*. Philadelphia: Hanley and Belfus.

Baudouin S, Blumenthal S, Cooper B, Davidson C, Davidson A, Elliott A, Kinnear W, Patron R, Sawicka E, Turner, L, British Thoracic Society Standard of Care Committee (2002). Noninvasive ventilation in acute respiratory failure. *Thorax* 57, 192–211.

Jeffrey AA, Warren PM, Flenley DC (1992). Acute hypercapnic respiratory failure in patients with chronic obstructive lung disease: risk factors and use of guidelines for management. *Thorax* 47, 34–40.

Rochester DF (1991). The diaphragm in COPD. Better than expected but not good enough. *New England Journal of Medicine* 325(13), 917–923.

Tuberculosis

Introduction

The World Health Organisation (WHO) declared tuberculosis (TB) a global health emergency in 1983. Targets have since been set to bring down TB rates at global, national, and local level.

It is estimated that a third of the world's population has TB infection; one-tenth of those infected are expected to develop the disease.

Mycobacterium Tuberculosis (MTB) is part of a family of mycobacterium which includes *Mycobacterium bovis*. *M. bovis* is uncommon in humans, although it frequently affects cattle and badgers.

MTB can affect any organ in the body; this chapter will concentrate on the diagnosis, treatment and prevention of pulmonary MTB in adults in the UK.

Key facts

- TB is a notifiable disease
- All TB patients should have a named caseworker. The caseworker must be contacted immediately, by telephone if necessary, regarding any change in anti-tuberculosis medication
- All patients should be under the care of a respiratory or infectious diseases physician, accustomed to treating TB
- Drug-resistant TB should be discussed with the local microbacteria reference laboratory, or a recognized expert in the field
- Never introduce a single agent into a failing regime, discuss with the local microbacteria reference laboratory or recognized expert.

Epidemiology and pathophysiology

- Improvements in sanitation, followed by the discovery of TB treatments, resulted in falling rates of TB at the start of the twentieth century. However, TB rates have increased year on year since the late 1980s; over 8000 new cases of TB were notified in 2006
- TB is more prevalent in cities, with London having the highest rates
- The majority of TB is found in the non-UK-born population; among the UK born, TB is likely to be found in certain high risk groups
- It is very important not to rule out TB from the list of differential diagnosis—as TB can affect anyone.

Risk factors

High risk of TB infection:
- Anyone who has close, prolonged and repeated contact with someone who has infectious TB and is coughing
- People from high TB burden countries, these can be found on the WHO website
- Those who have spent time in prison
- Homeless people.

High risk of developing TB disease if infected:
- Immuno-compromised patients
- Patients receiving steroid treatment
- Drug and alcohol users
- Those who have spent time in prison
- Homeless people.

Signs and symptoms

- Cough—lasting more than three weeks, particularly if unresolved by antibiotics
- Haemoptysis
- Weight loss
- Night sweats
- Loss of appetite
- Flu-like feeling
- Chest pain.

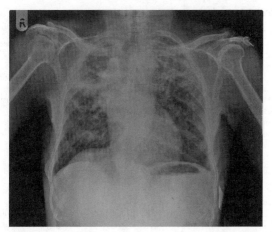

Fig. 22.1 AP chest X-ray showing a large cavity in the right upper zone: this is also associated with volume loss, indicating fibrosis. There is air space shadowing seen throughout the rest of the lungs, this is in keeping with TB, and the air space shadowing suggests that there is active disease.

Reproduced with permission from Stephen Ellis, Radiology Department, Barts and the London NHS Trust

Clinical assessment and history taking as well as a CXR are important when reviewing a patient with a pulmonary disease.

Investigations

- At least three sputum specimens for acid-fast bacilli (AFB)
- A patient is classed as infectious if the bacilli in the sputum can be seen under light microscopy—this is known as smear positive
- Failure to see the bacilli does not rule out TB
- All sputum should be sent to a laboratory for culture in liquid medium, subsequent growth is referred to as smear negative, culture positive
- If the patient is unable to produce sputum then a bronchoscopy must be performed to obtain samples
- Induced sputum must take place in a suitable environment—such as a negative pressure room
- Blood tests including:
  - ESR and CRP
  - Liver function tests (LFTs)—will be needed as a baseline if the patient commences anti-tuberculosis treatment.

Until sputum samples have been sent to the laboratory, anti-TB treatment should not commence, unless the patient is gravely ill.

Initial sensitivities are very important if there is a resistant organism. Without initial sensitivities it would be guess work changing medication.

Treatment phase

- Patients should be assessed for issues which may make them unable to complete treatment (see the section on Directly observed therapy).
- LFTs must be repeated 2 weeks after the start of treatment and at any signs of liver toxicity
- The patient's baseline colour vision should be tested within 2 weeks of starting ethambutol
- Failure of the sputum to grow AFB's does not rule out TB. Patients who have responded clinically should remain on treatment for 6 months
- If AFB's are not cultured and there is no improvement in either the chest X-ray (cxr) or symptoms, consider drug resistance or a different diagnosis
- Patients who are diagnosed with TB should be offered an HIV test
- Side-effects of medication can usually be treated symptomatically, inform the caseworker if you intend to do this but never reduce treatment without authority from the TB consultant in charge of the patient's care. Under prescribing can lead to drug resistance
- If patients have severe side-effects such as liver toxicity, uncontrollable vomiting or a florid rash all over their body, medication can be stopped
- In the event of severe side-effects, refer urgently to a consultant in charge of the patients' care.

Standard drug therapy

NICE Guidelines (2006) recommend all new TB patients start on quadruple therapy.

Combination drugs can be used as part of the 4-drug regime.

Drug	Body weight	Dose
Rifater® (rifampicin, isoniazid, pyrazinamide)	Under 40kg	3 tablets daily
	41–49kg	4 tablets daily
	50–64kg	5 tablets daily
	65kg or more	6 tablets daily

For 4-months continuous phase

Drug	Body weight	Dose
Rifampicin	Under 50kg	450 mg daily
	50kg and over	600 mg daily
Isoniazid		300 mg daily

Or combination drug

Drug	Body weight	Dose
Rifinah® (rifampicin, isoniazid)	Under 50kg	3 tablets daily of Rifinah®—150
	50kg and over	2 tablets daily of Rifinah®—300

Drug resistance can be caused by under-prescribing of anti-tuberculosis medication and if there is any doubt specialist advice should be sought regarding the regime.

Pyridoxine (Vitamin B6) is normally given to patients on isoniazid as prophylaxis against peripheral neuropathy.

Directly observed therapy (DOT)

DOT is when a patient, for whatever reason, is required to be supervised taking their anti-TB medication.

Patients who have drug and alcohol issues, mental health issues, ex-prisoners and people who live alone, should be monitored very closely and offered DOT if appropriate. DOT should be patient-centred and not service-centred.

For the 2-month initial phase

Drug	Body weight	Dose
Pyrazinamide	Under 50 kg	2g 3 times a week
	50 kg and over	2.5g 3 times a week
Isoniazid		15 mg/kg (max 900 mg) 3 times a week
Rifampicin		600–900mg 3 times a week
Ethambutol		30 mg/kg 3 times a week

For 4-months continuous phase

Drug	Body weight	Dose
Isoniazid		15 mg/kg (max 900 mg) 3 times a week
Rifampicin		600–900mg 3 times a week

Drug-resistant TB

Mono-resistant TB

Most common is resistance to isoniazid in 5–10% of patients.

Multi-drug resistant TB (MDRTB)

MDRTB is when the TB organism is resistant to the two most important first-line drugs, rifampicin and isoniazid. Extreme drug-resistant TB (EDRTB) is when the TB organism is resistant to all four first-line drugs, and streptomycin.

Anti-TB medication regimes for any of the above must be decided in collaboration with an expert in TB.

Patients can acquire drug-resistant TB by:
• Being infected with a resistant organism (primary infection)
• Inappropriate prescribing of anti-TB medication—not in line with NICE TB guidelines
• Non-adherence or poor adherence to TB medication.

Pregnancy

- TB cannot be transmitted to the fetus
- There are no known risks to the fetus from TB medication
- All pregnant patients should be on pyridoxine
- Streptomycin should not be used
- Rifampicin reduces the efficacy of the combine oral contraceptive pill so alternative methods should be used
- Breastfeeding should be discussed with an expert, although in most cases some breastfeeding will be acceptable.

Nursing care

NICE guidelines stipulate that all patients with TB should have a named key worker who is easily contactable. In most cases this will be a TB nurse specialist who will provide support to the patient on all aspects of their care, throughout the duration of treatment. The patient must be put in contact with that person as soon as they are diagnosed with TB.

Unless it is clinically indicated patients do not need to be admitted to hospital. If there are small children the patient may be admitted to hospital to avoid further exposure of vulnerable children at home, but separating a mother and baby may well do more harm than good. Infectious patients should be advised to stay at home for the first 2 weeks of treatment, after which they will no longer be infectious.

Patients should be considered for admission if they are from one of the high non-compliance risk groups—this will enable them to be stabilized on medication and a plan made for supervision after discharge.

All pulmonary TB patients should be nursed in a side room. Patients with suspected or known MDRTB and XDRTB should be nursed in a negative pressure room.

If a patient is required to leave the side room then a mask must be worn whilst outside the room.

NICE TB guidelines support the use of high-performance masks for staff caring for patients with suspected or known MDRTB. These guidelines do not support the use of masks for infectious pulmonary TB patients. Trusts may consider that not using masks and working over a prolonged period of time in certain areas will increase the risk to staff.

Contact tracing

All household contacts of patients with pulmonary disease should be assessed in accordance with Figure 22.2 below.

Where the index case (the person with infectious pulmonary TB) is a school pupil, a college student or an employed person, and if he/she has recently travelled on an airplane or been an inpatient in an open ward in a hospital, the local Health Protection Agency should be informed, and contact tracing should be undertaken in accordance with NICE TB guidelines.

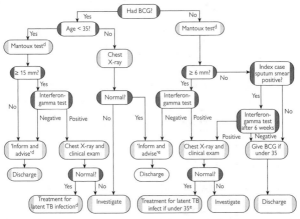

Fig. 22.2 Testing and treating asymptomatic household and other close contacts of all cases of active TB.

Reproduced from the National Collaborating Centre for Chronic Conditions. Tuberculosis: clinical diagnosis and management of tuberculosis, and measures fot its prevention and control, London. Royal College of Physicians 2006. ©2006, Royal College of Physicians.

References

NICE (2006). *TB Guidelines*. NICE, London.

Further reading

Davies PDO (2003). *Clinical Tuberculosis*. Arnold, London.

Links

http://www.nice.org.uk/guidance/CG33/niceguidance/pdf/English, full version
http://www.nice.org.uk/guidance/CG33/quickrefguide/pdf/English, quick reference version

Palliative care

Palliative care is the active, total care of patients whose disease is not responsive to curative treatment. The goal of palliative care is the best quality of life for patients and their families.

(National Council for Hospice and Specialist Palliative Care Services 1998)

The importance of palliative care

Although there are respiratory diseases that are acute and respond well to treatments, unfortunately many end in what could be termed an essentially palliative or terminal phase. Many respiratory disease processes are essentially chronic in nature and some patients could be considered palliative from diagnosis. The management of many chronic respiratory conditions is amelioration of symptoms rather than active treatment, so for these patients progressive decline is inevitable, bringing with it the problems faced by all patients dealing with end-stage disease.

There is an increasing body of evidence that patients with end-stage lung disease experience declining heath, anxiety, depression, fatigue, coping difficulties, and somatic preoccupation, and if this is unrecognized then there is a potential for basic needs to remain unmet.

Inequalities in health care and palliation

The ethos for palliative care grew out of the hospice movement and the founding of St Christophers, a centre for palliative patients primarily with cancer in the 1960s. Palliative care is the approach taken to managing patients with progressive and incurable disease and this would certainly seem applicable for numerous patients with respiratory disorders. It is an interdisciplinary approach and seeks to care holistically, including emotional physical, social, and spiritual aspects.

Traditionally palliative care provision has largely been provided for patients with cancer-related diagnoses and there has been little provision for patients with other disease processes, however amenable they would be to palliation. A major challenge for health care provision is to channel finite resources to all that may benefit, and how best to deliver palliative care to all patients with life-limiting disease.

Care and management 1

The care and management of respiratory patients requiring palliative care should focus on the issues, symptoms, and needs of the individual patient. These may vary at different times of the disease trajectory but may include:

Breathlessness/dyspnoea

Breathlessness or dyspnoea is often the overriding symptom for most patients, and in the later stages of respiratory diseases additional and alternative treatments may need to be considered. The experience of breathlessness is very individual and has little correlation with the severity of the underlying lung disease, but is complicated by perception, coping mechanisms and so forth. The use of a fan, which acts on the sensory receptors in the face, may help to alleviate breathlessness and anxiety.

For those patients who would benefit, bronchodilators in the form of inhalers or nebulized medication should be optimized. Codeine either in linctus or in tablet form may reduce breathlessness and is also useful in treating cough. Opiates have been shown to be effective for both breathlessness and cough, especially morphine oral solution but cause some side-effects particularly constipation. There is little evidence for nebulized morphine, oral is the recommended route of administration. Constipation may be of particular concern to patients, causing additional stress and strain, and laxatives may be used alongside codeine or morphine.

Respiratory depression is a consideration that merits discussion with both patient and relatives, but should not be seen as a problem for patients at the end-stage of their disease. Some practitioners may worry about addiction, but for patients with a chronic progressive disease it is probably of little consequence.

Using the Medical Research Council (MRC) dyspnoea scale provides an objective tool to measure exercise tolerance and correlates well with perceived breathlessness (Table 23.1).

Many of the other management strategies detailed below are also useful in treating breathlessness.

Smoking cessation

Smoking is implicated in the majority of respiratory diseases and smoking cessation is relevant to avoid deteriorating lung function. This is a sensitive issue in end-stage disease where the benefits of stopping may be perceived by the patients to be negated by the effects of withdrawal. This is an issue that needs to be handled sensitively, especially when considering other treatment options such as oxygen therapy.

Table 23.1 The Medical Research Council dyspnoea scale

Grade	Degree of breathlessness related to activity
1	Not troubled with breathlessness only with strenuous exercise
2	Short of breath when hurrying on the level
3	Walks slower than contemporaries of the same age on the level because of breathlessness or has to stop for breath when walking at own pace on the level
4	Stops for breath after walking 100 yards or after a few minutes on the level
5	Too breathless to leave the house or breathless when washing or undressing

Medication

At all stages of the disease trajectory medication should be optimized. As the disease progresses it is often worth reviewing all medication, considering alternatives and removing those that are no longer beneficial. Patients may have concomitant disease and may be on multiple medication regimens. Treatment should be individualized and each patient's response monitored. Obviously as disease progresses some treatments may need to be increased; some treatments may be no longer effective and may be withdrawn without significant effect.

Relaxation and breathing exercises

Teaching the patient simple breathing exercises or relaxation techniques may help to control feelings of breathlessness and panic. When patients are anxious about their condition they tend to hyperventilate, and fast shallow breathing decreases alveolar ventilation and can enhance breathlessness. Exercises can be also be undertaken sitting down and adapted for bed-bound patients. They are also useful techniques for carers to learn so that they feel involved and able to help, which may lessen their own anxieties.

Chest clearance

If a patient is able to effectively clear their chest then they are likely to reduce breathlessness and have less chest infections. The 'active cycle' of breathing may help (🕮 p.330). An adequate fluid intake will be important to help keep secretions loose and is an important factor in respiratory diseases, where fear of breathlessness means patients often restrict their fluid intakes so they do not have to move around to the bathroom as often. Other options include the use of steam inhalations, nebulized saline or flutter valves, although the latter may be considered a more active treatment. Suction should be avoided if at all possible as it can be very distressing to the patient. Medication such as hyoscine could be used to dry up excessive secretions.

Care and management 2

Anxiety and depression management

Anxiety and depression are almost always present in end-stage disease and can be treated effectively with anxiolytics and antidepressants. Tricyclics have antimuscarinic effects and cause sedation, both of which could be beneficial in selected patients with end-stage disease. Buspirone is also of value in reducing anxiety and depression. Studies on depression and anxiety in respiratory disease are inconclusive, but it would appear that these problems are often are not recognized and more often not treated.

Pain

For some patients pain may be a distressing symptom. This is commonly chest pain, which may be due to respiratory muscle hypoxia, and/or musculoskeletal problems, which are generally more common in inactive elderly populations. The full range of analgesics may be used to alleviate pain, but pain is often overlooked in respiratory disease. Codeine may be useful both for pain and for reducing the sensation of breathlessness and cough, although the side-effect of constipation may deter some patients.

Non-pharmacological management of pain may involve positioning, mobility aids, immobilization, the use of heat therapy, transcutaneous nerve stimulation (TENS) or in more extreme cases local nerve blocks or spinal analgesia. In some instances physical assistance for the patient can help to reduce pain levels.

Oxygen

Oxygen therapy has a proven benefit in some of the respiratory disorders and careful monitoring for need and provision should be integral to care. There are clear indications for oxygen use and ordering, however, it may be relevant to use oxygen as palliation in the end stages of respiratory diseases where patients would not normally meet the criteria for its usage, although there is little evidence for this and limited studies in palliative disease show air is just as good. The use of oxygen should be balanced against the patient's own wishes for this therapy.

Cough

Cough is often distressing for patients and may respond to codeine or morphine.

Nutritional status

Weight loss is a good indicator of a poor prognosis in respiratory disorders. This may be due to a poor appetite, breathlessness, a dry mouth or the generalized muscle wasting and cachexia associated with end-stage disease. Small frequent meals may be advocated and meal supplements suggested, although there is no good evidence that any intervention is effective

Oral hygiene

In respiratory diseases many patients mouth breathe, and as a consequence the mouth can be very dry and prone to infections. Good oral hygiene will avoid this distressing consequence.

Social issues

Patients may require help with benefits such as disability living allowance or attendance allowance, and a DS1500 can be filled in for those with less than 6 months to live. House adaptations may be needed as disease progresses or practical solutions such as moving beds downstairs or closer to toilet facilities. These interventions need to be timely as they are often a prolonged process: problems need to be recognized and addressed early.

Ventilation

The issue of whether ventilation is appropriate either invasive or nasally should be discussed with patients, preferably before the situation arises so that the patient's wishes can be taken into account. This is a difficult topic to bring up at an appropriate time, especially if patients have benefited from these interventions before; also patients' wishes may change when they are actually faced with a crisis situation.

Complementary therapies

Patients may wish to use complementary therapies and there should be open and frank discussion to ensure that these do not conflict with any current treatments.

End of life/after care

Although with some of the respiratory diseases the end stage is not easy to determine, at some time patients, and carers if appropriate, may appreciate an honest discussion about prognosis and end of life wishes. In primary care the use of the 'Gold Standards Framework' covers the last 6–12 months of life and allows for a clear plan of patients' wishes and treatment options to be available for all those involved in patient care.

Nursing care

Patients with end-stage respiratory disease have needs which could be regarded as palliative in nature. Advanced respiratory disease has a poor prognosis and the uncertain nature of the condition means that patients can live in a declining state of poor health for variable lengths of time, although these may be punctuated with intermittent acute episodes. There is a growing recognition of the problem of palliation in respiratory disease and of the perceived disparity in provision, but little formalized care in place for this group of patients. Recognition of the problem and relatively simple interventions may make the palliative phase of the illness easier to deal with for patients and their carers.

Patients who are essentially dying deserve good care and support regardless of the setting and cause of the disease.

The nurses' role may include:
- Information giving
- Symptom control
- Coordination of care
- Support
- Needs assessment
- Liaison with other health and social care professionals
- Patient advocate.

Key points
- There are many respiratory diseases that are chronic in nature and that are responsible for a sizeable burden of morbidity and mortality
- Best supportive care for respiratory patients includes meeting physical, psychological, social, and emotional needs
- Both pharmacological and non-pharmacological measures may be important in providing good palliative care
- Treatment should be individualized for each patient at the relevant stage of their disease
- A palliative care approach is appropriate for respiratory patients
- Palliative care should be available for all end-stage patients regardless of diagnosis.

Further reading

Gore JM, Brophy CJ, Greenstone MA (2000). How well do we care for patients with end stage chronic obstructive pulmonary disease (COPD) ? A comparison of palliative care and quality of life in COPD and lung cancer. *Thorax* 55, 1000–1006.

Hill KM and Meurs MF (2000). Palliative care for patients with non-malignant end-stage respiratory disease. *Thorax* 55(12), 979–981.

National Council for Hospice and Specialist Palliative Care Services (1998). *Occasional Paper 14. Reaching Out: Specialist Care for Adults with Non-Malignant Diseases*. NCHSPCS. London

Rushby I, Scullion J (2004). Managing dyspnoea in end-stage chronic obstructive pulmonary disease (COPD). *Primary Health Care* 14(1), 43–49.

Simonds AK (2003). Ethics and decision making in end-stage lung disease. *Thorax* 58(3), 272–277.

Skilbeck J, Mott L, Page H, Smith D, Hjelmeland-Ahmedzai S, Clark D. (1998). Palliative care in chronic obstructive airways disease: a needs assessment. *Palliative Medicine* 12(4), 245–254.

The National Collaborating Centre for Chronic Conditions (2004). Chronic Obstructive Pulmonary Disease. National clinical guidelines on management of chronic obstructive pulmonary disease in adults in primary and secondary care. *Thorax* 59(Suppl. 1), 1–232.

Pulmonary rehabilitation

Introduction

Pulmonary rehabilitation is an important component in the management, care, and treatment of patients with chronic lung disease, particularly with COPD. There are a number of definitions of pulmonary rehabilitation; one of the most widely used is the American Thoracic Society's definition which states:

> Pulmonary rehabilitation is a multidisciplinary programme of care for patients with chronic respiratory impairment that is individually tailored and designed to optimize physical and social performance and autonomy.

Pulmonary rehabilitation is an organized programme of exercise and education, prescribed on an individual basis for patients disabled by their symptoms. It aims to improve physical fitness and social well-being, and to help the patient gain some control of the disability, impairment and handicap that lung disease causes.

The aims of pulmonary rehabilitation are to:
- Enhance functional performance
- Improve quality of life
- Promote physical independence
- Improve psychosocial well-being.

These aims combine to restore the patient to the highest level of independent functioning.

Why is pulmonary rehabilitation necessary?

The most common presenting symptom for many patients with lung diseases, especially those with COPD, is breathlessness. This is a symptom of the underlying lung disease as the lungs are not working efficiently enough to give the patient sufficient oxygen for their body's needs. As a result of this breathlessness, many patients restrict their activities and become less fit, essentially deconditioned. Patients then do less, which results in breathlessness at even lower levels of exercise and further de-conditioning. This process continues, bringing with it other problems such as social isolation, depression, and anxiety, known as the cycle of breathlessness (Figure 24.1).

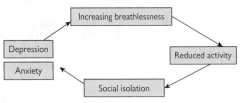

Fig. 24.1 The cycle of breathlessness

Most patients present with breathlessness when it is having a significant effect on their lives. Initially breathlessness may be associated with physically demanding activities like exercise, gardening or housework, and patients can compensate for this by reducing their physical activity. Eventually, breathlessness interferes with more basic activities of daily living, and this may prompt a person to seek help. The patient's condition steadily worsens as a result of breathlessness, which is associated with both the respiratory disease and reduced levels of fitness. As a patient becomes more incapacitated, they can become socially isolated, and often anxious and depressed.

Pulmonary rehabilitation aims to reverse this spiral of decline.

The second most common symptom reported by patients with COPD is fatigue, thought to be due in part to the effort of breathing, deconditioning and other factors, e.g. poor sleep patterns. Fatigue also increases the feelings of depression and social isolation.

Who benefits from pulmonary rehabilitation?

Patients with all levels of disease severity benefit from pulmonary rehabilitation, although those with the motivation to improve their lives are likely to do better. The ethos of rehabilitation presumes that any patient experiencing breathlessness impacting on their lives is likely to benefit (Table 24.1).

It is increasingly recognized that the severity of the lung function has very little correlation with an individual's perception and experience of breathlessness. Breathlessness is very much what the patient says it is; it is not easy to define purely on objective spirometric lung measurement. A useful measure is the Medical Research Council (MRC) Dyspnoea Scale. This allows the patient to rate their degree of disability and it gives some indication of their exercise tolerance. Generally, patients at stage three and above on the MRC dyspnoea scale appear to benefit from pulmonary rehabilitation (Table 24.2).

Patients should be optimally medically and pharmacologically managed and their condition should be clinically stable prior to commencing pulmonary rehabilitation. Rehabilitation provides benefit for all patients with varying degrees of disability, including smokers. There are no grounds for selection against patients who require oxygen, provided there is access to O_2 in the sessions. Patients not suitable include those in whom significant comorbidity would prevent them undertaking the programme.

Patients who are committed to completing the programme and who wish to improve their lives are likely to achieve the most from pulmonary rehabilitation. It is also essential that the patient takes the advice to exercise on board and is motivated to undertake and continue the programme of exercise at home. This will be essential to maintain fitness levels when the formal programme ends. Programmes should take into account what the patient wants out of the programme when planning their training schedule (Table 24.3).

Table 24.1 Suitability for pulmonary rehabilitation

No barrier	Barrier
FEV$_1$	Comorbidity
Age	Transport problems
Gender	Geographical location
Level of disability	Language difficulties
Oxygen-dependent	Lack of motivation
Current smoker	

Table 24.2 The Medical Research Council Dyspnoea Scale

Grade	Degree of breathlessness related to activity
1	Not troubled by breathlessness—only with strenuous exercise
2	Short of breath when hurrying on the level or walking up a slight hill
3	Walks slower than contemporaries of the same age on the level because of breathlessness or has to stop for breath when walking at own pace on the level
4	Stops for breath after walking about 100 yards or after a few minutes on the level
5	Too breathless to leave the house or breathless when dressing and undressing

Table 24.3 What patients may want

Increased mobility
Reduction in disability
Freedom from symptoms
Stable disease
Increased knowledge
A consistent approach to care
Control

What should a programme entail?

Pulmonary rehabilitation traditionally consists of two elements:
• Physical exercise
• An educational component.
Although these may be distinct components they can complement each other.

Assessment

Before starting the course, the patient's exercise tolerance, health status, psychological status and ability to complete activities of daily living should be assessed. There are a variety of tools available to assist in this process. Spirometry may be performed to identify the patient's degree of impairment—although as COPD is irreversible, spirometry would not be expected to improve after rehabilitation.

The physical exercise component

The evidence for rehabilitation shows benefits for patients who undertake lower-limb aerobic activity such as cycling, stepping or walking. The benefits of upper limb exercise are not as evident; but low-intensity, peripheral muscle training has been shown to be beneficial. Patient exercise levels are prescribed at around 60–80% of an individual's peak capacity, that is, at a high enough level to provoke a physiological training response. There is some evidence to show that training at a higher intensity may be even more effective. To establish an individual's exercise tolerance a formal laboratory-based exercise test can be performed, or a field exercise test, such as a corridor-walking test.

All exercise should be individually prescribed. This possibly explains why patients do not benefit as much from classes where exercise is done on a group basis.

Education

The educational component of pulmonary rehabilitation may vary between courses, but a multiprofessional approach appears to work well. This may not be possible in some settings, and programmes undertaken with relatively few health care professionals are still beneficial and effective.

Patient education in pulmonary rehabilitation covers a wide range of subjects delivered informally and in more practical sessions. The educational component of pulmonary rehabilitation does not appear to be effective on its own, without the exercise component of the rehabilitation course.

Outcome measures for pulmonary rehabilitation may include improvements both in exercise tolerance and health status.

Exercise tolerance may be measured by:
• The 6-minute walking test—where patients are instructed to cover as much ground as possible in 6 minutes
• The shuttle walking test—which measures maximum capacity and which has two forms:
  • The incremental shuttle-walking test—a paced and incremental test where patients walk between two cones 10 m apart at speeds dictated by sounds from a tape cassette. The speed of walking is

increased every minute and stresses the patient to maximal performance which is symptom limited
- The endurance shuttle-walking test—sets the workload at a constant pace and the patient walks at this pace until their symptoms limit their performance.

Health status may be measured by a variety of validated questionnaires, for example:
- The St George's Respiratory Questionnaire
- Short Form 36 Health Survey (SF 36)
- The Chronic Respiratory Disease Questionnaire
- The Hospital Anxiety and Depression Scale (HADS).

However, health status has only a weak correlation with functional capacity.

Where should pulmonary rehabilitation take place?

Pulmonary rehabilitation originated within the hospital setting, but the location of the course is of less importance than the actual content. Both primary and secondary care locations have advantages and disadvantages. In primary care the location may be easier for patients to get to, but facilities and personnel may be more limited than in secondary care.

What is clear is that in order to demonstrate a physiological training effect, patients need to exercise:

• For between 4 and 12 weeks
• For a minimum of two occasions per week
• For around 20–30 minutes at a time.

Follow-up

Patients that take on the ethos of pulmonary rehabilitation and who continue to exercise after the course ends fare better than patients who complete the course and then return to an inactive lifestyle. Patients should be encouraged to maintain their levels of fitness; short top-up programmes could be a way of doing this.

Patient's should be encouraged to join support groups such as Breathe Easy, after rehabilitation, so that the confidence they have gained during the programme is maintained.

Joining an exercise referral scheme may also help patients maintain their exercise levels after a rehabilitation programme.

Pulmonary rehabilitation enables an individual to adjust to having a chronic condition, whilst encouraging maximum functioning and independence. However, it is an essentially palliative process in the management of disease, aimed at ameliorating symptoms and assisting individual coping mechanisms. Rehabilitation programmes also appear to reduce the burden of the disease upon the individual and their family, with positive consequences for the NHS.

Key points
- Pulmonary rehabilitation combines exercise, education and support
- The location of the programme is less important than the content
- The programme may be delivered by a team, although it can be delivered by an individual.

Further reading
American Thoracic Society (1999). Pulmonary rehabilitation. *Am J Respir Crit Care Med* 159, 1666–1682.
British Thoracic Society (1997). Guidelines on the management of COPD. The BTS Standards of Care Committee. *Thorax* 52(Suppl. 5), S1–S28.
Troosters T, Gosselink R, Decramer M (2000). Short- and long-term effects of outpatient rehabilitation in patients with chronic obstructive pulmonary disease: a randomized trial. *Am J Med* 109(3), 207–212.

Public health

Introduction

Public health practice is focused on enhancing the health of the population as a whole, rather than treating individual patients. This chapter defines a population as all those with respiratory disease; it aims to examine a variety of approaches to promoting the health of respiratory patients.

There are many determinants that influence health including:

- Individual influences—lifestyle factors such as smoking, diet and exercise
- Influences from the social, economic and physical environment—quality of housing, access to health care, access to good food, levels of air pollution. For example, it has been accepted for some time that there is a direct relationship between deprivation and poor health. Poorer people tend to die at a younger age than those who are more affluent.
- Wider social, economic, and physical environment—pricing policy on tobacco and alcohol, effects of greenhouse gases and global warming.

Much of the work of the respiratory disease practitioner involves the promotion of health. The role of the respiratory nurse includes preventative care and health promotion. This chapter will look at how the wider nursing team contributes to the health and well-being of the respiratory patient.

The facts about smoking

Around 13 million adults in the UK are smokers, despite public knowledge about the ill effects of smoking. Most smokers take up the habit as teenagers. Reasons for starting are varied and include:

- Low education attainment
- Low socio-economic status
- Peer pressure
- Living with other smokers
- Weight control in girls.

There are over 4000 chemicals in each cigarette, 600 of which are known carcinogens (📖 p.544). The majority of smokers know that it is harmful, and an estimated one in three smokers want to stop. Over half of smokers will eventually be killed by their habit. Smokers have a much higher incidence of lung cancer and chronic obstructive pulmonary disease (COPD). Stopping smoking is the single most important intervention in COPD, and the only thing that significantly alters the natural history of the disease. (📖 p.249)

Tobacco addiction

Nicotine is highly addictive, and smokers quickly become adept at adjusting their smoking to satisfy their need for tobacco. It is a powerful stimulant, acting on the pleasure centres of the brain.

Following the inhalation of cigarette smoke, nicotine is absorbed through the lining of the lung, and high concentrations reach the brain in 7–10 seconds: faster than if nicotine was injected intravenously. This gives the smoker an instant hit and is an important factor in causing dependency. As nicotine levels start to fall, smokers experience symptoms of withdrawal including irritability, restlessness, and lack of concentration; they crave another 'hit'.

Nicotine is addictive, but it is relatively harmless. It is this addiction to nicotine that makes it difficult for smokers to stop. Other factors that make it difficult to stop include:

- 20 cigarettes smoked a day equals up to 250 daily hand to mouth movements
- Smoking is associated with pleasurable everyday activities such as relaxing after a meal, social occasions and pleasurable memories
- Fear of failure in an attempt to quit
- The loss of an 'old friend' that might have been part of the smoker's life for many years
- Fear of gaining weight.

The physical addiction and the habit of smoking mean that breaking the habit can be very difficult.

The physiological effects of smoking on the respiratory system

Toxic components of tobacco smoke

When the tobacco leaf is burnt, the smoker is exposed to over 4000 chemicals. Tobacco smoke contains chemicals in the form of particulate substances and gases. A number of the substances found in tobacco smoke are known to cause cancer. These include:

- Benzene
- Vinyl chloride
- Ethylene oxide
- Aromatic amines
- Arsenic
- Nickel
- Chromium
- Cadmium
- Radioactive element.

Smoke is divided into gas and particulate phases. Most of the carcinogenic components are in the particulate phase that forms the tar. The introduction of low tar cigarettes has been a response to this finding. Smokers are known to compensate when they change from high to low tar cigarettes. This compensation is driven by the need to achieve a required amount of nicotine. To achieve this smokers take deeper and more frequent puffs or smoke more of the cigarette or even by covering the ventilation holes in the cigarette.

Many of the constituents of the gas phase of smoking are also very damaging to the respiratory tract. For example, carbon monoxide is the main gas formed when a cigarette is lit. Carbon monoxide binds to haemoglobin more readily than oxygen and this means that the blood can carry less oxygen. Other constituents of the gas phase include:

- Acetone
- Ammonia
- Acrolein
- Carbon monoxide
- Nitrogen
- Hydrogen
- Methane
- Phenol
- Formaldehyde
- Benzene.

Mechanisms of damage

The constituents of tobacco smoke cause damage throughout the respiratory tract. This includes:

- Loss of cilia and mucous gland hypertrophy occur in the upper airways
- Inflammation, epithelial changes, fibrosis and secretory congestion in the peripheral airways
- Alveoli are destroyed with the loss of the gas exchange surface area and airway flexibility
- Vascular changes to the small arteries and capillaries of the bronchioles and alveoli
- Inflammation of the cells of the bronchial tree leading to squamous metaplasia (a pre-cancerous condition), smooth muscle hypertrophy and fibrosis.

Lung disease and smoking

The two most common respiratory diseases caused by smoking are lung cancer and COPD. In Western countries smoking is the major risk factor for these two diseases, and the increased mortality risk from both diseases has an approximately straight-line relationship with the numbers of cigarettes smoked per day.

COPD

Smoking is the major cause of COPD, responsible for 80–90% of cases: 25% of smokers show a more rapid and greater falling-off of lung function than non-smokers or non-susceptible smokers (📖 p.249). The changes induced by the irritant tobacco smoke produce the recognizable symptoms of COPD including persistent productive cough, regular chest infections requiring antibiotics, and shortness of breath.

Lung cancer

Like COPD, over 80% of all lung cancer deaths are caused by smoking. Inhaled carcinogens from cigarette smoking play a major part in the development of all lung cancers (squamous cell, adenocarcinoma, small cell, and undifferentiated carcinomas) (📖 p.323).

Asthma

It has been known for some time that passive exposure to tobacco smoke increases the frequency and severity of asthma attacks in both children and adults. It is unclear whether exposure to tobacco smoke increases the risk of developing asthma in adults (📖 p.147).

Pneumonia

The risk of pneumonia is increased by the irritant effect of smoke inhalation accompanied by mucous gland hypertrophy and damage to the immune system. Pneumonia is not only more common among smokers, but it is also more likely to be fatal (📖 p.455).

Other non-respiratory diseases caused by smoking

- Cardiovascular disease
- Aortic aneurysm
- Crohn's disease
- Gastric and duodenal ulcers
- Cataracts and age-related macular degeneration.

Smoking cessation

Smoking cessation should be an integral part of the management of all patients with respiratory diseases and have a high priority: they have a greater and more urgent need to stop smoking than the average smoker.

It is important to take a proactive role in motivating patients to stop. People who have been smoking for many years may be reluctant to stop. Others, for example people with severe COPD, may see stopping as futile, as the damage already done to their lungs is irreversible.

People are unlikely to stop smoking if they cannot identify any benefits from stopping; they have to want to stop smoking. The practitioner needs to remember that the road from contented smoker to serious quitter is long and hard.

Health professional concerns

Many professionals have difficulty talking to patients about their smoking behaviour. Some health professionals believe that it is pointless and not worth the effort. Attitudes are changing, and addiction to nicotine is now viewed as a chronic disease, like diabetes or hypertension. The subject needs to be dealt with sensitively and in a non-threatening way.

Approximately 70% of smokers, when asked, want to stop smoking. The health practitioner is in an excellent position to offer constructive advice, encouragement, and support to move the patient from the contemplative stage to being a successful quitter.

A censorious approach is not helpful, and may make the patient even more resistant to stopping smoking. It may even prevent the patient attending the clinic or surgery for fear of being reproached. A helpful approach involves getting people to identify what personal benefits they would get from stopping smoking. These may include:
• Health benefits
• Financial savings
• Smelling nicer
• Cleaner home and car
• Less social stigmatization.
Table 25.1 illustrates the general benefits to health of stopping smoking.

Brief smoking cessation advice provided by a health practitioner is simple and effective, although practitioners often say that lack of time is a barrier to offering this advice. For every 40 patients given brief advice there will be one extra quitter. Every consultation is an opportunity to make an impact, and continued or follow-up advice can assist in sustaining quit rates.

All health professionals managing patients with respiratory disease should have appropriate training in smoking cessation to give the patient the best chance of stopping permanently.

Table 25.1 Health benefits of smoking cessation

Time	Health benefit
20 minutes	Blood pressure returns to normal Circulation improves in hands and feet, making them warmer
8 hours	Oxygen levels in the blood return to normal Chances of a heart attack start to fall
24 hours	Carbon monoxide is eliminated from the body Mucus and other debris starts to clear from the lungs
48 hours	Nicotine is no longer detectable in the body The ability to taste and smell improves
72 hours	Breathing becomes easier as the bronchial tubes relax and recover Energy levels increase
2–12 weeks	Circulation improves so walking becomes easier
3–9 months	Breathing problems such as cough, shortness of breath and wheeze improve with lung function increasing by about 5–10%
5 years	Risk of heart attack falls to about half of that of a smoker
10 years	Risk of lung cancer falls to half that of a smoker Risk of heart attack similar to a never-smoker

Pharmacological treatments for smoking cessation

Given the highly addictive nature of nicotine, smokers find it difficult to quit. To be successful in stopping, smokers need to be motivated to want to stop: the higher their motivational levels, the more likely the person is to stop. Although motivation is crucial, it is unlikely that willpower alone is sufficient to enable a smoker to stop.

Many patients fail in their attempt to stop smoking because of physical nicotine withdrawal symptoms such as irritability, nervousness and cravings. Fear of reliving these symptoms stops some smokers from making further attempts to quit.

Patients should understand that nicotine withdrawal has behavioural elements as well as physical elements. Smoking cessation treatment should include pharmacological treatment combined with behavioural support.

Pharmacological therapies that can help patients to minimize these symptoms are recommended and have been shown to double the short-term success figures for those who use them. The National Institute for Health and Clinical Excellence recommends that therapies should only be prescribed for a smoker who commit to a target stop date. Therapy to aid smoking cessation should be based on:

- Smoker's likely compliance
- Availability of counseling and support
- Previous experience of smoking cessation aids
- Medical contraindications and adverse effects of the products
- The smoker's preference
- Intention and motivation to stop.

The initial supply of therapy should be sufficient to last only two weeks after the target stop date. A second prescription should only be issued if the smoker has demonstrated a continuing attempt to stop.

Nicotine replacement therapy

Nicotine replacement therapy (NRT) is recommended for those patients smoking more than ten cigarettes a day. It has been shown to increase the chances of success for smokers trying to quit. NRT minimizes many of the withdrawal symptoms experienced, and increases the likelihood of abstinence. NRT gives smokers the chance to break their addiction to nicotine by gradually reducing the nicotine levels in the body.

NRT is available on prescription. This is important for patients on a low income who may not be able to afford to buy it. It is also available over the counter from pharmacies and supermarkets.

NRT is available in a range of preparations, including:
- Transdermal nicotine patches
- Inhalators
- Nasal spray
- Sublingual tablets
- Lozenges
- Chewing gum.

Table 25.2 illustrates the appropriate form of NRT according to smoking habit. Patients should not smoke while receiving NRT.

Adverse effects associated with NRT
- Nausea
- Dizziness
- Headache
- Gastrointestinal disturbances
- Blood pressure changes
- Mouth ulcers (inhalator, gum, sublingual tablets)
- Skin reactions (patches)
- Nasal irritation (nasal spray, inhalator).

Cautions
- Severe or unstable cardiovascular disease (severe arrhythmias, recent myocardial infarction, recent cerebrovascular accident)
- Uncontrolled hyperthyroidism
- Diabetes mellitus (monitor blood sugars closely).

Patients for whom NRT is contraindicated may be at particular risk from the adverse effects of smoking, so the risks and benefits should be considered carefully in each individual case.

Table 25.2 NRT and smoking habit

Preparation	Smoking habit	Strength	Comments
Inhalator		10mg	• Inhale when urge to smoke occurs • Initially use between 6–12 cartridges daily for up to 8 weeks • Reduce number of cartridges by half over next 2 weeks then stop
Chewing gum	<20 cigarettes/day >20 cigarettes/day	2 mg 4 mg	• Initially chew one piece for 30 min when urge to smoke occurs • Withdraw gradually over 3 months • Sugar-free, mint, and liquorice flavours available
Patch*	>10 cigarettes/ day <10 cigarettes/day	15–21 mg 10–14 mg	• High-strength patch for 6 weeks then reduce to medium strength for 2 weeks • Medium strength patch for 6 weeks then reduce to low strength for 2 weeks
Lozenge	>30 cigarettes/day <30 cigarettes/ day	2 mg 1 mg	• Suck one lozenge every 1–2 hours when urge to smoke occurs • Maximum 30 mg daily • Withdraw gradually after three months
Sublingual tablets	<20 cigarettes/day >20 cigarettes/day	2 mg 4 mg	• Place one tablet under the tongue every hour • Maximum dose 80 mg/day
Nasal spray		500 mcg/ metered spray	• One spray into each nostril • Max. 64 sprays/day

* These dosages are a guide, consult product literature.

Non-nicotine-based pharmacotherapy

There are two other therapies available to help smokers quit in addition to NRT: these are buproprion and varenicline. They are only available on prescription and they are recommended for use alongside motivational support.

Buproprion

Buproprion was initially developed as an antidepressant drug. It is not fully understood how it works as far as being an adjunct to smoking cessation, but it is believed to modify dopamine levels and noradrenergic activity. This reduces the cravings and the withdrawal symptoms associated with quitting smoking.

Dosage

An agreed quit date is set at about 10–17 days into the course of treatment and the smoker can continue to smoke until then. One buproprion 150 mg tablet is taken for 6 days, then one twice daily, at least 8 h apart, for the remainder of the 2-month course. The smoker stops smoking on the designated quit date but continues to take the buproprion for the full eight weeks.

Adverse effects of buproprion

Buproprion is generally well tolerated and any adverse effects are usually mild; they normally stop when the treatment is stopped. Adverse effects include:

- Insomnia
- Dry mouth
- Headache
- Agitation
- Generalized rash.

Contraindications/cautions include:

- Current or past seizures
- Current or past eating disorders
- History of bipolar disorder (manic depression, psychosis)
- Severe hepatic cirrhosis
- Brain tumour
- Patient undergoing withdrawal from alcohol or benzodiazepines.

Interactions

Buproprion should be administered with extreme caution to patients receiving other medication known to lower the seizure threshold. It can interact with antidepressants, antiepileptics and antivirals.

Varenicline

Varenicline is a new drug developed specifically for smoking cessation. It has been available in the UK on prescription from December 2006 and has a different mode of action to buproprion. It is a nicotinic acetylcholine receptor partial agonist, and is thought to work by reducing the strength of the smokers' urge to smoke, and relieving withdrawal symptoms. If a patient smokes a cigarette while using varenicline, it can diminish the sense of satisfaction associated with smoking.

Dosage

Treatment with varenicline starts one week before the quit date. During this week the dose is titrated until it reaches the treatment dose of 1 mg twice daily which is continued for 11 weeks, ie. total treatment course of 12 weeks.

If the patient has stopped smoking at the end of the 12 weeks but is not confident of remaining abstinent, the clinician can consider whether a further 12-week course is justified.

Adverse effects of varenicline

The main adverse effect is nausea; patients should be advised to drink plenty of water when taking the tablet. A few patients have reported insomnia and disturbed dreams, and these patients should be advised to take the second pill with their evening meal rather than at bedtime. No serious side-effects have been found. As Varenicline is a new drug, patients should be encouraged to report any adverse effects.

Contraindications/cautions

Varenicline has been licensed for all patients over the age of 18 except those with severe renal impairment or pregnant or breastfeeding women. As varenicline has not been tested on patients with psychiatric illness, it should be used with caution.

Interactions

There are no known interactions with varenicline.

Smoking cessation services

Smoking cessation services provide locally focused support for smokers who want to quit. Registered smoking cessation advisors offer group and individual support depending on local policies and patient preference.

Most advisors are practice nurses or pharmacists who have been specially trained in the role.

Smoking cessation services are now offered by most primary care trusts (PCTs), these offer support to smokers who can self-refer or who are referred by other health professionals. Many services also run clinics in GP surgeries, work places, acute hospital trusts, and in community settings.

The role of the nurse in smoking cessation

Nurses have a key role to play in influencing the health of patients. Regardless of where the nurse is based, they are ideally placed to encourage patients to stop. Even the most basic intervention by a nurse can have a profound effect; either encouraging a smoker to stop or to seek help in stopping.

Nurses should be given sufficient theoretical and practical training to enable them to offer opportunistic advice, encourage cessation, and offer advice on pharmacological treatments.

Practice nurses are ideally positioned to provide advice on quitting whenever they see a patient who smokes. As the recording of smoking status is an essential part of the quality indicators of the General Medical Service (GMS) contract, there are now even stronger reasons for proactively raising the issue of smoking cessation in the primary care setting.

It is highly recommended that nurses in secondary care settings should be part of systems that record the smoking status of outpatients and inpatients, and ensure that these records are kept up to date. This will enable suitable advice to be offered to patients. Many hospitals now offer local smoking cessation services, and these should be made available to inpatients: advisers should offer cessation counselling to inpatients.

Many nurses smoke themselves, and they may feel uncomfortable or hypocritical talking about smoking with a patient. However, it is vital to view smoking cessation information as professional advice and to treat the subject non-judgementally. Nurses who smoke will be familiar with a smokers' life experience and are well placed to be able to advise on the NHS smoking cessation services and treatments available.

Exploring motivation and confidence

Asking the following questions can promote a discussion and move the client on to the action stage—planning to stop. (0 is not motivated, 10 is very motivated)

- On a scale of 0–10 how motivated are you to give up smoking?
- What brings you to this point?
- What needs to happen to make you more motivated?
- What needs to happen to make it seem more important?
- How confident are you that you could give up smoking?
- What needs to happen for you to choose a higher number?
- How do you feel about your smoking?
- Do you have any concerns?
- How ready do you feel to stop smoking?

A contented smoker should not be pushed or nagged into stopping, but they should know that if they change their mind they will be offered support to quit.

Further information

http://www.doh.gov.uk/smoking
http://www.ash.org.uk

Smoking cessation support

A good approach is the 'four As' recommended by the Royal College of Nursing in 2001:[1]

- Ask patients about their smoking status and assess their motivation to stop
- Advise patients on the benefits of stopping
- Assist patients in stopping by helping them to plan and prepare for it
- Arrange for them to use professional help and advice from the smoking cessation service.

If the nurse feels that the patient is ready to change, they should be referred to the appropriate smoking cessation service. The offer of one-to-one support may be more suitable for some, while others may gain greater benefit from group sessions.

Group sessions

Group sessions are usually facilitated by a trained smoking cessation advisor but are very interactive. Practical sessions on how to stop smoking and advice from smokers attending the group can help smokers maintain interest and be rewarding for the participants and the nurse involved.

The effectiveness of a group session depends on two factors: the skill and enthusiasm of the nurse or facilitator, as well as the commitment of the attendees. For a nurse working in a small practice it may take some time to gather enough patients to start a group, and it is inevitable that some will drop out. Small numbers may make group dynamics difficult, and may affect the cohesiveness of the group.

The group approach to smoking cessation is cost-effective, as a number of patients can be helped in far less time than it would take in individual consultations. Other advantages to the group approach are:

- A sense of belonging and being valued
- A discovery that problems are not unique
- A feeling of satisfaction and motivation—the patient can be of help to others in the group
- The benefits of hearing the experiences of other group members.

Transport to the location of the group setting may be a problem for some patients, and those who work irregular hours are not always able to make the same time each week. Others may find attending a group daunting, and this may create a barrier to their quit attempt. Some patients with severe disease may be too unwell to travel to the group setting and one-to-one support may be the best choice.

One to one support

Group interventions are not always appropriate for a variety of reasons and individual support may be a patient's preference. Individual support should cover the same ground as group support, but is obviously much less time-effective for the nurse.

Relapsing

Even though there are many ways to help a smoker to quit, individuals may have to make several attempts before they eventually succeed. It may take months or years for a smoker to achieve their goal. It is not only nicotine addiction that causes the smoker to relapse, but also other factors such as stress or depression.

Many quitters relapse in the first month. The brain has to become used to the absence of nicotine surges and the smoker has to learn how to cope with external stimuli such as drinking alcohol, socializing, emotional upsets, stress, or boredom. Before quitting, many smokers associated these stimuli with a cigarette.

As part of smoking cessation support, the nurse should help the quitter identify their particular triggers to smoking and help them identify risky situations and how to cope with them. If the smoker does relapse, the nurse should reassure the patient that a previous failure does not mean it is not worth trying again. They should be reminded that relapse is common and that the next attempt will be easier and more likely to be successful.

1. Royal College of Nurses. 2001. *Clearing the air 2. Smoking and tobacco control—an updated guide for nurses* RCN London.

Respiratory health surveillance in the workplace

Health surveillance is about putting a systematic and appropriate procedure in place to detect early signs of work-related ill health among employees exposed to certain health risks. It is appropriate for all employees significantly exposed to respiratory sensitizers.

Respiratory sensitizers are substances that have the potential to cause a sensitization (allergy) such as rhinitis and occupational asthma (📖 p.147). In workplaces where there is a risk of exposure to airborne allergens, respiratory health surveillance is vital.

Health surveillance can take many forms:
- Self-assessment
- A responsible person making basic checks for signs of disease
- Clinical/psychological assessments of individuals by a specialist that involves a screening process.

Types of health surveillance

Health surveillance can be planned according to known hazard and risk, and to any statutory imperatives; or unplannned.

Unplanned health surveillance

This can be as a result of:
- Employees reporting symptoms of concern
- Employers becoming aware of symptoms of concern, either through individual reports or through monitoring of medical certificates
- Potential risk or exposure situation.

Planned surveillance

Respiratory surveillance must comply with statutory requirements. In the UK the main applicable regulation is the Control of Substances Hazardous to Health (COSHH).[2] To comply with COSHH the employer needs to:
- Assess the risks to health arising from work with respiratory sensitizers
- Decide what precautions should be taken to prevent or control the risk
- Ensure control measures are used and maintained properly
- Monitor work exposure
- Provide health surveillance as appropriate
- Inform, instruct and train workers about the risks and precautions needed.

Awareness

Before providing respiratory health surveillance, individual employees should be made aware of the reason for and nature of the surveillance. They should also be made aware that:
- Statutory health records will be kept for 40 years
- Access to their own health record is available under the Data Protection Act
- Feedback will be given to employees and employers if the surveillance results indicate a requirement for further assessment of them or their work.

As a result of health surveillance, modifications to the workplace or to the job may need to be made. Properly informed staff must comply with this legal requirement, or cease working in that environment.

Respiratory health assessment

Those who work with respiratory sensitizers are required to undergo a respiratory health assessment unless their risk of exposure is extremely low. This will be determined by a risk assessment carried out in accordance with the COSHH regulations.

The health assessment is usually carried out by an occupational health nurse or doctor. A typical baseline assessment may involve:

- Completion of a questionnaire to assess health history and the presence of any respiratory symptoms
- An assessment of lung function (spirometry)
- A physical examination
- Educating the employee to report any new respiratory symptoms which may indicate sensitization.

The health assessment should be carried out before any exposure or potential exposure occurs and should be repeated annually. Occasionally, where there is a higher level of risk, additional surveillance should be carried out 6 weeks and 6 months after initial exposure or potential exposure, as this is the riskiest time for development of sensitization. Additional surveillance should also be arranged if there is an unexpected increase in exposure, for example following an incident.

2. http://www.hse.gov.uk/coshh

Housing and respiratory health

The quality and nature of housing has an important impact on health. When considering mortality rates, housing tenure (owner-occupier or rented accommodation) has largely been accepted as a useful indication of several dimensions of an individual family's social class. Owner-occupiers have been shown to have a lower mortality rate than council or other tenants.

Poor housing can lead to a number of respiratory conditions, and there are a range of housing-related factors which impact on health. These include the following:

Damp

Dampness is associated with a higher prevalence of poor health. One of the ways that damp housing poses a risk to health is through the effects of house dust mites and moulds. Allergic reactions and infections develop with repeated exposure: children, older people and those with existing illnesses are most at risk. House dust mites and airborne mould spores can cause or exacerbate respiratory conditions such as asthma as well as other symptoms such as wheeze. Children who sleep in damp homes are twice as likely to suffer from wheezing and coughs than those who sleep in dry homes.

Cold homes

Many homes have inefficient heating systems; so the presence of a central heating system does not necessarily mean a warm home. Issues of affordability and fuel efficiency are important when considering the health implications of cold housing. Those experiencing fuel poverty, defined as needing to spend over 10% of their income on energy to maintain an adequate standard of warmth, are likely to be particularly vulnerable. The ability to keep the home warm enough in winter, and the worry associated with such concern, has been shown to be associated with poor health outcomes. Colder temperatures in winter are also linked to excess winter deaths. The biggest cause of these winter deaths is cardiovascular and respiratory conditions, such as pneumonia, particularly for older age groups.

Overcrowding

The health risks of overcrowded housing were recognized as long ago as the nineteenth century when such conditions were associated with the spread of infectious diseases such as tuberculosis, and led to an extensive slum clearance programme. Overcrowding is still recognized as a risk to health and has been associated with the spread of infectious diseases and asthma.

Homelessness

Those living on the street are especially vulnerable to many respiratory disorders, amongst them tuberculosis and pneumonia

Nursing homes

Pneumonia can be transmitted quite rapidly amongst residents of nursing homes because of the close proximity of residents. The elderly are at risk, and prophylaxis in the form of vaccination against influenza and pneumonia is recommended.

Prisons

The respiratory health of the prison population is unknown, but is likely to reflect the prevalence in the wider community although it is possible that there is under-diagnosis, resulting in under-treatment.

Indoor pollutants

Domestic indoor air pollution poses a risk to health. The greatest risk is associated with hydrothermal conditions (humidity and temperature), radon, house dust mites, environmental tobacco smoke, carbon monoxide and biomass fuels used for cooking purposes.

Air pollutants tend to be most detrimental to asthmatics and older people. Increased levels of domestic allergens have been linked to the increased risk of asthma in children: exposure to such allergens may trigger asthma attacks.

Asbestos

The inhalation of asbestos fibres causes two main kinds of cancer: mesothelioma and lung cancer. It can also cause asbestosis, diffuse pleural thickening and benign asbestos pleural plaques.

There are many sources of asbestos which may contribute to non-occupational exposures and many asbestos materials are present in homes. The risk of exposure will be related to the release of asbestos fibres, for instance during home renovations or repairs, or when building surface materials have been damaged or have deteriorated. The link between exposure to non-occupational sources of asbestos and lung diseases highlights the importance of using asbestos free materials in the home.

Environment and pollution

Environmental pollutants are chemical substances of human origin found in air, water, soil, food, or the home environment. Air pollutants are the main environmental cause of respiratory disease; globally they are responsible for high incidences of lower respiratory tract infections and COPD.

The extent to which environmental pollutants contribute to respiratory disease is unclear. Attempts have been made to estimate the environmentally attributable burden of disease globally, focusing on health outcomes for which there is strong evidence of an association with pollutants.

Air pollution

Air quality in the UK has improved since the urban smogs of the 1950s, caused mainly by the burning of coal. This is because of the Clean Air Act and subsequent environmental health legislation.

However, the nature of air pollution has changed: some pollutants have decreased, others have increased.

The main cause of air pollution today is vehicle exhaust emissions. Both nitrogen dioxide and particulates are related to acute and long-term respiratory health problems. Weather conditions can exacerbate the pollution problem by trapping polluted air at ground level, and preventing the air rising and dispersing into the atmosphere. Trees, particularly along roadsides, help to clean the air by absorbing pollution and filtering dust. The wide-scale burning of fossil fuels for heating, machinery, and equipment used in businesses and households, also release pollutants into the air. This contributes significantly to global air pollution and climate change in particular.

Air pollution may have a long-term effect on a child's lung function. It is believed that air pollution may reduce lung development in children from 10 to 18 years old. Lung development is usually complete at 18, and therefore unlikely to recover. Asthma is thought to be aggravated by airborne pollutants such as diesel particulates. It is not known whether there is a causal association between the prevalence and incidence of asthma and air pollution in general, but it is believed that there is an association between asthma and living in close proximity to traffic. The respiratory health of children, especially those with asthma, will benefit substantially from a reduction in air pollution, especially from motor vehicle exhausts.

Table 25.3 Health and environmental effects of air pollution

Pollutant	Source	Health and environmental effects
Sulphur dioxide	Burning of coal and oil	Reacts with water in the atmosphere to form sulphuric rain (acid rain). Can irritate the respiratory system
Nitrogen dioxide and nitrogen oxide	Burning of fuels	At high concentrations, nitrogen oxide produces inflammation of the airways
Carbon monoxide	Vehicle exhausts	Can prevent the blood taking up oxygen from the lungs
Particulates	Diesel vehicle exhausts, industry	Can penetrate deep into the lungs and cause respiratory symptoms, asthma and excess deaths in people with existing lung and disease
Lead	Vehicle exhausts, industry	Less lead in air now due to lead-free petrol. Can affect the nervous system
Ozone	Secondary pollutant	Irritates respiratory system
Benzene	Petrol car exhausts, petrol stations, industry	Carcinogenic at very high levels

Income and respiratory disease

A person's level of income has been found to be correlated with a wide range of health indicators; many of the measures that are used to look at social disadvantage are proxies for income.

People that cause the most concern are those on the lowest incomes and living in poverty. Poverty is generally regarded as the most important determinant of health, and also one of the most difficult areas in which to achieve change. Levels of disposable income affect the way patients live, the quality of their home and work environment, and the ability of parents to provide the kind of care for their children they would want. Some of the most obvious effects of health inequality are seen in:

- Premature mortality and morbidity—strongly related to indicators of low income. There is evidence that this gap in health between the most and least well-off is increasing
- Infant mortality rates—tend to be higher in the more deprived communities. Figures include stillbirths, neonatal deaths and infant mortality
- Low birthweight—inappropriate nourishment or smoking can reduce infant and pre-natal development. Slow early growth is associated with a range of respiratory health problems in later life
- Mental health problems—stress and depression reduce a patients' ability to cope with diseases such as COPD and TB
- Health-related behaviours—smoking, poor diet and lack of exercise may be more common in lower income social groups. Increasing the opportunities for healthier lifestyles is one way to achieve significant long-term health gains
- Emergency admissions to hospital—these are higher in patients with COPD who are on a low income
- Communicable diseases such as TB tend to be higher amongst families in poor-quality housing.

Social inequalities

Social inequalities cause a higher proportion of deaths in respiratory disease than any other disease area:

- Almost a half of all deaths (44%) are associated with social class inequalities compared with 28% of deaths from ischaemic heart disease
- Men aged 20–64 employed in unskilled manual occupations are around 14 times more likely to die from COPD and 9 times more likely to die from tuberculosis than men employed in professional roles.

Nutrition in respiratory disease 1

Patients with respiratory disease have many problems that affect their ability to maintain a healthy diet. These may include:

Breathlessness

A breathless patient may find that the effort of chewing and swallowing reduces the amount of food they eat, and the enjoyment they get from eating. Eating small, regular meals may help and using their bronchodilator inhaler (p.391) prior to eating may help.

Oxygen therapy

Wearing an oxygen mask can make eating and drinking difficult. This can be overcome by using a nasal cannula to deliver the oxygen (p.359). This allows the patient to receive oxygen and eat and drink at the same time.

Oral problems

There are several factors that can cause oral problems, all of which can make eating difficult. These include:
- Patients who are breathless, who are receiving oxygen therapy, or who are using anticholinergic drugs, have an increased risk of a dry mouth
- Patients on high-dose inhaled corticosteroids may develop oral candidiasis leading to a sore mouth and throat
- Patients who have lost a lot of weight may have ill-fitting, loose dentures.

Good oral hygiene, plenty of fluids and regular dental care can help individuals maintain an adequate diet.

Posture

It is important that the patient is in a suitable position to be able to eat and drink. A physiotherapist or an occupational therapist (OT) can offer help and advice on positioning, aids and appliances to enable a patient to eat and drink in comfort.

Mobility

Poor mobility can affect a patient's ability to shop, prepare and cook a meal. The nurse or physiotherapist can give the patient information and advice on energy conservation (p.330) which can help the patient to cope. Social services may also be able to help with shopping and meal preparation.

Economic factors

Many patients with respiratory disease come from a lower socio-economic group. Lack of money can prevent them from accessing good-quality food, either because of lack of affordable transport or because of the high cost of fresh food.

Malnutrition

Many patients with chronic lung disease are malnourished. This is common in patients with COPD, tuberculosis, cystic fibrosis, and lung cancer. The malnutrition in these patients can be progressive, leading rapidly to a cachexia-like syndrome.

Malnutrition is clinically significant. This is especially so in patients with COPD, where it is has been shown to be a predictor of mortality: individuals who have lost weight have a higher morbidity and mortality rate than those whose weight is within predicted values.

Malnutrition can:
- Affect the composition and function of respiratory muscles
- Impair skeletal muscle function
- Increase impairment and disability by affecting exercise performance.

Respiratory patients may also experience an increase in calorie expenditure. This can be caused by:
- Increased work and an increase in the energy cost of breathing
- Increased energy cost of physical activity
- Systemic inflammation or infection
- Metabolic effects of medication.

The body mass index (BMI) is a useful method of identifying patients who are underweight ([] p.75). A BMI of <20 or a weight loss of 5% in the preceding 6 months are indicators of a poor and deteriorating nutritional status.

Management of malnutrition

Identification of a malnourished patient is the first step towards appropriate management of nutritional problems. Identification involves measuring a patient's BMI and asking them about any history of weight loss. A range of interventions have been studied and these show that:
- Nutritional supplements given in an unsupervised form produce little improvement in body weight. This is because patients take the supplements instead of eating their meals
- Nutritional supplements given in combination with an anabolic stimulus such as exercise, together with education on dietary interventions are more successful.

Nutrition in respiratory disease 2

Obesity

Obesity is classified as a BMI >30. People who are obese are more likely to develop:

- Obstructive sleep apnoea
- Hypoventilation of obesity syndrome (Pickwickian syndrome).

Obesity is a problem for some respiratory patients. It may be aggravated by intercurrent disease such as diabetes or by corticosteroid therapies. It may also be caused by lack of mobility due to breathlessness.

Many respiratory patients who smoke are encouraged to stop. Stopping smoking brings about a decrease in the rate of energy expenditure and an increase in food intake, which are associated with weight gain.

What may be only a minor degree of obesity in a normal patient will increase the work of breathing in a respiratory patient causing greater levels of exertional breathlessness. Obesity also results in reduced exercise capacity and activity levels with a resultant increase in symptoms.

Management of obesity

A weight-reducing diet is required ideally in combination with an exercise programme (📖 p.531), however significant weight reduction in respiratory patients is often difficult to achieve. Patients have to agree a common goal for weight reduction and be motivated. Attending a slimming club may offer peer support.

Nutritional support for respiratory patients

- Assessment
- Access to a respiratory dietician
- Education
- Practical advice on dietary supplements or weight-reducing diets
- Occupational therapy referral for kitchen adaptations
- Goal setting in conjunction with the patient
- Review of respiratory medication.

Sex, sexuality and breathlessness

Introduction

Sex and sexuality are an integral part of human relationships. A discussion of these issues should be an important part of a holistic patient assessment, but the subject is often avoided by healthcare professionals.

Patients with a variety of respiratory conditions may require advice and support on sexual matters. This can range from infertility issues for male patients with cystic fibrosis, contraceptive issues for patients on anti-tuberculosis medication, and a range of problems for other patients experiencing symptoms and adapting to their disease processes.

The physical act of making love may be problematic for people with respiratory diseases; some may find it difficult to participate fully in what can be a strenuous activity. Apart from the actual sexual act what may be more important is sustaining a relationship in the face of illness.

Sexuality and chronic disease

People who are chronically ill are often regarded as non-sexual adults. They are subject to certain fixed views and beliefs; it is either assumed that they do not or cannot have sex, or that if they have a sex life it is dysfunctional and unsatisfying.

These views are often based on ageist stereotypes, because sex is associated with the young and physically attractive. Such stereotyping and misinformation may lead many professionals to adopt a negative or indifferent attitude towards sexual relationships in the chronically sick.

If it is accepted that sexual expression is a natural and important part of human life (Box 26.1), then denying sexuality and the sexual act for people with chronic disease denies them a basic right of expression.

> **Box 26.1 Sexual expression**
>
> | **Sex** = biology | **Sexuality** = the total person |
> |---|---|
> | Facts | Attitudes |
> | Male/female | Maleness/femaleness |
> | Genitalia | Personality |
> | Physical pleasure | Intimacy |
> | Doing | Being |
> | Self-orientated | Relational |
> | What we do | What we are |

Sex and respiratory symptoms

Breathlessness is perhaps the most common reason for the referral of respiratory patients, who have a variety of illnesses and disease processes. The experience of breathlessness can be extremely distressing and is often accompanied by panic and anxiety.

The spectrum of breathlessness ranges from slight to life-threatening, with symptoms from the trivial to the very severe. Breathlessness is a major symptom of lung disease, but there have been studies showing that this is not a major problem unless there is dyspnoea at rest. Therefore patients should be reassured that sexual activity is still possible with breathlessness as a symptom.

Patients with some respiratory disorders may be mouth breathers; they often have a dry mouth and can be embarrassed by kissing or close contact. Those producing sputum may not feel good about their oral hygiene, or may be embarrassed.

What is evident is that despite effective medical management and pulmonary rehabilitation, there is a group of patients who experience considerable handicap as a result of their respiratory disease. Chronic disease impacts on physical, psychological, social, and emotional functioning. As physical function decreases so does confidence, and this will have an effect on an individual's relationships and well-being.

Many patients are unable to distinguish between physical and psychological functioning, and the impact of their condition on their psychosexual functioning is rarely addressed by healthcare professionals.

Patients cannot change the lung disease that causes breathlessness, but they can reduce some of the overwork it can cause, for example by breathing exercises and breathing control. Patients should aim to reduce, where possible, the work of breathing and save energy. If they have only a limited amount of energy they can be encouraged to save it for the important things in life. This energy can then be used in whatever area of their life that they wish which may be for sexual activity.

Nursing care

The nursing role has expanded in recent years, but basic skills such as listening and seeing the patient not merely the illness can be just as important to a patient's well-being as advanced nursing practices.

Issues relating to sex and sexuality and sexual relationships are highly relevant to nursing practice, and nurses are uniquely placed to help individuals experiencing difficulties. They can offer patients appropriate information, help reduce their anxiety, and where appropriate, reassure them that sexual activity is not harmful.

If a patient makes a disclosure about a sexual issue, a nurse may be inclined to divert them by cracking a joke, or even pretending not to have heard. This can leave the individual feeling exposed, misunderstood, betrayed, angry or embarrassed.

As healthcare professionals it is our duty to acknowledge the sexuality of our patients. Comments such as 'not applicable' or 'has had hair done' or 'not menstruating' under the 'Sexuality' heading in a patient's care plan does little to offer the patient a truly holistic service.

Ethically, confidentiality is of paramount importance, and this should be made clear to the patient. Nurses should maintain professional boundaries at all times; they should be cautious about probing too deeply, exceeding their personal limitations and, as a consequence, distressing the patient (Box 26.2).

The difficulty in dealing with patients' sexual needs should not be underestimated; dealing comfortably with sexuality can require people to resolve complex cultural and emotional issues. The Royal College of Nursing accepts that providing support for patients' sexual health needs is part of nursing practice, and believes that nurses need better education about sexuality at all stages of training. The ways in which nurses can learn to be more adept at tackling sexual issues are listed in Box 26.3.

Sexual assessment

The purpose of a sexual assessment is to obtain physical, medical and psychological information in order to plan appropriate nursing care. The Royal College of Nursing suggests that nurses should also assess the patient's level of understanding of the body and how it works, along with their knowledge and awareness of their own sexuality and sexual health.

Whilst there are no formalized assessment tools in this area relevant to everyday practice, perhaps an easy way of assessing if a patient has concerns in this area is simply to state that you understand that illness can affect relationships and is everything alright? This is unthreatening and allows the patients to express any concerns they may have. If a patient feels there is an understanding they may disclose their worries or they may simply let the opportunity pass. Another opener is when discussing medication. Stating that many medications can cause problems with libido or may cause impotence again allows the patient to verbalize any concerns.

Caution is needed if embarrassment and offence are to be avoided. Permission must always be sought from the patient, before starting to discuss sexual matters. Most adults are quite willing to talk about sexual issues if the discussion is respectful, confidential and professional, and most patients feel it is appropriate for nurses to discuss sexual concerns with them.

Nurses are often reluctant to carry out a sexual assessment. Reasons identified for this avoidance include:
- Feeling that the patient's sexual history is not relevant
- Inadequate training
- Embarrassment
- Fear of offending.

Even an experienced nurse may be afraid of undertaking sexual assessment because of concerns such as:
- 'Will I make it worse? Will I open a can of worms?'
- 'How will I keep my own views and feelings out of it?'
- 'Do I really want to get mixed up in something so intimate?'
- 'How can I contain unpredictable feelings and issues?'
- 'What can I actually do about it?'

Box 26.2 Guidance on undertaking sexual assessments

Three cautions:
- Be aware of your own limitations
- Be sensitive to your role
- Know how far to go and when to ask for help.

Box 26.3 Useful tips

- Be open
- Be non-judgemental
- Give practical suggestions/advice
- Be prepared
- Be available
- Be responsive
- Introduce the subject of sex and sexuality
- Communicate acceptance
- Have educational materials
- Be sex positive, accept that sex and sexuality are an important part of some people's lives
- Use open-ended questions
- Do not categorize or stereotype
- Use comfortable terminology
- Be a good listener
- Encourage and support
- Be useful.

Sexual expression and the respiratory patient

Sexual intercourse is for many people an expression of human love, and one of the key factors in relationships. Clearly people with lung disease may find it difficult to participate fully in sexual relations. Some patients perceive kissing to be harmful, as they consider that it may hinder breathing. An individual whose illness causes acute episodes of breathlessness may be over-cautious about sexual activity. People with respiratory cancers, their partners or carers may be afraid of catching the disease or of passing it on.

In spite of some patients' anxiety about dying during sex, sudden death during intercourse is rare. Although breathing effort will be increased during sex, the ensuing increase in the breathing rate and shortness of breath is entirely normal. If such breathlessness can be tolerated, it should cause little concern.

If the concern is about stamina, many studies have shown that the energy used during sexual activity, including orgasm, is equivalent only to that expended by climbing a small flight (up to 14 steps) of stairs. This may be an impossibility for some patients, but achievable for many, especially if they go at their own pace.

It is not only shortness of breath that limits sexual activity. Low self-esteem and fear of failing to meet a partner's needs also play a part. The fears of the non-respiratory partner should also be considered. He or she may falsely believe that abstaining from sexual activity is in the patient's best interests, when quite the contrary may be true. Resuming intimacy and closeness with their partner can help to counteract the loneliness and isolation felt by a person who is diagnosed with a chronic disease.

Adverse effects of medication

Great strides have been made in developing medication to treat lung disease, but these same medications can have profound effects on libido and sexual performance.

Common therapies such as bronchodilators can intensify existing problems in some patients by causing nervousness and anxiety. Steroids can cause side-effects, such as weight gain, mood swings and depression, which may lessen the desire for sex. Other medications that can affect sexual activity are listed in Box 26.4.

Practical suggestions

Respiratory patients may need specific ideas for improving lovemaking, and the nurse can make several simple, practical suggestions. For example:

- Take adequate rests before sexual activity
- Practice a controlled cough in private before embarking on sexual activity
- Use your bronchodilator medication prior to any activity
- Use your normal amount of oxygen via a nasal cannula during any lovemaking
- Don't try to have sex after a heavy meal or after alcohol
- Keep the room temperature comfortable
- Have your partner assume a more active role if possible
- Avoid allergenic elements in the atmosphere such as perfumes
- Choose your sexual position carefully.

Advising the patient to avoid alcohol is important because alcohol may inhibit sexual arousal. A discussion of the normal ageing process can help dispel any myths or fears the older, chronically ill person may have.

Choosing a sexual position to limit energy expenditure can help to reduce effort during lovemaking, while maximizing pleasure. For the patient with lung disease it may be that their partner will need to take more of the weight or using pillows for support may help. One easy position is spooning. Masturbation either singly or mutually, and the use of sex aids may help patients to continue a varied and active sexual relationship, despite a diagnosis of respiratory disease. This may also be important if there is comorbidity, for example arthritis may further limit sexual positions.

Box 26.4

Impotence	**Decreased libido**
Diuretics	
Antihypertensives	Antihypertensives
Anticholinergics	
Antipsychotics	Antipsychotics
Antihistamines	Antihistamines
Antidepressants	Antidepressants
Sedatives	Sedatives
Alcohol/cigarettes	Alcohol

Points to remember

Sexual problems are common among those with long-term respiratory disease, and the way in which a person deals with sexual issues is an integral part of that person's personality and self-image.

Nurses, perhaps because of their own uncertainties, worries and anxieties, don't always make it easy for patients to talk about sexual problems. This is despite the fact that sexuality, sexual problems, and problem resolution are, at least in part, within the remit of nursing care.

Sexuality is an important health concern for all those with long-term respiratory disease; it should therefore be acknowledged in sensitive and responsive health practices. It is imperative that nurses allow patients the opportunity of open and genuine communication about sexual matters. In this way a foundation of acceptance for the whole person is established which is, of course, what nursing is all about.

In brief...

- Sex and sexuality are an integral part of a life
- Breathlessness is the major presenting complaint of patients with many respiratory diseases and most commonly of those with COPD
- Chronic disease can impact on patients emotional and psychological functioning and can ultimately affect their relationships
- Relationship problems are rarely addressed in caring for patients with respiratory disease
- Respiratory disease does not preclude the desire for an active sex life
- Discussions with patients about sexuality should when appropriate form part of a routine nursing assessment
- The skills that nurses need to offer simple sexual counselling interventions to respiratory patients are openness and good listening skills alongside an empathetic approach. Recognizing that there may be a problem can go a long way to solving it
- There are practical suggestions that can be made to help respiratory patients enjoy a fulfilling sex life. At the very least booklets addressing the issue may be made available.

The multidisciplinary team

Introduction

Respiratory services should be delivered in an integrated way, taking into account the overlap in patient population and in the personnel providing care. The majority of patients with respiratory disease are cared for by a team of health professionals from both primary and secondary care.

There is a considerable skill base in the primary healthcare community, as well as in secondary care. By providing all these skills within a multi-disciplinary team (MDT), patients will have the potential to receive a better quality of care, in a place more convenient to them, reducing the burden of disease on the patient, the health service, and society as a whole.

Respiratory nurses work as part of the MDT. This team includes doctors, ward-based and outpatient nurses, physiotherapists, occupational therapists, lung function technicians, community pharmacists, social services and, of course, the patient.

Role of the respiratory nurse specialist

Respiratory nurse specialists make an invaluable contribution to the services offered by respiratory units and to the quality of those services. Respiratory nurse specialists undertake many roles, including:

- Running asthma and COPD clinics
- Providing education for patients with asthma and COPD
- Liaising with GPs and nurses in the community
- Supervising the domiciliary nebulizer service
- Assisting in the assessment and monitoring of patients requiring long-term domiciliary oxygen.

In some units, respiratory nurse specialists have the primary role in supervising patients with COPD who are selected for hospital at home care, and in running the pulmonary rehabilitation service.

They may be employed full-time to supervise patients requiring domiciliary non-invasive ventilation (NIV) and continuous positive airway pressure (CPAP) for sleep-related breathing disorders.

In small units, respiratory nurse specialists may undertake many of these tasks together, whereas in large units one or more respiratory nurse specialists may be required for each service.

Tuberculosis nurse specialist

The tuberculosis (TB) nurse specialist is the interface for a fully integrated individualized patient-focused service for patients with TB. They ensure continuity of care to patients and carers, and help promote individual and public health. The TB nurse specialist is generally responsible for:

- Supporting and educating patients diagnosed with TB
- Detecting medication side-effects
- Supervising treatment to ensure it is taken correctly
- Following up patients discharged home either through home visits, follow-up clinics, or telephone helplines
- Screening close contacts of patients with infectious TB
- Organizing and conducting contact tracing
- Offering a BCG clinic for those at risk of TB
- Carrying out education, research and audit. (📖 p.507).

Lung cancer nurse specialist

Lung cancer nurse specialists provide an invaluable counselling service to patients and their relatives when a diagnosis of lung cancer is made. They also advise patients and other healthcare workers on the general management of symptoms caused by lung cancer.

They may visit patients at home, or they may liaise with other nurses who provide the domiciliary service. The role involves:

- Providing emotional and social support to patients and carers
- Providing continuity for patients
- Facilitating improved communication with patients and between healthcare teams
- Working across traditional and organizational boundaries to provide a seamless service
- Guiding patients through the system
- Education, research and audit. (📖 p.323).

Nurse bronchoscopist

The nurse bronchoscopist offers a nurse-led, standardized, patient-centred service. They ensure that patients receive a comprehensive plan of care when undergoing a bronchoscopy. The role involves:

- Explaining the risks, benefits and alternatives of the procedure and gaining informed consent from patients
- Administering sedation
- Writing formal reports, describing clearly the areas of the lung being investigated
- Taking biopsies to enable other members of the multidisciplinary team to make decisions about disease management
- Communicating results to patients.

Cystic fibrosis nurse specialist

The cystic fibrosis (CF) nurse specialist works with patients, their families and the staff that are involved in their care (📖 p.297). Once the diagnosis has been confirmed, the CF specialist nurse will give a full explanation of the condition, and provides individual clinical and psychological care for each patient and their family. The role includes:

- Advocacy for the patient and their family
- Decision-making and monitoring of care, ensuring that each patient receives optimum care for their individual needs
- Acting as a link between patient and family, community services and the hospital multidisciplinary team
- Advising and supporting patients and their families, and professional colleagues
- Educating the patient, families and carers on the disease process and the medication prescribed
- Research into aspects of CF
- Management of CF nursing teams
- Intravenous antibiotic prevention.

Other specialist roles

Other roles such as bronchiectasis nurse specialists and thoracic nurse specialists have been developed to work with specific patients. Many nurses work on specialist respiratory wards, managing patients with an acute exacerbation of their respiratory disease, and in outpatient respiratory clinics.

Role of the community nurse

The community respiratory nurse specialist takes a leading role in providing treatment, care and the management of individuals, groups and communities with respiratory disease. They can be employed either by an acute trust or by the primary care trust (PCT).

The community nurse usually liaises closely with chest and respiratory physicians, General Practitioner (GP), practice nurses and other health professionals. Their key role is to ensure a high level of intermediate care for all patients, children or adults, with respiratory disease.

Much of the care given by the community nurse is in the home. These specialist nurses have been shown to reduce hospital admissions and outpatient waiting lists through assessment, monitoring, education, and support of the patient and their carers.

Practice nurse/nurse practioner

Most GPs now employ practice nurses, and in many surgeries, a dedicated nurse may be responsible for the care of patients with asthma and COPD. This nurse may hold nurse-led clinics or work alongside the GP. It is also common for the nurse to see patients at general clinics. Many of these nurses are qualified as non-medical prescribers.

Community matrons

The community matron works as a member of an established integrated nursing team, managing patients with complex chronic disease in the community.

Community matrons are expected to:

- Work collaboratively with health professionals, carers and relatives to understand all aspects of the patients' physical, emotional, and social situation
- Teach patients, their carers and/or relatives to recognize subtle changes in the patient's condition that could lead to an acute deterioration in health
- Develop a personalized care plan with the patient, carers, and their relatives, based on a full assessment of medical, nursing, and social care needs, including contact numbers
- Monitor patients regularly, by home visits or telephone contact
- Ordering tests, or prescribing appropriate medication as required
- Maintain medical records, and inform other relevant health professionals about changes in the patient's condition
- Undertake a regular medicines usage review, including inhaler and nebulizer technique
- Liaise with other agencies, such as the fast response team, social services and/or the voluntary community sector, to mobilize resources as and when they are needed.

Hospital at home services

Many types of nurse-led service have been developed, including home-care teams, early supported discharge teams and acute respiratory assessment services. These services have been designed to prevent hospital admissions, or shorten the length of hospital stay.

Hospital at Home (HaH) is a service that enables patients with respiratory disease to be discharged from hospital as soon as possible. The patient is assessed in hospital by a member of the HaH team; and if appropriate they will be discharged for treatment at home.

Criteria for admission to HaH service

Local hospital and primary care trusts have their own protocols for the type of service offered, and the inclusion/exclusion criteria. The following would generally enable a patient to have the HaH service:

- Patient assessed as clinically stable
- Adequate family and social support
- Able to cope at home
- Normal blood pH (7.35–7.45) (📖 p.75)
- A stable blood pressure and pulse
- The patient, their doctor and family happy for discharge
- Be prescribed medication to treat their respiratory condition.

The following would generally exclude a patient from the HaH service:

- An impaired level of consciousness
- Acute confusion
- Blood pH <7.35
- Acute changes on chest X-ray (malignancy, pneumothorax)
- A concomitant medical problem requiring inpatient stay
- Insufficient social support
- No access to a telephone
- Patient's home geographically removed from HaH team.

The HaH team

The HaH team consists of health care professionals with expertise in respiratory disease, including nurses, physiotherapists, occupational therapists, and generic health workers. The patient will be visited at home, by one of the team, on a daily basis—or as required—to assess their progress, provide treatment, advice, and support. The patient will be provided with medication and any equipment they may need, such as a nebulizer. The patient will be given advice on:

- Medication
- Breathing techniques
- Relaxation
- Diet and nutrition
- Mobility.

The team has direct contact with the hospital respiratory consultants for any further specialist advice. Once the patient is feeling better (usually within 10 days) they will be discharged back to the care of their GP.

Advantages of HaH

- Patients are treated in their home environment
- Patients should get better rest in their own bed with fewer distractions
- Patients have a lower risk of hospital-acquired infections
- The team can make treatment more individual and practical
- The patient and their family or carers can work closely with the team and learn how to manage their lung disease and symptoms more effectively.

Role of the respiratory nurse consultant

The role of nurse consultant was proposed by Tony Blair at the 1998 Nurse Awards. It arose from a national consultation, intended to inform a new strategy for nursing, and responded to a broad consensus about the need to strengthen clinical leadership, and to improving career paths and opportunities.

The document *Making a Difference*,[1] launched in 1999 and the NHS Plan in 2000 set a target of 1000 nurse consultant posts by 2004.

A small but growing number of consultant nurses currently work in the respiratory field, either leading or developing nurse teams with the aim of raising standards of care across the interface.

Expert practice

The workload expectation for a consultant nurse is that 50% of the nurses' time will be spent in expert/clinical practice. It is sometimes difficult to determine what is meant by expert practice, but one interpretation is to keep the expert working clinically.

Once medical needs have been addressed and pulmonary rehabilitation undertaken, there may still be ongoing problems for many patients with respiratory disease. Nurses may play an important part in symptom control, preventing deterioration, preventing complications, palliation, and improved health status.

Professional leadership and service development

The present focus is on new ways of working and on the interface between primary and secondary care. The role of the consultant nurse allows the crossing of traditional barriers between primary and secondary care, working under the strictures of clinical governance and balancing patient need with service requirements. Many consultant nurses develop services for patients in areas where little was previously provided.

Training and education

The consultant nurse role requires a masters' level qualification, and the practitioner must continue to work towards a doctorate. It is envisaged that this will increase the body of nursing knowledge whilst improving the individual skills and knowledge.

The consultant nurse role also incorporates the teaching of others. This can be either formal or informal, and may involve affiliation to the local university or to a specialist centre.

Research and evaluation

Any new role has to be both clinically and cost-effective, the consultant role needs to be subject to both audit and evaluation. The evaluation of a role can be problematic if the service is a new development.

If no service has been provided previously for patients with chronic respiratory disease, then there are cost implications that may be difficult to quantify. The identification of unmet need is important but it often comes at a price.

Research also has a place within the role of the nurse consultant; they will often develop a body of research pertinent to their own areas of expertise that is likely to be both pragmatic and patient focused.

The role of consultant nurse or midwife can be developed in any speciality where it can be shown that they will provide better outcomes for patients by improving services and quality.

In respiratory disease both acute and chronic disease contribute to the disease burden. Many respiratory diseases are chronic in nature, although patients have acute episodes. The consultant nurse aims to address the situations and problems arising resulting from the disease process, and not just the problems arising from the medical diagnosis. Whilst early recognition and treatment of respiratory problems is fundamental to patient care, it is perhaps the burden of chronic disease that is most amenable to nursing intervention.

1. Department of Health (1999). *Making a difference.* http://www.doh.gov.uk

Role of the paediatric respiratory nurse

The prevalence of paediatric respiratory disease has increased in recent years. This has given nurses the opportunity to grow with the specialty and become a provider of high-quality care. Because of the increasingly complex diagnostic investigations now available, nurses must be educated and trained both in practical skills and in supporting parents and young people.

Respiratory disease can affect all ages, but advances in neonatal intensive care have resulted in a group of children who have persistent respiratory disease into early life. The incidence of asthma continues to rise, and can affect children of any age, and children with CF are increasingly surviving into adulthood.

Paediatric respiratory nurses work in a variety of hospital and community settings. An acutely ill child will require hospital care delivered by trained and experienced paediatric nurses, but the development of paediatric ambulatory care and community services means that inpatient stays are reduced to a minimum. Children are frequently nursed at home wherever possible, but they still need support and information if they are to get the best from community care.

Paediatric respiratory nurse specialists offer a comprehensive respiratory service for their patients. This includes:

- A nurse-led asthma clinic providing information and support for patients and carers
- Training and liaison with other professionals involved with the child
- Lung-function testing including body pleythsmography, spirometry and exercise testing (☐ p.75)
- Establishing protocols and guidelines to support good practice
- Skin-prick testing for allergen advice
- Home visits
- A resource for other health care professionals
- Multidisciplinary team working.

The ability to empower carers to manage their child's respiratory condition effectively is fundamental to specialist practice. This demands many different skills of the specialist nurse including:

- An ability to work autonomously but as part of a multidisciplinary team
- Management, teaching, communication and listening skills
- Time and ability to talk with the family is vital to establish their health beliefs and concerns.

Children and their parents often feel more comfortable talking to a nurse, who may be able to offer more time than medical colleagues. This allows the nurse to build up a rapport with the child and family. The nurse specialist often becomes the team member providing a consistent approach to the child's care, liaising with other professionals to promote best practice and continuity of care.

It is also important to recognize the limits of professional practice and to have a robust and supportive referral system for children who do not respond to treatment, or those who require further intervention.

Role of the pharmacist

Pharmacists specialize in drugs and medicine. They work in a variety of settings including hospitals, community pharmacies and in GP surgeries. Some pharmacists work for PCTs as advisors on medicine management.

Community pharmacist

Patients with chronic long-standing diseases, or their carers, usually see their community pharmacist more often than their GP, whether it is to simply collect a prescription or to seek advice.

Community pharmacists are ideally placed to identify individuals with respiratory disease or those with poorly managed disease. People may present at the pharmacy with laboured breathing and constantly purchase over the counter (OTC) cough medicines to treat their 'smokers cough' or who collect prescriptions for repeated courses of antibiotics; these individuals may have mild to moderate COPD. People diagnosed with chronic conditions that collect repeat prescriptions, but constantly complain that the treatment has little beneficial effect, can be advised to attend for a respiratory review.

Early identification of these individuals may facilitate appropriate disease management and lifestyle changes, such as smoking cessation and exercise, before the end stage of the illness when there is substantial disability.

Other key services offered by the pharmacist

Health education

Health education is an important factor in the outcome of many chronic respiratory diseases. A lack of understanding of their condition is likely to adversely affect disease management, and this may result in poorer quality of life for the individual concerned. Most community pharmacists are aware of the patient's family background and social circumstances and can use this knowledge to provide relevant personal care and information.

Health promotion

The role of the pharmacist is in helping to prevent chronic disease through health promotion. Pharmacists have been active in this area for many years, especially in smoking cessation. They are often the first port of call for those wishing to stop smoking, and have a key role in providing advice as well as providing nicotine replacement therapy.

Medication reviews

Through clinical medication reviews, pharmacists can identify problems that patients are having with their medicines, and help to resolve these before they become serious, preventing unnecessary hospital admissions.

The pharmacist can ensure that patients are receiving the appropriate level of pharmacological intervention for the severity of their disease and guarantee that the patient's medication is reviewed frequently.

The choice of inhaler device should be individualized to ensure its acceptability, and its effectiveness in practice. It is important to ensure that the patient is able to manipulate their device. People often require reinforcement of technique by repeated advice and encouragement. The community pharmacist can provide this support when the patient collects their inhaler device from the pharmacy.

Over the next few years, other new drugs may reach the UK. Pharmacists must work with their local GP practice or hospital to ensure that appropriate patients are prescribed these new therapies, outcomes are monitored, and patients are educated on how and when to use them.

Hospital respiratory pharmacist

Hospital pharmacists have a role in ensuring that patients are discharged on appropriate safe medicines, and that effective communication about an individual's medicines takes place with colleagues in nursing homes or primary care.

Some hospital pharmacists have disease-specific roles, and work extensively with respiratory patients. This involves:
- Monitoring of drug levels such as theophylline (📖 p.391)
- Checking sputum samples to investigate antibiotic sensitivity (📖 p.75)
- Optimizing and rationalizing all the patient's medication prior to discharge
- Checking concordance and the patient's understanding of their medication
- Ensuring that the patient can use the inhaler device prescribed
- Smoking cessation advice
- Advice on influenza and pneumococcal vaccinations
- Intravenous antibiotics, for example patients with CF or bronchiectasis
- Supporting early discharge or hospital at home schemes
- Advice and support to other members of the MDT.

Role of the respiratory physiotherapist

Physiotherapists bring advanced clinical reasoning and assessment skills to the care of respiratory patients, and have a solid background in physiology. Some physiotherapists have extended their assessment skills with techniques such as arterial or capillary earlobe blood gas sampling, and can request and review chest X-rays and/or sputum sample cultures. These build on existing assessments, including chest X-ray interpretation, simple spirometry, auscultation, and reviewing nutritional and functional status.

The work of a respiratory physiotherapist includes the following:

- Working as a member of the MDT, assessing and treating patients with respiratory disability (including complex cases), and maintaining accurate and comprehensive patient records
- Acting as a clinical lead for the respiratory physiotherapist service including critical care, acute medicine, and outpatients
- Working closely with the respiratory consultant in leading the development of the respiratory physiotherapy service
- Managing and organizing the specialist respiratory outpatient service, pulmonary rehabilitation and the on-call respiratory physiotherapy service
- Providing formal and informal ongoing training and education to physiotherapy staff, doctors, other healthcare professions, and students.

Physiotherapy techniques

Physiotherapy techniques may help by reducing the work of breathing, aiding mucociliary clearance, and increasing exercise capacity.

Reducing the work of breathing

The normal breathing pattern can be lost in the breathless patient, and the use of the accessory muscles of respiration increases the work of breathing.

Breathing control—patients are encouraged to relax their upper chest and shoulders, while breathing gently using their lower chest. This often helps to relieve breathlessness by reducing the work of breathing.

Positioning—positions that encourage the use of breathing control include:

- Sitting in a relaxed manner, leaning forward
- Lying on one side with the upper body propped up and supported by pillows
- Standing upright, leaning forward supporting the arms on a chair back or a banister, for example.

These positions alter the length tension status of the diaphragm and allow it to work more efficiently, allowing movement of the lower chest and abdomen.

Practising breathing control techniques may dramatically increase exercise capacity. Many people with chronic breathlessness hold their breath and rush what they are doing in order to complete their task. This limits any activity that they can achieve. By teaching the person to walk more slowly, to relax their shoulders and upper body, and to use breathing control, activities that would normally induce breathlessness may become achievable.

Mucociliary clearance

Physiotherapists use a number of techniques to help patients' clear excessive bronchial secretions. Excess secretions can lead to breathlessness and infection.

Postural drainage

Postural drainage is the use of gravity-assisted positions, often with the patient lying head down in a tipped position. Postural drainage combined with chest percussion and/or vibration can help to clear excessive secretions and enable the patient to breathe more easily again. The treatment is combined with techniques which encourage the patient to develop lung expansion and mobility of the thorax.

Humidification

Humidification may ease the removal of mucus when combined with physiotherapy, and can be given as steam inhalation or nebulized saline.

Active cycle of breathing technique (ACBT)

ACBT consists of controlled breathing, deep breathing (three or four relaxed deep breaths) followed by a 'huff'. A huff is a forced, but gentle, expiration with an open mouth that uses abdominal contraction to expel the air. The huff requires less effort than a cough.

Non-invasive positive pressure ventilation (NIPPV)

Many physiotherapists take the lead within an acute trust for the NIPPV service. As NIPPV improves ventilation it seems logical that physiotherapists will be involved in its administration. They have all the prerequisite skills and knowledge to administer and monitor NIPPV, and can teach other health professionals how to become competent (📖 p.494).

Pulmonary rehabilitation

The physiotherapist plays an important role in pulmonary rehabilitation (📖 p.531). This can take place either in the community or in secondary care. The main role of the physiotherapist is in reducing patients' fears of exercise and breathlessness.

Role of the respiratory occupational therapist

The role of the respiratory occupational therapist (OT) focuses upon enabling adaptations and promoting daily living. The OT plays an essential role in encouraging respiratory patients to take responsibility and ownership for their health. Through a combined approach of education and rehabilitation, they aim to help patients to manage their condition with the least distress and disruption to their daily life.

OT interventions

OTs provide patients with information and strategies on how to improve their functional ability, thereby limiting the impact of the disease on their life. They help patients develop coping strategies by:
- Balancing work, rest and play activities
- Using energy conservation methods
- Applying pulmonary rehabilitation strategies
- Using stress management techniques.

The OT assessment includes gathering information on how the patient and their family are managing with the disease at home. It covers three main areas.

Impact of the disease upon the patient's life
The OT will look at the extent to which daily life is affected by the respiratory disease. This part of the assessment will focus on:
- What specifically triggers any exacerbations
- How long an exacerbation generally lasts
- If there are any residual problems
- If the severity of symptoms varies throughout the day
- Which symptoms cause the most distress.

Coping strategies used
Most respiratory patients live with their disease for a long time, and many will have adapted their daily life accordingly. Patients will employ a mix of positive and negative coping strategies and the OT will ascertain what techniques the individual is using.

Assessment of occupational performance
The OT will assess how the respiratory disease affects the following:
- Work—what activities the patient undertakes, including self-care tasks
- Rest—when does the patient rest, including sleep patterns?
- Play—what does the patient enjoy doing socially? Are they involved in any leisure pursuits?

The OT gains a clear picture of how the disease affects the individual's daily life by performing a thorough assessment. The main areas examined are:
- Intensity of breathlessness
- Activity tolerance
- Fatigue
- Pain
- Recovery rates.

OT interventions

Energy conservation

Many respiratory patients experience chronic symptoms, which limit their physical tolerance to activity and their occupational performance. Many of the individuals affected are older people who have other problems associated with ageing, such as comorbidities and a reduced range of movement. For some of these people the effort to remain independent is outweighed by the physical cost.

The OT can help the patient to perform activities in a more efficient way.

Prioritization

The OT will help the patient make a list of occupational areas, including work, rest, and play. The list will be rated in order of importance to the patient.

Planning

Once activities have been prioritized, each activity is analysed to determine the actions needed to perform it and the physical cost of undertaking it. The OT will then suggest adaptive techniques, or the use of adaptive equipment to enable the patient to perform the tasks in a less energy-consuming, but efficient way.

Pacing

The OT will show the patient how to gain a balance between activity and rest. Pacing gives the body time to recover from physical and mental exertion. The inclusion of regular rest periods into the day can increase the level of activity achieved by many patients.

Coping with fear

Many patients find breathlessness frightening. Fear makes people avoid activity, and prevents them attending pulmonary rehabilitation, contributing to further deconditioning. The OT can help patients to recognize the fear-driven aspects of breathlessness, and their cause and effect relationship, in order to break the cycle of fear.

Some OTs use approaches such as cognitive behavioural therapy, neuro-linguistic programming, relaxation, and even hypnotherapy.

Role of the respiratory physician

Most respiratory physicians working in district general hospitals and teaching hospitals have a commitment to general medicine in addition to caring for patients with respiratory disease. This commitment varies from hospital to hospital, depending on local practices and staffing levels. Approximately one-third of all acute medical admissions have respiratory problems.

Inpatient work

The inpatient work of the majority of respiratory physicians predominantly involves the investigation and management of patients admitted acutely, but it also includes some patients admitted electively. Many units are able to offer a self-admission policy to patients with conditions such as CF, lung cancer or asthma.

Respiratory physicians undertake a considerable amount of referral work for patients under the care of other specialists in the hospital.

Respiratory physicians caring for patients with lung cancer attend weekly MDT meetings with oncologists, thoracic surgeons, pathologists, and radiologists. Some consultants have close links with the intensive therapy unit (ITU) and attend regular meetings. Consultants offering other specialist services such as transplantation assessment and follow up have close links with thoracic surgeons.

General medical clinics

Respiratory physicians working in district general hospitals may see new general medical referrals, and most see follow-up general medical patients following discharge from hospital.

Specialist investigative and therapeutic procedure services

Bronchoscopy

Most respiratory physicians perform bronchoscopies (📖 p.75). They are a diagnostic test performed to help the consultant confirm or rule out the cause of the patient's symptoms.

Sleep-related breathing disorders

This is a rapidly developing subspecialty. Many units are able to offer a basic overnight oximetry service even if they do not hold dedicated clinics. Some units now offer a comprehensive sleep service and hold dedicated clinics for patients with sleep-related breathing disorders, both for diagnosis and monitoring of patients receiving continuous positive pressure airway pressure (CPAP) treatment (📖 p.494). The provision of a comprehensive sleep service requires the provision of one to two sleep rooms and a funded supply of CPAP machines.

Domiciliary assisted ventilation service

This is provided by specialist centres and, increasingly, in large district general hospitals. With the introduction of domiciliary NIV for patients with COPD, plus the use of this therapy for patients with neuromuscular disorders, it is likely that the number of consultants offering this service will increase significantly.

Occupational lung diseases

Relatively few units have consultants who offer a comprehensive occupational lung disease investigation service.

Specialist services within the respiratory specialty

Lung cancer

Most respiratory physicians investigate and provide supportive care for patients with lung cancer. The lead lung cancer physician spends some of their time coordinating services such as chemotherapy.

NIV for acute respiratory failure

NIV is rapidly being established as a routine service in most hospitals. The service is largely provided by trained nursing staff and physiotherapists, but consultant supervision of this service is essential.

Role of the GP with a Specialist Interest (GPwSI)

General Practitioners with a special interest (GPwSIs) challenge traditional models of specialist care and are a key component of the UK National Health Service (NHS) modernization agenda.

The emphasis is on maintaining a family care perspective, while developing defined specialist competencies to meet local healthcare needs. This results in improved access and healthcare nearer the patient's home, as more patients are treated for specialist complaints without having to visit a consultant in hospital.

The role of the respiratory GPwSI is a relatively new one. Respiratory problems are the most common reason to visit a GP, and the role has evolved as part of a government initiative to reduce hospital admissions for patients with respiratory disease. The GPwSI will already be a competent and experienced generalist, and will have undertaken further accredited training in respiratory medicine.

Core activities of a GPwSI in respiratory medicine

The core activities of a GPwSI service will vary, depending upon local needs and resources. They are likely to focus on asthma and COPD, but may also cover allergies and respiratory tract infections.

The key role of a GPwSI in respiratory medicine is as a clinical lead within primary care organizations (PCO); providing clinical expertise along with the necessary leadership, negotiating and coordinating skills needed to develop an integrated respiratory service.

Clinical role

Patients are referred to the GPwSI by other practitioners within the PCO for advice on the diagnosis and clinical management of defined respiratory problems. The scope of such advice depends on the individual expertise of the GPwSI, on agreements made with local secondary care specialists, and should depend on locally negotiated agreements about clinical responsibility.

The GPwSI may also be involved in the development of specialized community-based services to manage respiratory disease. Examples could be:
- Pulmonary rehabilitation
- Home oxygen service
- Immunotherapy for allergic disease
- Intermediate care beds
- Palliative care.

The GPwSI will also be involved in:
- Monitoring of quality standards of care
- Benchmarking quality performance with other GPwSI providers and providing feedback to primary and intermediate care health professionals.

Education and liaison

The GPwSI will develop the competence and the confidence of professional colleagues, to enable an optimal service to patients with respiratory disease. This will involve:
- Liaison with other health professionals in the PCO
- Advising on cost-effective prescribing

- Giving advice on matters of respiratory medicine within the PCO, including commissioning
- Determining service provision in conjunction with PCO managers, secondary care providers, nurse specialists and expert patients, after an assessment of local needs
- Liaison with local patient groups, e.g. Breathe Easy groups, to provide advice on service needs and provision
- Advising on developing uniform disease registers in respiratory disease across the PCO
- Liaison with secondary healthcare providers to agree service levels and provide integrated care pathways for disease management, such as the management of acute exacerbation of COPD, asthma or pneumonia.

Role of the clinical respiratory physiologist

The role of the clinical respiratory physiologist is to support the respiratory team in the diagnosis and management of the patient's condition by providing accurate reproducible and reliable data on various aspects of a patient's lung function. They have a vital role in the diagnosis and management of a patient's respiratory condition, and help the respiratory physician to monitor, evaluate, and measure the patient's lung function.

The range of tests performed by clinical respiratory physiologists reflects the wide range of respiratory conditions that require an assessment of lung function. A clinical respiratory physiologist sees patients of all ages, with conditions that include:
• COPD
• Sarcoidosis
• Interstitial lung disease
• Cystic fibrosis
• Asthma
• Extrinsic allergic alveolitis
• Pre-operative screening
• Allergy testing
• Sleep breathing disorders.
They work with computers linked to sophisticated respiratory equipment. Measurements made typically include:
• Lung volumes and forced expiratory flows
• Respiratory gas exchange
• Response to treatment such as bronchodilators
• Breathing patterns and oxygen measurements during sleep
• Allergy testing
• Physiological responses to exercise.
The information obtained is used to assist in the diagnosis of disease, to identify treatment regimes, to measure the effects of treatment and to estimate the likely risks during surgery.

Depending on local PCT policies, some physiologists also perform more complex tests including:
- Bronchial challenge testing
- 6-minute walk tests
- Full cardiopulmonary exercise testing
- Respiratory muscle weakness assessment
- Fitness to fly assessment
- Long-term oxygen therapy assessment
- Arterial and capillary blood gases
- Domiciliary nebulizer assessment
- Hyperventilation studies.

These practitioners are responsible for the maintenance and calibration of all equipment, including therapeutic/diagnostic equipment issued for use in the patient's home.

Some clinical respiratory physiologists work in research centres. Their role may involve investigations to discover new information about disease, and work towards cures and improved treatments.

Further information

Association of Respiratory Technicians and Physiologists

Role of the 'expert patient'

One of the defining trends in modern healthcare is the growing interest of patients in their own well-being. With the spread of healthcare information via the Internet, the emergence of powerful patient advocacy groups, such as the British Lung Foundation, and a general awareness of healthy living, the patient has ceased to be simply a passive recipient of healthcare advice.

It is now well recognized that patients should be involved in decision-making about their treatment. This is particularly important where potentially harmful drugs may be used; for example in the treatment of lung cancer, but also in the use of oral steroids and other immunosuppressant drugs in respiratory disease. The involvement of the 'expert patient' is likely to be extremely helpful in the development of self-care and support for patients and families, where chronic respiratory conditions are a problem.

The role of the expert patient

The patient who has received education, training, and support will be better able to manage their respiratory disease. Asthma self-management plans, including written personalized action plans, have been shown to improve health outcomes for people with asthma. The evidence for self-management plans for patients with COPD is not conclusive, but the limited data does suggest that patients with a management plan use less health services and have less hospital admissions, resulting in lower costs for the NHS.

The expert patient can be a valuable teacher in nursing and medical training programmes. Patients with chronic respiratory conditions may be involved in:

- Giving feedback about interpersonal, communication, and physical examination skills
- Developing and enhancing the quality of teaching
- Patient narratives to capture the patient experience
- Curricula development in undergraduate and postgraduate education and training.

The expert patient can be involved in developing new services, such as the home oxygen service, developing guidelines and pathways, and in peer review processes.

The expert patients programme

Set up in 2002, the Expert Patients Programme (EPP) is a training programme providing opportunities for people who live with long-term chronic conditions such as COPD, to develop new skills to manage their condition better on a day-to-day basis.

The EPP is based on research over the last two decades, showing that people living with chronic illnesses are often in the best position to know what they need in managing their own condition. It aims to empower patients, showing that if they have the necessary self-management skills, they can make a tangible impact on their disease and quality of life.

Structure of the programme

EPP groups tend to have between 8–16 participants, with a mix of different long-term conditions. The group meet over six weekly sessions and are led through a structured course by trained tutors, who are also living with a long-term condition. Each session (lasting two-and-a-half hours) looks at ways to manage the effects of these chronic conditions, such as:

- Dealing with pain and extreme tiredness
- Coping with feelings of depression
- Relaxation techniques and exercise
- Healthy eating
- Communicating with family, friends and health professionals
- Planning for the future.

There is a strong emphasis on participants setting practical, achievable goals, which are monitored each week. Core skills such as problem-solving, decision-making, being resourceful and behavioural changes are also developed throughout the course. The EPP does not provide health information or treatment, nor does it look at clinical needs. The aim of the EPP is to give participants the confidence to take responsibility for their own health, while also encouraging them to work in partnership with health and social care professionals.

Support organizations 1

British Lung Foundation

The British Lung Foundation (BLF) provides support to patients and improve treatment and care for people affected by lung disease. The BLF helps people to understand their respiratory condition by providing information in the form of leaflets, a website, and in the form of a telephone helpline. The BLF is also involved in research and fundraising.

Breathe Easy groups

Breathe Easy is the BLF's nationwide support network. It provides a network of friends, advisers, events, and activities that support and empower people affected by lung disease.

Baby Breathe Easy

Baby Breathe Easy provides information, support and telephone advice to parents and carers who are looking after children with a lung condition. The helpline is manned by a paediatric respiratory nurse specialist.

Information and publications

BLF publications cover a range of lung conditions and related topics that respond to the needs of people affected by lung disease.

BLF nurses

BLF nurses aim to improve the health status of people with severe respiratory disease. They deliver this by providing a customized service of care that would otherwise be unobtainable.

The nurses provide information to people with lung disease and their carers, to help manage their disease better. They also share their expertise with other health professionals, through delivery of tailored training programmes.

Asthma UK

Asthma UK is a charity dedicated to improving the health and well-being of everyone whose life is affected by asthma. They work with people with asthma, health professionals and researchers to develop and share experiences, to help increase understanding and reduce the effect of asthma on peoples' lives.

Asthma UK has a range of services and activities including:
- A telephone advice line staffed by asthma nurse specialists
- Funding for research
- Health information leaflets
- Influencing government and policy
- An asthma magazine
- Organizing holidays for children with asthma.

British Thoracic Society

The British Thoracic Society (BTS) was formed in 1982. It is a registered charity and its membership includes doctors, nurses, scientists, and any professional with an interest in respiratory disease.

Its core objectives are:
- The relief of sickness of people with respiratory and associated disorders, by the promotion of the highest standards of clinical care
- Research into the causes, prevention and treatment of respiratory and associated disorders, and disseminating the results of such research
- The provision of information in matters concerning respiratory and associated disorders and how they might be prevented.

The key activities of the BTS include:
- Acting as a representative of respiratory medicine in the UK, raising the profile and understanding of respiratory disease
- Publishing scientific papers in respiratory disease and management
- Organizing regular scientific meetings
- Organizing medical education for respiratory practitioners
- Producing and disseminating guidelines on the treatment and management of a range of lung diseases
- Promoting clinical research, educational and organizational links between the Royal College of Physicians, Royal College of Nursing, and other representative bodies
- Advising on, and contributing to, the education of trainees in respiratory medicine
- Supporting professionals facing a changing health service by providing information, critical analysis and support.

Support organizations 2

Association of Respiratory Nurse Specialists

The Association of Respiratory Nurse Specialists (ARNS) evolved in 1997 as a specialty nursing forum for respiratory nurse specialists and is now affiliated with the BTS. Its purpose is:

- To provide a supportive network for this group of nurses
- To promote specialty practice through education and professional development
- To influence the direction of nursing and respiratory care
- It is the only group in the UK that caters specifically for respiratory nurse specialists and consultants in primary and secondary care. ARN's objectives are:
  - To provide a supportive network for ARNS members, to encourage information sharing, best practice and research collaboration
  - To develop opportunities to enable collaboration between primary and secondary care services and other agencies
  - To support and promote a quality seamless service for patients with respiratory disease and their carers. To initiate and drive forward innovatitive projects influencing practice to improve patient care
  - To cooperate and collaborate with other multidisciplinary respiratory specialist groups to influence improvements and developments in respiratory care
  - To participate in raising the standard of respiratory nursing and clinical effectiveness in conjunction with the relevant government policies
  - To support the role of the RNS, in an ever-changing political climate
  - To support and promote patient self care.

Royal College of Nurses Respiratory Forum

The Royal College of Nurses (RCN) Respiratory Forum provides support, advice and disseminates specialist knowledge as well as promoting respiratory nursing. They organize respiratory conferences and issue newsletters to their members.

General Practice Airways Group

The General Practice Airways Group (GPIAG) is an independent charity representing primary care health professionals interested in delivering the best standards of respiratory care. It is dedicated to achieving optimal respiratory care for all through:

- Representing primary care respiratory health needs at policy level
- Promoting best practice in primary care respiratory health through education, training and other services
- Supporting the development of primary care health professionals in respiratory medicine
- Facilitating and leading primary care respiratory research.

IMPRESS (IMProving and Integrating RESpiratory Services in the NHS)

IMPRESS is a collaboration between the BTS and GPIAG. Their aim is to drive high quality patient-centred care across the traditional boundaries of secondary and primary care, integrating and improving the services for people with respiratory disease.

Further information

http://www.lunguk.co.uk
http://www.asthma.org.uk
http://www.brit-thoracic.org.uk
http://www.arns.co.uk
http://www.brit-thoracic.org.uk/impress
http://www.gpiag.org

Flying, altitude and diving

Atmospheric pressure and altitude

Up to an altitude of approximately 30,000 feet, the composition of the gas in the air we breathe remains almost constant. Atmospheric pressure decreases exponentially with altitude. This means that although the gas composition at high altitude remains the same, the air is less dense, resulting in less available oxygen for gaseous exchange. Hypobaric hypoxia therefore develops as a result of low atmospheric atmosphere.

Altitude sickness

Altitude sickness can occur in some people as low as 8,000 feet, but serious symptoms do not usually occur until over 12,000 feet. Even then it is not the height that is important, but rather the speed at which the person ascends to that altitude.

It is difficult to determine who may be affected by altitude sickness as there are no specific factors such as age, sex, or physical condition that correlate with susceptibility. Most people can ascend to 2,500 metres (8,000 feet) with little or no effect. Acute mountain sickness (AMS) is more common in fit young men because they are more likely to attempt a rapid ascent up the mountain.

The causes of altitude sickness

The percentage of oxygen in the atmosphere at sea level is about 21% and the barometric pressure is around 760 mmHg. As altitude increases, the percentage remains the same but the number of oxygen molecules per breath is reduced. At 3,600 metres (12,000 feet) the barometric pressure is only about 480 mmHg, so there are roughly 40% fewer oxygen molecules per breath and the body must adjust to having less oxygen.

In addition, high altitude and lower air pressure causes fluid to leak from the capillaries in both the lungs and the brain, which can lead to fluid build-up. Continuing on to higher altitude without proper acclimatisation can lead to the potentially serious, even life-threatening altitude sickness.

Acclimatization

The main cause of altitude sickness is going too high too quickly. Given enough time, the body will adapt to the decrease in oxygen at a specific altitude. This process is known as acclimatization and generally takes 1–3 days at any given altitude.

Several changes take place in the body which enable it to cope with decreased oxygen:
- The depth of respiration increases
- The body produces more red blood cells to carry oxygen
- Pressure in pulmonary capillaries is increased, 'forcing' blood into parts of the lung which are not normally used when breathing at sea level.

Periodic breathing

Above 3,000 metres (10,000 feet) most people experience a periodic breathing during sleep known as Cheyne–Stokes respirations. The pattern begins with a few shallow breaths and increases to deep sighing respirations then falls off rapidly, even ceasing entirely for a few seconds, then the shallow breaths begin again. During the period when breathing stops, the person often becomes restless and may wake with a sudden feeling of suffocation. This can disturb sleeping patterns, exhausting the climber. This type of breathing is not considered abnormal at high altitudes.

Acute mountain sickness (AMS)

AMS is very common at high altitude. At over 3,000 metres (10,000 feet) 75% of people will have mild symptoms. The occurrence of AMS is dependent upon the elevation, the rate of ascent, and individual susceptibility. Many people will experience mild AMS during the acclimatization process. The symptoms usually start 12–24 hours after arrival at altitude and begin to decrease in severity around the third day.

Mild AMS

Mild AMS is due to hyperventilation provoked by the hypoxia. Symptoms include:
- Headache
- Nausea/vomiting and anorexia
- Numbness/tingling of extremities
- Fatigue/light-headedness
- Shortness of breath
- Disturbed sleep/insomnia
- Periodic ventilation during sleep
- General feeling of malaise.

Symptoms tend to be worse at night and when respiratory drive is decreased. Mild AMS does not interfere with normal activity and symptoms generally subside within 2–4 days as the body acclimatises. As long as symptoms are mild, ascent can continue at a moderate rate. Climbers should be advised to communicate any symptoms of illness immediately to others on their trip, as the symptoms may also indicate the early development of moderate or severe AMS.

Moderate AMS

The signs and symptoms of moderate AMS include:
- Severe headache that is not relieved by medication
- Nausea and vomiting, increasing weakness and fatigue
- Shortness of breath
- Decreased coordination (ataxia).

Normal activity is difficult, although the person may still be able to walk on their own. At this stage, only advanced medications or descent can reverse the problem. Descending only 300 metres (1,000 feet) will result in some improvement, and 24 h at the lower altitude will result in a significant improvement. The person should remain at lower altitude until all the symptoms have subsided, which may take up to 3 days. At this point, the person has become acclimatised to that altitude and can begin ascending again.

The best test for moderate AMS is to have the person walk a straight line heel to toe just like a sobriety test. A person with ataxia would be unable to walk a straight line. This is a clear indication that an immediate descent is required. It is important to get the person to descend before the ataxia reaches the point where they cannot walk on their own, as this would necessitate a stretcher evacuation.

Severe AMS

Severe AMS is due to the hypoxia itself. It can develop rapidly, and tends to occur more in those with a lower hypoxic drive. Severe AMS requires immediate descent of around 600 metres (2,000 feet) to a lower altitude.

Symptoms include:

• Shortness of breath at rest
• Inability to walk
• Decreasing mental status.

There are two serious conditions associated with severe altitude sickness; high altitude cerebral oedema (HACE) and high altitude pulmonary oedema (HAPE). Both of these happen less frequently, especially to those who are properly acclimatized. However, when they do occur, it is usually in people going too high too fast or going very high and staying there. In both cases the lack of oxygen results in leakage of fluid through the capillary walls into either the lungs or the brain. Both conditions are potentially fatal.

Management of AMS

The only cure for mountain sickness is either acclimatization or descent.

Preventative medications

Acetazolamide (Diamox): This is the most tried and tested drug for altitude sickness prevention and treatment. This drug does not mask the symptoms but actually treats the problem. It seems to works by increasing the amount of bicarbonate excreted in the urine, making the blood more acidic. Acidifying the blood drives the ventilation, which is the cornerstone of acclimatization. Temazepam has also been shown to reduce the periodic breathing at night, and does not appear to worsen the hypoxia.

A trial course is recommended before going to a remote location where a severe allergic reaction could prove difficult to treat if it occurred.

Mild AMS

Symptoms of mild AMS are likely to resolve spontaneously over a few days. Simple, symptomatic treatment, analgesics, and plenty of hydration is all that is usually required.

Moderate and severe AMS

The climber should have their inspired oxygen tension increased by rapid descent, extra inspired oxygen, or by using a portable hyperbaric chamber (such as a Gamow bag).

The Gamow bag is composed of a sealed chamber with a pump. The casualty is placed inside the bag and it is inflated by pumping it full of air, effectively increasing the concentration of oxygen and therefore simulating a descent to lower altitude.

The bag can quickly create an 'atmosphere' that corresponds to that at 900 to 1,500 metres (3,000 to 5,000 feet) lower. After two hours in the bag, the person's body chemistry will have 'reset' to the lower altitude. This acclimatization lasts for up to 12 h outside of the bag which should be enough time to get them down to a lower altitude and allow for further acclimatization.

Further information
http://www.high-altitude-medicine.com

Lung disease and flying 1

Air travel has become increasingly popular, offering a convenient form of transport for many. Given the ageing nature of Western populations, the age of air travellers is also likely to increase, with a greater risk of medical problems. Unfortunately, respiratory problems are a common cause of in-flight medical problems and emergencies, and the third most common reason for medical diversions.

Cabin pressurization

Although referred to as a pressurized cabin, an aeroplane cabin is pressurized only in relation to the outside air pressure, at a given flight altitude. This means that the partial pressure of oxygen in a pressurized aeroplane will be less than at sea level, on the ground, and this means less in-flight oxygen is available. In a healthy passenger, saturated oxygen (SaO_2) levels fall to between 85–91% (📖 p.75).

Cabin altitude is achieved by a pressurization system which draws air into the aircraft via the jet engines. The air is compressed, cooled and filtered by high-efficiency filters (HEF), and is then fed into the aircraft compartments. To maintain the cabin pressure, approximately 50% of the air is vented outside the aircraft, recycling the remaining 50% via the HEF. The HEFs remove almost 100% of the microbial load produced by passengers.

Passengers with impaired respiratory function may be especially susceptible to the ascent to the usual flight altitudes. This is particularly relevant to those passengers who are hypoxic at sea level.

Fitness to fly

Deciding on fitness to fly for those with pre-existing respiratory disease can be difficult. A combination of history, examination, pulmonary function tests and arterial blood gases may be needed in difficult cases, and when deciding on whether in-flight oxygen ought to be provided. People who are breathless at rest should not fly without oxygen.

A simple test that is often used to indicate sufficient respiratory reserve to cope with flying is the ability of a patient to walk 50 metres unaided at normal pace, or to ascend one flight of stairs. Many patients and doctors are poor at judging their distance walked in this context. It is wise to observe objectively the ability to walk this distance comfortably.

Anyone with an active exacerbation of respiratory disease would be wise to wait until their respiratory condition has improved before flying. In severe or complex cases it is often worth seeking the advice of a respiratory physician, and a formal pre-flight assessment performed.

Pre-flight assessment

Pre-flight assessments are performed in order to predict people who are at risk of developing complications. Currently there is little scientific evidence on which to base formal assessment guidelines. Recommendations have been produced by the British Thoracic Society (BTS),[1] which are based on expert opinion. The BTS recommend that the following groups should be assessed. Patients with:

- Severe COPD or asthma
- Severe restrictive lung disease, including chest wall and respiratory muscle disease
- Hypoxaemia and/or hypercapnia
- Cystic fibrosis
- History of air travel intolerance with respiratory symptoms (breathlessness, chest pain, confusion, syncope)
- Comorbidity with other conditions worsened by hypoxaemia (coronary artery disease, heart failure, cerebrovascular accident)
- Recent pneumothorax
- Risk of or previous venous thromboembolism
- Pre-existing requirement for oxygen or ventilator support
- Pulmonary tuberculosis.

Those patients with a sea-level SpO_2 of 92–95% and an additional risk factor should have a hypoxic challenge test. The patient breathes 15% FiO_2 (the equivalent to a cabin altitude of 8,000 feet) for 15 minutes, arterial or capillary bloods are then measured. The results are interpreted as follows:

- PaO_2 > 7.4kPa—oxygen not required
- PaO_2 6.6-7.4kPa—borderline. A walk test may be helpful
- PaO_2 <6.6kPa—in-flight oxygen required.

Patients who should not fly

Patients who should not fly include those with the following conditions:
- Infectious tuberculosis
- Pneumothorax
- Major thoracic surgery within the past two weeks.

Lung disease and flying 2

In-flight oxygen

Supplementary oxygen is usually prescribed at a rate of 2 L/min. It should be delivered by nasal cannulae. It need not be turned on until the plane reaches cruising altitude, and it should be switched off as the plane starts its descent.

People should be advised to book the oxygen from the airline as soon as the reservation is made. The airline medical department will issue a medical form for completion by the patient and their GP or hospital specialist. Information is required about the patient's medical condition and their oxygen requirements.

Other points that need to be considered are:

- Any need for oxygen at the airport and while changing flights
- Transportation in the air terminal
- Variation in fees for oxygen between airlines
- Provision of oxygen at the holiday destination.

Nebulizers

Battery-operated nebulizers can be used in flight with the exception of take off and landing.

Ventilators

Continuous positive airway pressure (CPAP) machines may be required by patients on long haul flights who have obstructive sleep apnoea (OSA). Dry-cell battery-powered CPAP machines are advised but some planes have laptop computer points available which CPAP machines can be plugged into. Medical clearance is not required for the carriage or use of CPAP machines as fitness to travel is not in doubt.

Ventilator-dependent patients should inform the airline of their requirements at the time of reservation, and provide a doctor's letter outlining the medical condition, equipment used and the ventilator settings provided. A medical attendant is likely to be needed.

Other precautions

- Patients with OSA and those at risk of venous thromboembolism should avoid excess alcohol before and during a flight
- Those not receiving oxygen should remain mobile
- Exercise without supplemental oxygen worsens hypoxaemia; patients should use oxygen when walking around the plane
- Patients should carry their inhalers in their hand luggage
- Patients should carry sufficient medication to cover the duration of their trip.

1. British Thoracic Society (2004). Managing passengers with respiratory disease planning air travel. London, BTS.

Diving 1

Diving has become a popular leisure pursuit, with an estimated 100,000 individuals participating in diving activities in the UK. Diving technology has evolved, allowing divers to dive in places previously not thought possible, and for divers to descend to greater depths.

The BTS Standards of Care Committee formed a Working Party to formulate national recommendations for assessing respiratory fitness to dive.[2] The recommendations provide practical evidence-based advice for healthcare professionals who may be asked to provide advice on respiratory aspects of fitness to dive.

Breath-hold dive

The simplest form of diving is breath-hold diving in which no equipment is used and the duration and depth of dive is determined by the individual's ability to sustain and remain functional during a single breath hold. A breath-hold dive is short enough to be performed on the air inhaled at the surface of the water. The air in the diver's lung is subjected to increased pressure, increasing the PaO_2. This extends the breath-hold time, particularly if the diver hyperventilates before submerging, as hyperventilating will reduce the $PaCO_2$. During the dive oxygen is used and the alveolar PO_2 falls. On ascent, the PO_2 falls to levels at which the diver may become unconscious, and be at risk of drowning. Standard advice is that four maximum breaths are allowed.

Snorkel dive

A snorkel dive is performed at a shallow depth of water. This means that connection with air can be maintained through a breathing tube (snorkel). The maximum lung pressure that the inspiratory muscles can generate is about 100 mmHg, equivalent to a depth of 1.2 m. This pressure cannot be maintained for longer than a few minutes, therefore the length of the snorkel is reduced to approximately 40 cm, thus reducing the dead space in the tube.

SCUBA dive

Most recreational diving is performed using breathing apparatus such as SCUBA (self contained underwater breathing apparatus) containing air. In recent years, gas mixtures containing varying concentrations of oxygen and nitrogen and, in some cases, other inert gases such as helium have been introduced to recreational diving. Closed and semi-closed circuit breathing apparatus are also used by a few recreational divers. During SCUBA dives, the gas is breathed through a regulated valve system from a pressure tank carried by the diver. There are problems with SCUBA dives at depths over 50 m because of increased density of the inhaled gas, increasing the work of breathing.

Diving-related illness

Any form of intercurrent acute illness may develop during diving. Trauma, oxygen toxicity, or hypoxia due to equipment malfunction or poor dive planning and hypothermia are also potential risks for the diver.

Pre-existing lung conditions

Individuals with pre-existing lung conditions may be recommended not to dive. These conditions include:

• Lung bullae or cysts
• Previous spontaneous pneumothorax unless surgically treated.
• Cystic fibrosis
• COPD
• Active tuberculosis
• Sarcoidosis
• Fibrotic lung disease.

Individuals who have a history of previous traumatic pneumothorax may be permitted to dive, if the pneumothorax has healed, and is associated with normal lung function, including flow-volume loop and thoracic CT scan (📖 p.75).

The British sub-aqua club (BSAC)[3] has made specific recommendations about asthma and diving. These include:

• Only well controlled asthmatics should dive
• Asthmatics may dive if they have allergic asthma but not if they have cold, exercise, or emotion-induced asthma
• Asthmatics should have normal spirometry (FEV_1 >80% predicted and FEV_1/VC ratio >70% predicted); and have a negative exercise test (<15% fall in FEV_1 after exercise)
• Asthmatics should not dive if they have required a therapeutic bronchodilator in the previous 48 h, or if they have had any other chest symptom
• During the diving season, the asthmatic should take twice daily PEFR measurements (📖 p.75). A deviation of 10% from best values should exclude diving until within 10% of best values for at least 48 h before diving
• A $ß_2$ agonist can be taken pre-dive as a preventative, but not to relieve bronchoconstriction at the time.

Diving 2

Barotrauma

Barotrauma is caused by compression or expansion of gas-filled spaces during descent or ascent, respectively. Compression of the lungs during descent may lead to alveolar exudation and haemorrhage. Expansion of the lungs during ascent may cause lung rupture. Divers with obstructive lung disease, such as asthma, can be predisposed to ruptured alveoli. Lung rupture can lead to pneumothorax, pneumomediastinum, and arterial gas embolism. Barotrauma is the second commonest cause of death in SCUBA divers.

Nitrogen narcosis

Nitrogen has high solubility in fat, and this solubility increases with increasing pressure. When divers breathe air under pressure, the inert nitrogen of the air diffuses into the various tissues of their body. This process continues and increases with the depth and duration of the dive. At approximately 100 feet, excess nitrogen is absorbed into the brain and interferes with the central nervous system. The more nitrogen present in the brain, the greater is the loss of performance. As depth increases, the problems get worse.

This narcosis effect poses a significant danger to divers because it might cause them to make decisions that place them at risk: A diver might not recognize a problem, or may not be able to respond to it. The greatest hazard of nitrogen narcosis is a total disregard for personal safety, which is identifiable when a diver acts abnormally. Symptoms of nitrogen narcosis include:

- Euphoria
- Mental confusion
- Impaired neuromuscular coordination
- Loss of consciousness.

To minimize these effects, divers who must dive to great depths typically breathe a special mixture of gases rather than regular air. Low concentrations of oxygen are used, diluted with helium or hydrogen rather than nitrogen, because helium and hydrogen do not produce narcosis.

Decompression sickness

Decompression sickness (also known as decompression illness, caisson disease, and the bends) is a disorder in which nitrogen dissolved in the blood and tissues by high pressure forms bubbles as pressure decreases. Because air under high pressure is compressed, each breath taken at depth contains many more molecules than a breath taken at the surface. Because oxygen is used continuously by the body, the extra oxygen molecules breathed under high pressure usually do not accumulate. However, the extra nitrogen molecules do accumulate in the blood and tissues. As outside pressure decreases during ascent from a dive, the accumulated nitrogen that cannot be exhaled immediately forms bubbles in the blood and tissues. These bubbles may expand and injure tissue, or they may obstruct the circulation—either directly or by triggering small blood clots. This blood vessel blockage causes pain. Nitrogen bubbles also cause inflammation, producing swelling and pain in muscles, joints, and tendons.

Tissues with a high fat content, such as those in the central nervous system, are particularly likely to be affected, because nitrogen dissolves very readily in fats.

The risk of developing decompression sickness increases with increasing pressure (that is, the depth of the dive) and with the length of time spent in a pressurized environment. Other risk factors include:

- Rapid ascent
- Fatigue
- Exertion
- Dehydration
- Cold water
- Obesity
- Older age.

Because excess nitrogen remains dissolved in the body tissues for at least 12 h after each dive, repeated dives within 1 day are more likely to cause decompression sickness than a single dive. Flying immediately after diving (such as at the end of a holiday) exposes a person to an even lower atmospheric pressure, making decompression sickness slightly more likely.

Hyperbaric re-compression therapy

Recompression therapy is a non-invasive medical treatment which involves breathing 100% oxygen for several hours at an increased atmospheric pressure, through the use of a hyperbaric chamber. The atmospheric pressure is gradually reduced back to normal atmospheric pressure over time. It is used to treat decompression sickness and arterial gas embolism.

The goals of recompression therapy are to increase oxygen solubility and delivery, increase nitrogen washout, decrease gas bubble size, and, in the rare case of diving-related carbon monoxide poisoning, decrease the half-life of carboxyhaemoglobin and reduce ischaemia.

Untreated pneumothorax requires a chest drain to be inserted before or during recompression therapy.

2. British Thoracic Society guidelines: http://www.brit-thoracic.org.uk/docs/diving.pdf

3. British Sub Aqua Club: http://www.bsac.com

Glossary

Accessory muscles: Muscles in the neck and shoulder which can be used to assist breathing in certain circumstances, such as severe exercise or respiratory failure

Acetylcholine: A parasympathetic neurotransmitter

Acidosis: Increased acidity/reduced pH of body fluids

Adherence: The extent to which the patient continues the agreed-upon mode of treatment

Adrenoreceptors: Receptors within the airway smooth muscle which respond to levels of adrenalin, which causes smooth muscle relaxation

Aeroallaegens: Allergens that are airborne, such as pollen, dust, or grasses

Aetiology: Study of disease causes

Aldosterone: A hormone produced by the adrenal glands

Allen's test: Test to assess the collateral arterial blood supply performed before obtaining an arterial blood gas sample

Allergens: Substances that cause an allergic reaction

α_1-**antitrypsin:** A protein produced in the liver, which blocks the action of trypsin and other proteolytic enzymes

Altitude: Elevation especially above sea level

Alveoli: Thin-walled sac-like structure at the end of each respiratory bronchiole where gas exchange takes place

Alveolitis: Inflammation of the alveoli

Aminophylline: A theophylline derivative that is used as a bronchodilator in the treatment of asthma and COPD

Anaerobic: Occurring in the absence of oxygen

Anaphylaxis: Severe allergic reaction to a foreign substance

Aneurysm: Weakness or injury to the wall of a blood vessel causing dilatation or ballooning

Angina: Chest pain due to an inadequate supply of oxygen to the heart muscle

Angiodema: Swelling similar to urticaria, but the swelling occurs beneath the skin instead of on the surface

Anoxia: Absence of oxygen in the tissues

Antibody: A soluble protein which is released in response to a specific antigen

Anticholinergic: An agent which blocks the normal cholinergic response and causes bronchodilation

Antigen: A protein which causes the production of an antibody, and reacts specifically with that antibody

Antihistamines: A class of medications used to block the action of histamines in the body and prevent the symptoms of an allergic reaction

Apnoea: Absence of breathing

ARDS: Form of lung failure that may result from any disease that causes large amounts of fluid to collect in the lungs

Arrhythmia: Irregular heartbeat

Arterial blood gas analysis: Measurement of the arterial pH, partial pressures of oxygen and carbon dioxide, and bicarbonate. Used to evaluate acid-base balance, and gas exchange

Asbestosis: Scarring of the lungs caused by inhaled asbestos fibres

Aspergillosis: Infection with the fungus *Aspergillus*

Aspergillus: A family of fungi commonly found in soil. Certain types may cause disease, especially in people who have suppressed immune systems

Asphyxia: A life-threatening condition in which oxygen is prevented from reaching the tissues by obstruction of or damage to any part of the respiratory system

Aspiration: Inhalation of any foreign matter, such as food, drink, saliva, or stomach contents (as after vomiting) into the airway below the level of the vocal cords

Asthma: A chronic inflammatory disorder of the airways. Inflammatory symptoms are usually associated with widespread but variable airflow obstruction and an increase in airway response to a variety of stimuli. Obstruction is often reversible, either spontaneously or with treatment

Atelectasis: Abnormal collapse of the distal lung parenchyma

Atopy: A genetic predisposition in particular individuals to develop immediate reactions to allergens

Autonomic nervous system: Controls involuntary actions such as respiration, the heart circulation, digestion, excretion, and temperature regulation

Bacteria: Living organisms, microscopic in size, which usually consist of a single cell

Barrel chest: Abnormal chest shape in which the chest appears round and bulging with a greater than normal front to back diameter

Basement membrane: A thin layer of connective tissue underlying the epithelium of many organs

Basophil: A type of white blood cell characterized by a pale nucleus and large granules

Beclometasone: Inhaled corticosteroid drug

Bibasal: At both bases

Bilateral: Affecting both the right and left side

Body mass index: A measure to determine if a person is underweight, normal weight, or overweight. It is defined as weight in kilograms divided by height in metres squared

Bradypnea: Decreased rate of breathing

Bronchi: Portion of the respiratory tree which divides to form the lobes and segments of the lungs

Bronchial breath sounds: Breath sounds heard next to the trachea, sounding loud, high-pitched, and discontinuous

Bronchiectasis: Chronic dilatation of the bronchi and destruction of bronchial walls

Bronchioles: Subdivisions of the bronchi, usually 2mm or less in diameter

Bronchiolitis: Inflammation of the bronchioles, or small airways often caused by a virus

Bronchitis: Acute or chronic inflammation of the bronchial tree

Bronchoconstriction: Narrowing of the airways due to contraction of bronchial smooth muscle

Bronchodilator: An agent which causes relaxation of the bronchial smooth muscle

Bronchoscopy: Direct inspection of the trachea and bronchi through a flexible fibreoptic or rigid bronchoscope

Bronchospasm: Abnormal contraction of the bronchial smooth muscle resulting in airflow disturbance

Budesonide: Inhaled corticosteroid drug

Bulla(e): Air-filled cysts within the lungs that take up space in the lungs, but have no ventilatory action

Cachexia: A dramatic weight loss and general wasting that occurs during chronic disease

Candidiasis: Fungal infection

Carbocisteine: A mucolytic medicine which breaks down some of the chemical bonds in mucus

Carbon monoxide: A colourless, odourless, highly poisonous gas formed by the incomplete combustion of carbon

Cardiomyopathy: An enlarged heart that no longer pumps effectively

Cartilage: Non-vasculated, firm, connective tissue made up from cells, fibres, and proteoglycans that hold it together

Chemotherapy: The use of chemicals or drugs to treat disease

Cheyne–Stokes respirations: Abnormal pattern of breathing consisting of progressively increasing, then progressively decreasing tidal volume, followed by apnoea at the resting expiratory level

Chronic: A long-term medical condition or symptom

Chronic obstructive pulmonary disease: A term used for a number of conditions; including chronic bronchitis and emphysema

Churg–Strauss Syndrome: A medium and small vessel autoimmune vasculitis, leading to necrosis. It involves mainly the blood vessels of the lungs (often beginning as a severe type of asthma), gastrointestinal system and peripheral nerves

Cilia: Motile hair-like structures that line the walls of the trachea and bronchi which help to expel foreign bodies, such as dust and bacteria caught in the mucus, up and then out of the respiratory tree

Clubbing: Angle of the fingernail entering the skin at an angle greater than or equal to 180°. Clubbing indicates long-term hypoxia

Collagen: Connective tissue found in muscles

Compensation: The body's attempt to maintain a normal pH level of arterial blood

Compliance: A measure of the ease with which the lungs and thoracic wall can be expanded

Compliance: A patient both agreeing to and then undergoing some part of their treatment programme as advised by their doctor or other health-care worker

Concordance: The patient and health professional discussing the options and reaching agreement about what treatment is required

Congenital: A disease, deformity, or deficiency existing at the time of birth

Consolidation: A clinical term for solidification into a firm dense mass

Continuous positive airway pressure: Mode of ventilation that maintains positive pressure in the airways throughout the patient's respiratory cycle

Cor pulmonale: Right-sided heart failure caused by enlargement of the right ventricle as a result of primary pulmonary disease

Corticosteroids: A natural or synthetic agent which has anti-inflammatory properties

Costochondral: Relating to the ribs and their cartilages

Cough: A sudden, forceful expulsion of air from the lungs; an essential protective response that serves to protect the lungs and airways from irritants and secretions and to prevent aspiration of foreign material into the lungs

Crackles: Intermittent non-musical explosive sounds heard on auscultation

Cyanosis: Blue discolouration of the skin and mucous membranes that result from lack of oxygen and the resulting deoxygenated haemaglobin

Cystic fibrosis: A recessive genetic disorder affecting the mucous lining of the lungs

Cytokines: Small protein hormones produced by lymphocytes and other cells to regulate immune response

Cytotoxic: An agent or process that is toxic to cells

Dead space: The area of the respiratory tract where there is no gas exchange

Degranulation: The release of granules from the mast cell as it breaks down

Deoxycorticosterone: A steroid hormone produced by the adrenal gland

Dermatitis: Inflammation of the skin—redness and often swelling, pain, itching, cracking. May be caused by an irritant or allergen

Desaturation: Less than normal amount of oxygen carried by haemoglobin in the blood

Diaphragm: Dome-shaped muscle that separates the abdomen from the thorax. The largest muscle involved in ventilation

Diffuse: Widespread

Diffusing capacity: The ability of the alveolocapillary membrane to transfer gas

Diffusion: The process by which atoms and molecules move through a semi-permeable membrane from an area of high to low concentration

Disability: A physical or mental incapacity, either congenital or resulting from an injury or illness

Distal: Away from

Diuretic: A medication that helps the kidneys to remove excess fluids from the body, lowering blood pressure as well as decreasing oedema

Diurnal variation: Variation in peak flow readings taken over a 24-hour period

Dyspnoea: Difficult or laboured breathing

Early phase: A demonstrable reduction in peak flow which occurs 15–30 minutes after exposure to an allergen or trigger. The reduction in peak flow lasts for approximately 3–4 hours before it returns to normal level

Eczema: A skin condition characterized by itchy, irritated, inflamed skin

Effort-dependent: A test or procedure which relies upon the effort of the patient in order to produce accurate results

Electrolytes: Minerals (such as sodium, potassium, magnesium, and calcium) found in the blood that must be maintained within a certain range to allow normal organ function

Emphysema: Irreversible disease of the lungs characterized by destruction of the alveolar walls. The damaged cells merge into larger sacs called bullae which are relatively inefficient for gas exchange

Empyema: Collection of pus within the pleural space

Endotracheal intubation: Oral or nasal insertion of a flexible tube through the larynx into the trachea to control the airway and mechanically ventilate the patient

Eosinophils: A type of white blood cell that can increase in allergy and other infections

Epithelial cells: Cells that cover the surface of the body and line its cavities

Equilibrium: Physical or chemical stasis

Erythema: A reddening of the skin

Erythrocytosis: High red blood cell count

Erythropoietin: A glycoprotein that stimulates production of red blood cells

Ethnicity: The cultural practices, language, cuisine and traditions used to distinguish groups of persons—not biological or physical differences

Exacerbation: Worsening of a condition, often acute in nature

Expectoration: The act of coughing up and spitting out sputum from the lungs, bronchi, and trachea

Expiration: Breathing out

Expiratory reserve volume: The volume from a tidal breath out to the point of residual volume

Extrinsic asthma: Asthma that is triggered by an allergic reaction, usually something that is inhaled

Exudate: Fluid with a high concentration of protein and cellular debris which has escaped from blood vessels and has been deposited in tissues, or on tissue surfaces, usually as a result of inflammation

FEV$_1$: The maximum volume of air a patient can exhale during the first second of a forced expiratory manoeuvre

Fibrosis: Abnormal formation of scar tissue

Fluticasone: Inhaled corticosteroid drug

Forced vital capacity: Amount of air than can be exhaled forcibly after maximum inspiration

Formoterol: Long-acting β_2-adrenergic receptor agonist drug

Functional residual capacity: The sum of the respiratory reserve volume and the residual volume

Gas exchange: The exchange of waste carbon dioxide produced by the body during respiration of oxygen from the atmosphere

Gastro-oesophageal reflux: A disorder where a backwash of gastric juices into the oesophagus lead to inflammation and pain

Goblet cells: The cells in the respiratory epithelium which secrete mucus

Granulocytes: White blood cells, granular in appearance, that attack and destroy foreign substances

Haemodynamics: The study of the forces and physical mechanisms concerned with the circulation of the blood

Haemoptysis: Spitting of blood from the lungs or bronchial tubes as a result of pulmonary or bronchial haemorrhage

Haemothorax: Accumulation of blood in the pleural cavity

Half-life: The time taken for the concentration of a drug to fall to half its initial value

Hilum: The depression in the medial surface of a lung that forms the opening through which the bronchus, blood vessels, and nerves pass

Histamine: Substance found in many cells, including mast cells, basophils, and platelets. It is released when the cells are injured and results in vasodilation, increased capillary permeability, and constriction of the bronchioles

Histology: The study of tissues and cells under a microscope

Homeostasis: The condition in which the body's internal environment remains relatively constant, within physiological limits

Hydrocortisone: A hormone secreted by the adrenal cortex which affects metabolism

Hypercalcaemia: Abnormally high level of calcium in the blood

Hypercapnia: High levels of carbon dioxide in blood

Hyperreactivity: A greater than normal response to a stimulus

Hypersecretion: Excessive secretion

Hypertension: Blood pressure that is above the normal range

Hyperthyroidism: Over active thyroid gland

Hypertrophy: An abnormal enlargement of an organ or thickening of its tissue

Hyperventilation: Excessive rate and depth of breathing

Hypobaric: Pressure lower than normal atmospheric pressure

Hypotension: Blood pressure that is below the normal range

Hypoventilation: Reduced gas exchange in the lungs resulting in low oxygen levels and high carbon dioxide levels

Hypoxaemia: Insufficient oxygen in the cells to meet metabolic need

Hypoxia: Reduction of oxygen in body tissues to below normal levels

Idiopathic: When the cause of a disease or process is not known

Immune response: The reaction of the immune system against foreign substances. When this reaction occurs against substances or tissues within the body, it is called an autoimmune reaction

Immune system: A complex system that normally protects the body from infections and environmental contaminants. It is comprised of groups of cells, the chemicals that control them, and the chemicals they release

Immunoglobulin: An antibody synthesised by plasma cells derived from B lymphocytes

Impairment: A loss of part or all of a physical or mental ability

Infiltrate: An abnormal substance that accumulates gradually in cells or body tissues

Inflammation: The body's reaction to injury or insult. In asthma, inflammation causes the airways to produce excess secretions, swelling, and bronchoconstriction of the airways

Inspiration: Breathing in

Inspiratory capacity: The volume of air in the lungs from a tidal breath out to maximum inspiration

Inspiratory reserve volume: The volume of air from the tidal breath in up to total lung capacity

Intercostal: Located or occurring between the ribs

Interstitial fluid: The extracellular fluid which fills the microscopic spaces between the cells of tissues

Intracellular fluid: Fluid located within the cells

Intrinsic asthma: A classification of asthma that means the asthma symptoms are not caused by exposure to allergens

Intubation: Insertion of a tube into the trachea for purposes of anaesthesia, airway maintenance, aspiration of secretions, lung ventilation, or prevention of entrance of foreign material into the airway

Ipratropium bromide: A short-acting anticholinergic drug

Kyphoscoliosis: Combination of kyphosis and scoliosis

Kyphosis: Excessive outward curvature of the spine, causing hunching of the back

Langerhans' cell histiocytosis: A generic term embracing a group of disorders characterized by proliferation of Langerhans' cells. Lesions affect the lungs, endocrine system and bone marrow

Larynx: Part of the respiratory tract between the pharynx and the trachea; commonly known as the voice box

Late phase: A demonstrable reduction in peak flow 8–12 hours after exposure to an allergen

Lateral: Sideways

Leucocytes: White blood cells

Leukotrienes: Inflammatory substances that are released by mast cells during an allergic response or asthma attack

Lobectomy: Surgical removal of one of the five lobes of the lung

Lobes: The segments of the lungs. The right lung has three lobes, the left lung two

Lumen: The space inside a tube

Lymphadenopathy: Any disease process affecting a lymph node

Lymphocytes: Cells which produce antibodies and cytokines as part of the immune response

Macrophage: Phagocytic cell derived from a monocyte

Mast cells: Cells found in the airways, which have many sites for binding of IgE. After binding has taken place degranulation occurs which releases mediators such as histamine

Mediastinum: Space between the lungs that contains the heart and pericardium, major vessels, oesophagus, and other structures

Mesothelioma: A malignant tumour of the mesothelium

Mesothelium: Membrane that lines the pleura

Metabolic: The complete set of chemical reactions that occurs in living cells

Metabolic acidosis: Condition resulting from excess acid retention or excess bicarbonate loss

Metabolic alkalosis: Condition resulting from excess bicarbonate retention

Metered dose inhaler: Device used to trigger the release of measured doses of aerosol drug from a canister

Mid expiratory flow: Measurement of rate of airflow over the middle half of a forced vital capacity

Minute volume: Amount of air breathed per minute

Morbidity: Ill health but not death

Mortality: Death

Mucolytic: An agent that breaks down mucous

Muscarinic receptors: Parasympathetic site, which when stimulated by acetylcholine causes smooth muscle to contract

Nebulizer: Device that uses compressed gas to convert liquid drugs into a fine aerosol for inhalation

Neurotransmitters: Chemicals that transmit nerve impulses across a synapse

Neutrophils: A type of white blood cell that is highly destructive of microorganisms

Nitric oxide: A free radical which is produced as a consequence of inflammatory processes

Non-rebreathe bag: Type of oxygen delivery device that involves a one-way inspiratory valve that opens on inhalation and directs oxygen from a reservoir bag into the mask. The patient breathes air only from the bag

Non-steroidal anti-inflammatory drugs: A group of drugs, such as aspirin and ibuprofen, used to reduce inflammation

Obstruction: A pattern of spirometry seen in diseases which affect the rate at which air can be expelled from the lungs

Obstructive sleep apnoea: A sleep disorder with symptoms of loud snoring and periodic pauses in breathing, for at least 10 seconds, after which breathing is resumed again with a snort

Oedema: Accumulation of an excessive amount of fluid in cells or tissues

Orthopnea: Shortness of breath when lying down

Osteoporosis: A disorder caused by the abnormal loss of bone density; bones become increasingly brittle, porous, and likely to fracture due to lack of calcium and other minerals

Oxygen-diffusing capacity: A measure of the rate at which oxygen diffuses from the alveoli into the blood

Oxyhaemoglobin: Haemoglobin with oxygen bound to it

Pack year: A measure of cigarette smoking history, calculated by multiplying the number of cigarettes smoked each day divided by 20 and multiplied by the number of years the patient has been a smoker

Palliative: A treatment that provides symptomatic relief but not a cure

Palpation: To examine or explore by touching

Parenchyma: The functional parts of an organ. For instance alveoli are part of the parenchyma of the lung

Partial pressure of arterial carbon dioxide ($PaCO_2$): Level of carbon dioxide in arterial blood

Partial pressure of arterial oxygen (PaO_2): Level of oxygen in arterial blood

Particulates: Fine liquid or solid particles such as dust, smoke, mist, fumes, or smog, found in air or emissions

Pathophysiology: The functional changes associated with or resulting from disease or injury

Peak expiratory flow: Maximum flow recorded on breathing out hard and fast into a peak flow meter

Percussion: Striking the chest with the fingers to evaluate the presence of fluid in a lung or collapse of part of a lung

Perennial: Lasting through the year or for several years

Perfusion: Blood supply to a tissue

pH: Measurement of the percentage of hydrogen ions in a solution

Phagocytes: Defence cells which ingest particulate matter such as microbes, cell debris and other matter

Pharmacodynamics: The study of how drugs act at target sites of action in the body

Pharmacokinetics: The study of the absorption, distribution, metabolism, and elimination of drugs

Pharynx: Upper portion of the digestive tract that links the mouth, nose, oesophagus and larynx

Phrenic nerve: The nerve supplying the diaphragm

Pickwickian syndrome: Hypoventilation of obesity syndrome

Placebo: A pill or injection made to appear exactly like a test medication, but without any of its active ingredients

Plethora: Term used to describe a red face

Plethysmography: Technique used to calculate alveolar air pressure and the volume of gas retained within the lungs

Pleura: Membrane that encloses the lungs or chest wall

Pleural effusion: Collection of fluid in the pleural space

Pleural rub: Low-pitched, rubbing sound heard on inhalation and exhalation

Pleurodesis: The artificial obliteration of the pleural space. It is done to prevent recurrence of pneumothorax or pleural effusion

Pneumococcus: A gram-positive bacterium (*Streptococcus pneumoniae*) that is the most common cause of bacterial pneumonia

Pneumoconiosis: Fibrosis and scarring of the lungs as a result of repeated inhalation of occupationally associated dust, such as silica, asbestos, and coal dust

Pneumocytes: Types of cell found in the lining of the alveoli

Pneumonectomy: The surgical removal of a lung

Pneumonia: Inflammation of one or both lungs with consolidation

Pneumothorax: Collapse of part or all of the lung due to air in the pleural space

Polycythaemia: Increased number of red blood cells in the blood. It occurs as a result of chronically low levels of oxygen in the circulation

Polyphonic: Multiple pitches and tones heard over a variable area of the lung

Precipitants: A substance that causes a precipitate to form when it is added to a solution

Prednisolone: Synthetic corticosteroid drug

Prognosis: The expected outcome of a disease and its treatment

Prophylactic: A medical procedure or practice that prevents or protects against a disease or condition (e.g., vaccines, antibiotics, drugs)

Prostaglandin: Potent substance that acts like a hormone and is found in many bodily tissues (and especially in semen); produced in response to trauma and may affect blood pressure and metabolism and smooth muscle activity

Proteases: Enzymes that aid in the breakdown of proteins in the body

Proximal: Near to

Pruritus: Itching of the skin, sometimes accompanied by a rash

Pulmonary embolism: Obstruction of a pulmonary blood vessel by foreign substance or a blood clot

Pulmonary hypertension: Chronically elevated pulmonary artery pressure higher than 30 mmHg and a mean pulmonary artery pressure higher than 18 mmHg

Pulmonary oedema: Abnormal fluid accumulation in the lungs

Pulmonary perfusion: Blood flow from the right side of the heart, through the pulmonary circulation, and into the left side of the heart

Pulse oximetry: A non-invasive diagnostic test used for detecting the percentage of haemoglobin that is saturated with oxygen

Pyrexia: Raised body temperature

RAST test: A blood test done to measure the amount of specific IgE antibodies in the blood to specific allergens

Reproducibility: A term used to check that spirometric tests are accurate to within 5% or 100mls of each other to eliminate error

Residual volume: Amount of air remaining in the lungs after forced expiration

Respiratory acidosis: Acidosis resulting from reduced gas exchange in the lungs; excess carbon dioxide combines with water to form carbonic acid which increases the acidity of the blood

Respiratory alkalosis: A rise in blood pH to above 7.45 due to excessive elimination of blood CO_2 as a result of hyperventilation

Respiratory failure: A clinical syndrome that is defined either by the inability to rid the body of carbon dioxide or establish an adequate blood oxygen level

Restriction: A pattern characteristic of a condition that affects the ability of the lungs to expand. There is a reduction in FVC and FEV_1 but the FVC/FEV_1 ratio is preserved

Reversibility: The improvement in FEV_1 a patient will experience following treatment with either a bronchodilator or corticosteroid

Rhinitis: Swelling or inflammation of the mucous membrane in the nose

Rhinorrhea: Persistent watery mucus discharge from the nose

Salbutamol: A short-acting β_2-adrenergic receptor agonist used for the relief of bronchospasm

Salmeterol: Long-acting β_2-adrenergic receptor agonist drug

Sarcoidosis: An inflammatory disease marked by the formation of granulomas (small nodules of immune cells) in the lungs, lymph nodes, and other organs

Scoliosis: A lateral curvature of the spine, either congenital or acquired by very poor posture, disease or muscular weakness due to certain conditions such as cerebral palsy or muscular dystrophy

Secretions: Mucus or phlegm from the respiratory passages

Sensitization: The development of a hypersensitive or allergic reaction upon re-exposure to a substance. The reaction may be immediate or delayed and may be of short-term or chronic duration

Sepsis: The presence of infection in the blood

Silicosis: Fibrosis of the lungs caused by the inhalation of silica dust

Skin prick test: An allergy skin test, used to identify the substances that are likely to provoke allergy symptoms

Spacer: Holding chamber device that attaches to the mouthpiece of an inhaler

Spirometer: A machine which measures air flow or lung volumes

Sputum: Material expectorated from a patient's lungs during coughing

Status asthmaticus: Emergency, life-threatening event resulting from an acute asthma attack where there is profound and intractable bronchospasm

Stridor: A high-pitched sound heard from the upper airway during inspiration

Sublingual: Underneath the tongue

Syndrome: Set of signs or a series of events occurring together that make up a disease or health problem

Synergistic: Working together to produce an effect that is better than the sum of the two individual effects

T cell: A type of lymphocyte that provides cell-mediated immunity

Tachycardia: Rapid beating of the heart, usually defined as greater than 100 beats per minute

Tachypnoea: Shallow breathing with increased respiratory rate

Tactile fremitus: Palpable vibrations caused by the transmission of air through the respiratory system

Tension pneumothorax: Air trapped within the pleural space

Terbutaline: A short-acting β_2-adrenergic receptor agonist drug

Theophylline: A methylxanthine drug used as a bronchodilator

Therapeutic range: Dosage range in which a drug exerts a therapeutic effect

Thoracentesis: Aspiration of pleural fluid to obtain a sample of pleural fluid for analysis

Thoracotomy: Surgical removal of all or part of a lung

Thromboembolism: Blockage of a blood vessel due to a blood clot

Tidal volume: Amount of air inhaled or exhaled during normal breathing

Tiotropium: Long-acting anticholinergic drug

Total lung capacity: The maximum volume of the lungs

Trachea: Tube linking the larynx with the bronchi

Tracheotomy: Surgical opening into the trachea to provide an airway

Transfer factor: Measurement of the lung's diffusion capacity

Transpulmonary pressure: The difference between the alveolar pressure and the pleural pressure

Tuberculosis: A highly contagious infection caused by the *Mycobacterium tuberculosis* bacterium

Unilateral: Affecting one side

Urticaria: Raised, itchy areas of skin that are usually a sign of an allergic reaction. Also known as hives

Vagal nerve: Either of the tenth and longest of the cranial nerves, passing through the neck and thorax into the abdomen and supplying sensation to part of the ear, the tongue, the larynx, and the pharynx, motor impulses to the vocal cords, and motor and secretory impulses to the abdominal and thoracic viscera

Vasodilation: Dilation of the blood vessels

Ventilation: The process of moving air into and out of the lungs

Venturi mask: Type of oxygen delivery system allowing a mixture of a specific volume of air and oxygen to deliver a highly accurate oxygen concentration

Vesicular sounds: Breath sounds heard over most of both lungs. They sound soft and low-pitched

Visceral pleura: The membrane which covers the outsides of the lungs

Viscosity: The measure of resistance to flow or 'stickiness' of a fluid

Vital capacity: The capacity of the lungs measured when the patient exhales slowly. Also known as relaxed, slow or expired vital capacity

Weal: A raised mark on the skin

Wheeze: High-pitched sounds heard on exhalation when airflow is obstructed

Useful contacts

Throughout the individual chapters in this book, references are made to useful contacts for specific disease areas, evidence-based guidelines, charities and support groups. The following list includes website addresses of organizations that may apply to the majority of readers.

Action on Smoking and Health (ASH)	http://www.newash.org.uk
Association of Respiratory Nurse Specialists	http://www.arns.co.uk
Asthma UK	http://www.asthma.org.uk
Association of Respiratory Technicians and Physiologists	http://www.artp.org.uk
British Lung Foundation	http://www.lunguk.co.uk
British Thoracic Society	http://www.brit-thoracic.org.uk
Education for Health	http://www.educationforhealth.org.uk
General Practice Airways Group	http://www.gpiag.org
Global initiative for chronic Obstructive Lung Disease (GOLD)	http://www.goldcopd.dk
National Institute for Health and Clinical Excellence	http://www.nice.org.uk
Respiratory Education UK	http://www.respiratoryeduk.com
Royal College of Nursing	http://www.rcn.org.uk

Index